Elderly Care Medicine
Lecture Notes

Claire G. Nicholl

MB FRCP
Consultant Physician and Associate Lecturer

K. Jane Wilson

MB FRCP
Consultant Physician and Associate Lecturer

Both of:
Department of Medicine for the Elderly
Addenbrooke's Hospital
Cambridge University Hospitals NHS Foundation Trust
Cambridge, UK

Eighth Edition

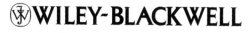

WILEY-BLACKWELL

A John Wiley & Sons, Ltd., Publication

This edition first published 2012 © 2012 by John Wiley & Sons, Ltd.
Previous editions: 1977, 1980, 1988, 1993, 1998, 2003, 2007

Wiley-Blackwell is an imprint of John Wiley & Sons, formed by the merger of Wiley's global Scientific, Technical and Medical business with Blackwell Publishing.

Registered office: John Wiley & Sons, Ltd, The Atrium, Southern Gate, Chichester, West Sussex, PO19 8SQ, UK

Editorial offices: 9600 Garsington Road, Oxford, OX4 2DQ, UK
The Atrium, Southern Gate, Chichester, West Sussex, PO19 8SQ, UK
111 River Street, Hoboken, NJ 07030-5774, USA

For details of our global editorial offices, for customer services and for information about how to apply for permission to reuse the copyright material in this book please see our website at www.wiley.com/wiley-blackwell.

Library of Congress Cataloging-in-Publication Data

Nicholl, Claire.
  Lecture notes. Elderly care medicine / Claire Nicholl, K. Jane Wilson. – 8th ed.
    p. ; cm.
  Elderly care medicine
  Includes bibliographical references and index.
  ISBN 978-0-470-65454-5 (pbk. : alk. paper)
  I. Wilson, K. Jane (Kathryn Jane) II. Title. III. Title: Elderly care medicine.
  [DNLM: 1. Geriatrics. WT 100]

  618.97–dc23

                                    2011049097

A catalogue record for this book is available from the British Library.

Wiley also publishes its books in a variety of electronic formats. Some content that appears in print may not be available in electronic books.

Set in 8.5/11pt Utopia by Thomson Digital, Noida, India
Printed and bound in Malaysia by Vivar Printing Sdn Bhd

2 2013

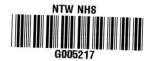
Elderly Care Medicine
Lecture Notes

Contents

Companion website

This book is accompanied by a companion website:

www.lecturenoteseries.com/elderlycaremed

The website includes:

- Key revision points for each chapter
- Appendices:
    1. Standards for long-term care
    2. The Barthel Scale
    3. CAGE questionnaire for alcohol problems
    4. The Abbreviated Mental Test (AMT)
    5. The Geriatric Depression Score (GDS)
    6. Fitness to fly
    7. Respiratory function in the elderly
    8. Malnutrition Universal Screening Tool (MUST)
    9. The Waterlow Score for pressure sores
- Extended content for specialty trainees
- Further reading

Preface

Unless you are planning to be a paediatrician or an obstetrician, this book is for you. 2011 was the year that the world population topped 7 billion (UN). Whilst population growth is still very rapid in some areas, in industrialized countries it is the ageing of the population that is having most effect on health and social needs. Because of the size of their populations, the greatest numbers of old people already live in China and India. By the end of the century it is estimated that the world population will be falling so the challenges of ageing will dominate worldwide.

Whatever career choice you make, with a few exceptions, the patients you look after during your career will be increasingly elderly and increasingly frail. Even in surgical specialties the majority of patients are old. A good understanding of the basics of managing this group with their fragile homeostatic mechanisms, multiple diseases and drugs, high prevalence of dementia and risk of delirium will make a difference to the outcome for your patient. Knowledge of the ways in which the multidisciplinary team can work with the patient and family and a grasp of the complexities of the social care system will also help you to put together the best package of care for an older person. This will reduce their length of stay in hospital, the risks of hospitalization and money wasted on inefficient care.

In the community, the limited time available for a GP consultation makes good medical management of older people with complex health problems difficult to achieve. If a specialist opinion is needed, frail older people are not easily managed by single-organ specialists, but elderly care medicine as a specialty remains poorly developed in much of Europe and North America. In the UK it is recognized that frail old people are the greatest users of the NHS and geriatric medicine is now the biggest specialty within the Royal College of Physicians. However, academic departments of medicine for the elderly have been in decline and the medicine of old age is often taught by non-specialists as an integrated part of medicine in the life cycle. This has the advantage that ageing is seen in the context of human development, but the time allocated to older people is not proportionate to what the student doctor will need to know as soon as they are qualified.

If you are still not convinced that a grasp of medicine for the elderly is essential, have a look at the medical or surgical 'take' list for the hospital where you are working. At Addenbrooke's the average age of the patients admitted on the medical take sometimes exceeds 75 years and the average age of the patients under the physicians here who specialize in elderly care is 86 years.

This book is aimed at medical students and junior doctors who may have had relatively little specialist teaching about older people. Therefore since the last edition, the content has been expanded as well as updated, particularly the chapters on dementia, stroke, falls and ethical issues. We hope that it is written in an approachable manner which would make it accessible to nurses and allied health professionals. The accompanying website gives key points for revision and more details particularly about health care provision, dementia and stroke. It also forms an initial refresher for trainees approaching their specialty examination to identify gaps in knowledge for appropriate supplementation from longer textbooks and papers.

You will need to learn the basics of medicine for the elderly – we are hoping to make it easier and to convince you that medicine for older people is interesting, varied and challenging. There is great scope for clinical acumen and decision making as the complexity of the patients makes guideline-driven medicine less relevant. Over recent years, geriatricians have expanded into orthopaedics, stroke medicine, acute medicine and community services and there is now demand for input into general surgery. As other specialties contract, a career in medicine for the elderly is well worth considering.

Claire G. Nicholl
K. Jane Wilson

Abbreviations

AA	Attendance allowance
AADC	aromatic amino acid decarboxylase
AAFB	acid and alcohol fast bacilli
ABG	arterial blood gas
ACA	anterior cerebral artery
ACE	angiotensin-converting enzyme
ACEi	ACE inhibitor
AChE	acetylcholinesterase
AChEi	acetylcholinesterase inhibitor
ACP	advanced care planning
ACS	acute coronary syndrome
ACTH	adrenocorticotrophic hormone
AD	Alzheimer's disease
ADH	antidiuretic hormone
ADL	activities of daily living
ADR	adverse drug reaction
ADRT	advance decision to refuse treatment
ADs	advance decisions
AED	anti-epileptic drug
AF	atrial fibrillation
AFO	ankle-foot orthosis
AIDP	acute inflammatory demyelinating polyradiculoneuropathy
AIP	acute interstitial pneumonia
AKI	acute kidney injury
ALD	alcoholic liver disease
ALL	acute lymphoblastic leukaemia
ALP	alkaline phosphatase
ALS	amyotrophic lateral sclerosis
AML	acute myelocytic leukaemia
AMPA	α-amino-3-hydroxy-5-methylisoxazole-4-propionic acid receptor
AMT	Abbreviated Mental Test
ANH	artificial nutrition and hydration
ANS	autonomic nervous system
AP	antero-posteriorally
APP	amyloid precursor protein
ARB	angiotensin receptor blocker
AMD	age-related macular degeneration
AS	Alzheimer's Society
ATN	acute tubular necrosis
AV	atrioventricular
AVP	arginine vasopressin
AXR	abdominal X-ray
BAFTA	Birmingham Atrial Fibrillation Treatment of the Aged study
BCC	basal-cell carcinoma
BMA	British Medical Association
BMD	bone mineral density
BMI	body mass index
BNF	British National Formulary
BNP	brain natriuretic peptide
BOOP	bronchiolitis obliterans organizing pneumonia
BP	blood pressure
BPH	benign prostatic hyperplasia
BPPV	benign paroxysmal positional vertigo
BPSD	behavioural and psychological symptoms of dementia
CAA	cerebral amyloid angiopathy
CAD	coronary artery disease
CADASIL	cerebral autosomal dominant arteriopathy with subcortical infarcts and leucoencephalopathy
CAPD	continuous ambulatory peritoneal dialysis
CBD	corticobasal degeneration
CBT	cognitive behavioural therapy
CCF	congestive cardiac failure
CCU	coronary care unit
CDAD	*Clostridium difficile* associated diarrhoea
CFH	complement factor H
CHARM	The Candesartan in Heart failure Assessment of Reduction in Morbidity and Mortality study
CHART	continuous hyperfractionated accelerated ratio
CHF	congestive heart failure
CI	confidence interval
CIDP	chronic inflammatory demyelinating polyradiculoneuropathy
CK	creatine kinase
CKD	chronic kidney disease
CLL	chronic lymphocytic leukaemia
CML	chronic myeloid leukaemia

CNS	central nervous system	EMA	endomysial antibodies
COHb	carboxyhaemoglobin	EMG	electromyogram
COMT	catechol-O-methyltransferase	EOFAD	early-onset familial Alzheimer's disease
COP	cryptogenic organizing pneumonia		
COPD	chronic obstructive pulmonary disease	ERCP	endoscopic retrograde cholangiopancreatography
COX-2	cyclo-oxygenase-2		
CPAP	continuous positive airways pressure	ESR	erythrocyte sedimentation rate
CPN	Community psychiatric nurse	ET	essential tremor
CPR	cardiopulmonary resuscitation	EVAR	endovascular aneurysm repair
CQC	Care Quality Commission	FAST	Face Arm Speech Time score
CRP	C-reactive protein	FBC	full blood count
CSF	cerebrospinal fluid	FDG	fluorodeoxyglucose
CT	computerized tomography	FEV_1	forced expiratory volume in 1 s
CTPA	computerized tomography pulmonary angiogram	FRAX	Fracture Risk Assessment tool
		FSH	follicle stimulating hormone
CTZ	chemoreceptor trigger zone	FTD	frontotemporal dementia
CVA	cerebrovascular accident	FTLD	frontotemporal lobar degeneration
CVP	central venous pressure	FVC	forced vital capacity
CXR	chest X-ray	GARS	glycyl-tRNA synthetase
DAN	diabetic autonomic neuropathy	GBS	Guillain–Barré syndrome
DBS	deep brain stimulation	GCA	giant-cell arteritis
DC	direct current	GDNF	glial cell-line derived nerve growth factor
DFLE	disability-free life expectancy		
DGH	District General Hospital	GDP	gross domestic product
DH	Department of Health	GDS	Geriatric Depression Score
DIC	disseminated intravascular coagulation	GFR	glomerular filtration rate
		GI	gastrointestinal
DIP	distal interphalangeal joints	GLP-1	glucagon-like peptide 1
DLB	dementia with Lewy bodies	GMC	General Medical Council
DM	diabetes mellitus	GORD	gastro-oesophageal reflux disease
DMARDs	disease-modifying anti-rheumatic drugs	GP	general practitioner
DNA CPR	do not attempt cardiopulmonary resuscitation	GSF	Gold Standards Framework
		GTN	glyceryl trinitrate
DNR	do not resuscitate	GU	genitourinary tract
DOLS	Deprivation of liberty safeguards	HCM	hypertrophic cardiomyopathy
DPLD	diffuse parenchymal lung disease	HLE	healthy life expectancy
DPP	dipeptidyl peptidase	HOOF	Home oxygen order form
DSPN	diabetic sensorimotor polyneuropathy	HRCT	high resolution computerized tomography scan
DVLA	Driver and Vehicle Licensing Authority		
		HSMN	hereditary motor and sensory neuropathy
DVT	deep vein thrombosis		
DXA	dual-energy X-ray absorptiometry	HUT	head-up tilt
ECG	electrocardiogram	IBS	irritable bowel syndrome
ECT	electroconvulsive therapy	IC	intermediate care
ED	Emergency department	ICA	internal carotid artery
EEG	electroencephalography	ICH	intracerebral haemorrhage
eGFR	estimated glomerular filtration rate	ICS	inhaled corticosteroids
		IHD	ischaemic heart disease
ELISA	enzyme-linked immunosorbent assay	ILD	interstitial lung disease

IM	intramuscular
IMCA	Independent Mental Capacity Advocate
INR	international normalized ratio
IPF	idiopathic pulmonary fibrosis
ITU	intensive therapy unit
IV	intravenous
IVU	intravenous urogram
JVP	jugular venous pressure
LABA	long-acting beta$_2$ agonist
LacI	lacunar infarct
LAMA	long-acting muscarinic antagonist
LBBB	left bundle branch block
LCP	Liverpool Care Pathway for the dying patient
LDH	lactate dehydrogenase
LE	life expectancy
LFT	liver function test
LH	luteinizing hormone
LHRH	luteinizing hormone-releasing hormone
LMN	lower motor neuron
LMWH	low molecular weight heparin
LOAD	late-onset Alzheimer's disease
LOC	loss of consciousness
LP	lumbar puncture
LPA	Lasting Power of Attorney
LTOT	long-term oxygen therapy
LUTS	lower urinary tract symptoms
LV	left ventricular
LVF	left ventricular failure
LVH	left ventricular hypertrophy
MAO-B	monoamine oxidase B
MAR	Medicines Administration Record
MCA	Mental Capacity Act
MCA	middle cerebral artery
MCCD	Medical Certificate of Cause of Death
MCI	mild cognitive impairment
MCV	mean corpuscular volume
MDRD	modification of diet in renal disease
MDS	myelodysplastic syndrome
MDT	multidisciplinary team
MGUS	monoclonal gammopathy of unknown significance
MHA	Mental Health Act
MI	myocardial infarction
MIBI	technetium ^{99} 2-methoxy isobutyl isonitrile
MMSE	Mini-Mental State Examination
MNA	Mini-Nutritional Assessment
MND	motor neuron disease
MPTP	1-methyl-4-phenyl-1,2,3,4-tetrahydropyridine
MR	magnetic resonance
MRC	Medical Research Council
MRCP	magnetic resonance cholangiopancreatography
MRI	magnetic resonance imaging
MRSA	methicillin-resistant *Staphylococcus aureus*
MS	multiple sclerosis
MSA	multiple system atrophy
MSU	midstream urine
MTP	metatarso-phalangeal joint
NAD +	nicotinamide adenine dinucleotide
NAFLD	non-alcoholic fatty liver disease
NBM	nil by mouth
NCS	nerve conduction studies
NCSE	non-convulsive status epilepticus
NG	nasogastric
NHS CC	NHS continuing care
NHS	National Health Service
NIA-AA	National Institute on Aging and the Alzheimer's Association (new criteria for diagnosis of AD)
NICE	National Institute for Health and Clinical Excellence
NIHSS	National Institutes of Health Stroke Scale
NIV	non-invasive ventilation
NMDA	N-methyl-D-aspartate
NOF	neck of femur
NPH	normal pressure hydrocephalus
NSAID	non-steroidal anti-inflammatory drug
NSCLC	non-small cell lung cancer
NSF OP	National Service Framework for Older People
NSIP	non-specific interstitial pneumonia
NSTEMI	non-ST-elevation myocardial infarct
OA	osteoarthritis
OGD	oesophago gastro duodenoscopy
OSAHS	obstructive sleep apnoea/hyponoea syndrome
OTC	over-the-counter
PA	pernicious anaemia
PACI	partial anterior circulatory infarct
PAF	paroxysmal atrial fibrillation
PBC	primary biliary cirrhosis
PBR	payment by result

PCI	percutaneous coronary intervention
PCR	polymerase chain reaction
PCT	Primary Care Trust
PD	Parkinson's disease
PDE	phosphodiesterase
PE	pulmonary embolism
PEC	percutaneous endoscopic colopexy
PEFR	peak expiratory flow rate
PEG	percutaneous endoscopic gastrostomy
PET	positron-emission tomography
PICC	peripherally inserted central catheter
PIP	proximal interphalangeal joints
PMR	polymyalgia rheumatica
PoCI	posterior circulatory infarct
POP	plaster of Paris
PPARγ	peroxisome-proliferator-activated receptor gamma
PPI	proton pump inhibitor
PPS	post-polio syndrome
PSA	prostate-specific antigen
PSP	progressive supranuclear palsy
PTCA	percutaneous transluminal coronary angioplasty
PTH	parathyroid hormone
PUVA	psoralen + UVA treatment
PV	polycythaemia vera
PVS	persistent vegetative state
QOF	quality and outcomes framework
RA	rheumatoid arthritis
RANKL	receptor activator of nuclear factor kappa-B ligand
RAS	renal artery stenosis
RCP	Royal College of Physicians
RCT	randomized controlled trial
RDW	red cell distribution width
RGSC	Registrar General's socio-economic class
ROSIER	Recognition of Stroke in the Emergency Room scale
RoSPA	Royal Society for the Prevention of Accidents
RPE	retinal pigment epithelium
rt-PA	recombinant tissue-type plasminogen
SABA	short-acting beta$_2$ agonist
SAH	subarachnoid haemorrhage
SAMA	short-acting muscarinic antagonist
SBOT	short-burst oxygen therapy
SCC	squamous-cell carcinoma
SCLC	small-cell lung cancer

SD	standard deviation
SE	status epilepticus
SERM	selective estrogen modulator
SHA	Strategic Health Authority
SIADH	syndrome of inappropriate antidiuretic hormone
SIGN	Scottish Intercollegiate Guidelines Network
SITS-MOST	Safe Implementation of Treatments in Stroke Monitoring Study
SIVD	subcortical ischaemic vascular disease
SLE	systemic lupus erythematosus
SN	substantia nigra
SNRI	serotonin and norepinephrine reuptake inhibitor
SOL	space-occupying lesion
SPA	state pension age
SPECT	single-photon emission computerized tomography
SSRI	selective serotonin reuptake inhibitor
STEMI	ST-elevation myocardial infarct
TACI	total anterior circulatory infarct
TAVI	transcatheter aortic valve insertion
TB	tuberculosis
TCC	transitional cell carcinoma
TDP	transactive response DNA-binding protein
TEDS	thromboembolic-deterrent stockings
TENS	transcutaneous electrical nerve stimulation
TFT	thyroid function test
TGA	transient global amnesia
TH	tyrosine hydroxylase
TIA	transient ischaemic attack
TLOC	transient loss of consciousness
TOE	transoesophageal echocardiography
tPA	tissue plasminogen activator
TSH	thyroid stimulating hormone
tTGA	tissue transglutaminase antibodies
TUIP	transurethral incision of the prostate
TUMT	transurethral microwave therapy
TUNA	transurethral needle ablation
TURP	transurethral resection of the prostate
TVT	tension-free vaginal tape
U&E	urea and electrolytes
UIP	usual interstitial pneumonia
UKPDS	United Kingdom Prospective Diabetes Study
UMN	upper motor neuron

UTI	urinary tract infection	VGCC	voltage-gated calcium channels
VA	visual acuity	VTE	venous thromboembolism
VaD	vascular dementia	WBC	white blood cell
VEGF	vascular endothelial growth factor	YAG	yttrium aluminium garnet laser

The world grows old

Introduction

The Western world turned grey in the 20th century and much of the rest of the world will follow this century. Improvements in housing, sanitation, nutrition and education, and smaller family size, higher incomes and public health measures such as immunization were the major factors driving this epidemiological transition. In many developed countries, this shift started in the mid-19th century and life expectancy increased as infant and maternal mortality and deaths from infectious diseases in children and young adults fell. Over the last 30 years, gains in life expectancy are also being made in middle age. In countries such as Japan the transition started later but proceeded more quickly. In many developing countries, the transition started even later and is still in progress.

In the West, the impact of an ageing population on the retirement age, pensions and the cost and practicalities of service provision has become an important issue. An increasingly small number of people of working age cannot fund the pensions of older people with ever longer retirements. Most older people are independent, but if they need help, family care is often not available; many of their daughters will be working, families are scattered geographically and options for care are less well developed than child care.

The common afflictions of old age are now accepted, not as a cause for shame, but as serious diseases. Examples include the public information about the dementia of ex-President Reagan of the USA and a dramatization of the same disease as it affected the famous philosopher and novelist Iris Murdoch and Margaret Thatcher. Middle-aged, middle-class articulate 'children' such as Michael Ignatief, Linda Grant and Margaret Forster have written in detail about the dementing process as it affected their parents, themselves and their families. Terry Pratchett, who has a form of Alzheimer's disease which initially affects visuospatial perception, discusses aspects of dementia in the media. *Still Alice*, a debut novel about Alzheimer's by neuroscientist Lisa Genova, became a *New York Times* bestseller in 2009.

The Human Rights Act 1998 (2000) has the potential to offer protection to vulnerable elderly people, especially Articles 2, 3, 8, 10 and 14 (see box below). This Act applies to all public bodies, i.e. the NHS and Local Authority Social Service Departments.

Human Rights Act 1998

Article 2	Right to life.
Article 3	Prohibition of torture and inhuman and degrading treatment.
Article 8	Right to respect for private and family life and home.
Article 10	Freedom of expression and right to information.
Article 14	Right not to be discriminated against.

Population trends

The United Nations report *World Population Ageing 2009* (United Nations 2009) describes four key points about population ageing:

1 **Unprecedented**, without parallel in the history of humanity.

Lecture Notes Elderly Care Medicine, Eighth Edition. Claire G. Nicholl and K. Jane Wilson.
© 2012 John Wiley & Sons, Ltd. Published 2012 by John Wiley & Sons, Ltd.

Table 1.1 The percentage of the population aged 60 years or older in a range of countries, with their world ranking for this statistic and median age of the population (UN 2009)

	Percentage aged 60+	World ranking (% 60+)	Median age (years)
World			28.1
Japan	29.7	1	44.4
Italy	26.4	2	43.0
Greece	24.0	7	41.3
UK	22.4	17	39.7
USA	17.9	42	36.5
China	11.9	65	33.9
Brazil	9.9	71	28.6
India	7.4	105	24.7
Nigeria	4.9	162	18.4

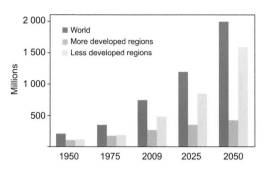

Figure 1.1 Population aged 60 and over: world and development regions, 1950–2050 (UN 2009). Reproduced with permission of UN.

2 **Pervasive**, affecting nearly all the countries of the world, the exceptions being African countries ravaged by HIV-AIDS and civil wars.

3 **Profound**, with major consequences and implications for all aspects of life.

4 **Enduring**, as short of a worldwide disaster, the trend will not be reversed.

In 1950, the proportion of the world population aged 60 and older was 8%; this had risen to 11% in 2009 and is expected to rise to 22% in 2050. Data from different countries are shown in Table 1.1.

Japan's population is the oldest in the world and most European countries have median ages of around 40 years. Population ageing is often thought of as a problem facing the developed world, but because the world's most populous countries are less developed, nearly two-thirds of older people already live in less developed regions. This proportion has increased from approximately 50% in 1950 and is predicted to rise to around 80% by 2050 (see Figure 1.1).

The greatest absolute numbers of older people live in China and India. An excellent online resource to look at demographic changes in different countries over time is Gapminder (http://www.gapminder.org/) – the trends with time, effects of war (e.g. France 1918, 1944; Japan 1945) and HIV (e.g. Swaziland) are readily seen.

Another important statistic for a country is its total dependency ratio, that is the number of under-15s plus the number of those aged $\geq$ 65 years per 100 people aged 15–64. In 2009, for the world, the sum of youth and old age dependency is around 50. In Africa the ratio is much higher due to the proportion of children. In Europe the ratio is similar to the world average but old age dependency exceeds youth dependency (see Figure 1.2).

There are marked differences in the **pace of population ageing** between developed and less developed countries, e.g. it took 115 years (1865–1980) for the proportion of older people to

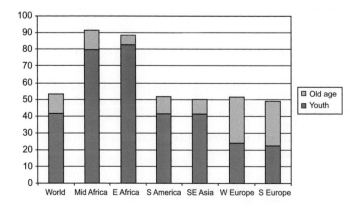

Figure 1.2 Youth and old age dependency ratios in world regions (UN 2009). Reproduced with permission of UN.

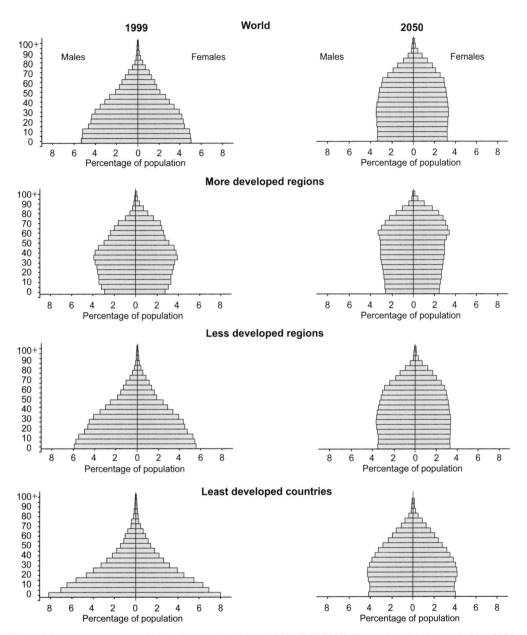

Figure 1.3 Population pyramids (age in years), 1999 and 2050 (UN 2009). Reproduced with permission of UN.

double in France (from 7 to 14%) whereas in China the proportion will have doubled between 2000 and 2027. The number of older people in the world is expected to exceed the number of children for the first time in 2045. By 2030 most countries will have a similar age structure, as can be seen from the population pyramids in Figure 1.3.

Developed countries

Demographic changes

- Death which was common in infancy and usual before 65 years is now rare in infancy and unusual before 65 years.

- Life expectancy continues to rise, partly due to improvements in medical care of conditions such as hypertension and ischaemic heart disease.
- The dramatic rise in the elderly population over the past 100 years is now slowing.
- However, the number of 'old old', i.e. those $\geq$ 80 years of age, is still increasing rapidly.
- The Commission on Global Ageing warns of the risk of 'ageing recessions' due to a fall in the size of the workforce (labour shortages) plus increased service demands (caring services). In 2010, China overtook Japan as the world's second largest economy, due in part to the ageing and shrinking population of Japan.

Medical services

- Sophisticated health systems are established with specialist services for the elderly.
- Population trends alone require increased health funding each year (estimated at 1% per year in the UK) in addition to inflation and costs due to technological development.
- Rising expectations of older people and their carers fuel rising health costs.
- Ethical dilemmas will be more pressing, e.g. the prolongation of death by technological intervention or medicated survival of the young chronically sick and acutely ill, and frail, elderly patients.
- Financial provision must be made to support the choices made. An elderly person costs the health services nine times as much as a young person.
- Medical training continues to concentrate on increasing specialization, so practitioners cannot cope with complex aetiologies (sociological, psychological and medical) and multi-pathology (co-morbidity), and the atypical presentations common in elderly patients, i.e. a mismatch between aspirations of young medics and the needs of their elderly patients.

Community services

- Community care is individually based and very varied. Comparison between provision in different countries is difficult because of political, socio-economic and demographic differences. It is easier to make comparisons with regard to institutional care, usually in residential or nursing homes. There used to be marked variation between countries, but figures are converging to 5–9% of the 65+ group being in care (5.5% in 2006 in England).

- The historical development of the patterns of care is similar. In all societies there has always been a heavy reliance on self-sufficiency and family care. The healthy and wealthy old have always faired the best. For the more disadvantaged, there has always been a need to rely on support from non-family members.
- In the 'Old World', non-family support was originally provided by the church or by occupationally related charities or guilds. In England, the state began to become more prominent in the 17th century with the first Poor Law Act, which provided workhouse care and 'outdoor relief'. This continued until the end of the 19th century. The 20th century saw the beginning of the welfare state – gradually growing in the first half of the century, reaching a peak mid-century and then declining towards the end of the 1980s. At the time of decline, the general move was away from the provision of services by the state to state regulation of services provided by other organizations. This regulation was gradually devolved and central control lost or weakened.
- From the 1980s onwards, an increasing number of nursing homes in the USA, and then Europe and Australia were run by profit-making organizations (increasingly large multinational companies). The for-profit companies had a worse record for staffing levels (20% less than non-profit-making institutions) and skill mix, and a higher incidence of violations of standards. There was concern that the regulatory arrangements were failing to improve or even maintain standards and costs were escalating.
- For example, in Australia, the proportion of for-profit nursing home beds was historically about 27%, but had risen to 55% by the year 2000. Between 1996 and 2000, the cost of public funding of private nursing homes rose from A$2.5 to A$3.9 billion. The cost of the regulatory system doubled, but unannounced inspections ceased, reports of inspections became more difficult to obtain and available sanctions were rarely used.

Less developed countries
Demographic changes

- Once people reached old age in developing countries, their life expectancy was not much lower than in the developed world and this remains the case (Table 1.2).
- Until recently the proportion of older people in the population was low, but as countries such as

Table 1.2 Mean life expectancy at different ages (UN 2009). Reproduced with permission of UN.

Country	At birth	At 60 years	At 80 years
More developed	76	22	9
Less developed	65	18	7
Least developed	55	16	6

China and India are so populous, over 60% of the world's elderly population already live in these countries.

- The population structure of these countries is changing very rapidly with falling birth rates as contraceptive policies become effective (or were imposed), infant mortality is reduced and to a lesser extent as survival in adult life improves.
- Population patterns are at risk of distortion by epidemics, e.g. HIV/AIDS, civil war and migration, e.g. sub-Saharan Africa.
- European studies show that the survival of babies with low birth-weight and reduced growth in the first year leads to poor adult health – especially regarding BP and blood sugar control. This is likely to have significant consequences in India and Southeast Asia.
- Potentially preventable disabilities acquired in youth will complicate old age.
- The poor will be unable to acquire sufficient wealth to provide for themselves in old age; therefore the total burden will either fall on the state or will be neglected.
- There are many pressing financial demands for expansion, e.g. education, housing and development of infrastructure.
- Many countries struggle with debt, and political instability is common.

Medical services

- Health services are often primitive, patchy and inappropriate to needs.
- 'High-tech' procedures for the few may be favoured over public health measures that would bring more benefit for the whole population.
- Doctors and nurses training in undeveloped countries will need expertise in elderly care because of the changing demography of their own countries. Depending on their country of origin, if they move to a developed country, they may find themselves confronted by very elderly patients for the first time.

- Development may be restricted by the tight macro-economic practices enforced by the International Monetary Fund which limit a government's ability to invest in health.
- Globalization via the World Trade Organization has resulted in conflict over the cost of drugs. High prices for patented drugs ensure financial profits for Pharma enabling development of new drugs but developing countries need access to cheap generic drugs, e.g. for the treatment of HIV, hypertension and diabetes.
- World trade tends to encourage bad health habits, e.g. smoking, excess alcohol and recreational drug abuse.

Community services

- The majority of the population continue to work as long as they are able and must rely on family support; retirement, at least for most people, is a concept of the developed world.

Ageing in India

India is in a rapid phase of transition. Life expectancy at birth has been increasing since the 1950s (Figure 1.4). As there are more children in India than China, by 2050 India is predicated to have overtaken China as the world's most populous country.

Life expectancy at the age of 60 in India has also increased for both men and women between 1961 and 2008 by 4–5 years and is now 16.3 years for men and 17.2 years for women. As a result, India's elderly population is growing rapidly.

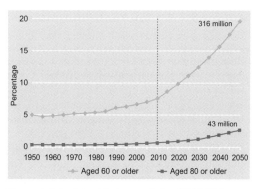

Figure 1.4 India's elderly population (UN 2009). *Source:* Bloom et al. (2010). Reproduced with permission of John Wiley & Sons, Inc.

Within India there is huge variation in health care, with very high standards in large centres but swathes of the country still lacking basic provision. The private sector accounts for over 80% of health care spending. The extremes are exemplified by cardiac centres which offer coronary surgery to health tourists and are feted by Western politicians. However, 10% of Primary Health Centres have no doctor. One approach had been the development of a 4-year Bachelor of Rural Health Care, but the lure of the city and practical problems with training remain a challenge.

Disease and disability in the over 60s in India

- Cardiovascular disease is the commonest cause of death in old age.
- There are 11 million elderly blind people – 80% due to cataract.
- Sixty percent have hearing impairment.
- Nine million have hypertension.
- Five million have diabetes.
- 0.35 million have cancer.
  (Source: WHO 1999.)

In 1999, the Government of India Ministry of Social Justice and Empowerment developed the 'National Policy on Older Persons'. This stressed the importance of setting up geriatric services and appropriate training, but implementation has been limited. Professional organizations are developing, including the Indian Academy of Geriatrics which publishes a quarterly journal, and the charity HelpAge India.

HelpAge India sponsored an economic and health survey of people aged 80 and older in eight cities in India, targeting mid or lower socio-economic groups. The results (2010) highlight the dependency of this group on their children for financial support (70%) and practical care. One-fifth of those interviewed reported abuse from their family. Half of the participants considered their health to be poor or very poor; the major problems were pain, poor vision, hypertension, arthritis and asthma. Most relied on a son to fund their health care.

Overall, 60–75% of elderly people in India are economically dependent on their families. The extended family is disappearing and the social status of elderly people is being eroded. Since 1992, an old age pension has been available for those over 65 with no means of support.

In 1997, there were only 354 old people's homes, usually organized by charities. The number of for-profit homes is now growing very rapidly, but provision is aimed at the emerging wealthier middle class.

Ageing in Africa

The pattern of ageing in Africa is different from the rest of the world due to the effects of AIDS and war, demonstrating how the unexpected can undermine projections. In 2009, the life expectancy at birth in Lesotho, Swaziland, Zambia and Zimbabwe was less than 47 years, and less than 50 years in a total of 13 other African countries. The only country with a lower figure currently is Afghanistan.

Sub-Saharan Africa has a more heavy burden of HIV-AIDS than any other region of the world, accounting for two-thirds of global cases. In 2008, around 1.4 million people died from AIDS and 1.9 million people became infected with HIV. Since the beginning of the epidemic, more than 14 million children have lost one or both parents to HIV/AIDS. Most AIDS deaths occur among young adults, with a devastating effect on families, communities and economies. The head of the family in 43% of Zimbabwean families with AIDS orphans is a grandmother. As their children and grandchildren die, the older generation are left with no carers for themselves. Older people do contract HIV infection, and it may run a more rapid course in this age group, but the incidence is unknown.

The response to HIV has been variable. Political denial of the problem was a major factor in the slow response in South Africa. Botswana began a national treatment programme, 'masa' (dawn), in 2002. It has better infrastructure than many countries in the region and after a slow start has now reached 90% coverage in terms of retroviral therapy.

Forty percent of the world's armed conflicts rage in Africa, with over a thousand fatalities in 2010. Most deaths due to direct violence are in those aged between 15 and 45. Indirect factors including movement of refugees, rape, famine, poverty and failure of infection control programmes, e.g. for TB, kill thousands more and limit sustainable economic development. For example, in over 10 years of war in the Democratic Republic of the Congo an estimated 350,000 people have died in combat but an estimated 5.4 million people have died as a result of the conflict, the vast majority from malnutrition and disease. Out of 50 African countries, 11 were considered to be involved in some form of armed conflict in 2010. However, since the African Union declared 2010 the Year of Peace and Security, the number of conflicts has fallen and there may be more willingness to criticize and take action against other African countries.

Ageing in Brazil

Brazilians' life expectancy has shot up to near Western European levels from just 37 years in 1940, while the number of births per woman has fallen to 1.8 from near 6 in 1970. In 1990 it was predicted that HIV-AIDS would have a major impact, but strategies including widespread promotion of condom use, educating prostitutes, needle exchange programmes and most controversially the manufacture and provision of cheap generic antiretroviral drugs were remarkably successful in containing the threatened epidemic. Disability rises with increasing age and the prevalence of difficulty walking and performing personal care is similar to that found in the UK (especially in men). Those with less education and wealth were almost twice as likely to suffer from disability compared with their peers. Urban dwellers were also more disabled than those in rural areas.

Global warming

The Kyoto protocol came into force in 2005. It is predicated that if greenhouse gas emissions are not reduced the health burdens of climate change are likely to double by 2020 (Kovats and Haines 2005). The experience from France in the 2-week summer heat-wave of 2003 indicates that older people are the most vulnerable. Most deaths occur in people over 70 and within the first few days of a heat-wave. The estimated number excess death in August 2003 was 13,600. The deaths were not due to hyperthermia but stress on already strained cardiac and respiratory systems. Preventative measures should be taken when a heat-wave is forecast.

There is also a fear that food poisoning may become more frequent with higher environmental temperatures. Frail elderly people are unable to withstand severe and prolonged diarrhoea. Other factors will include increased air pollution. Mosquito-borne diseases may spread; mosquitoes that can carry dengue fever virus were previously limited to elevations below 3,300 ft but recently appeared at 7,200 ft in the Andes in Colombia. Malaria has been detected in new higher-elevation areas in Indonesia and Africa.

Global warming is also associated with more unpredictable climatic events. Oxfam reports that the number of natural disasters, e.g. floods and cyclones, has quadrupled in the last two decades, and the number of people affected has increased from around 174 million to over 250 million a year. Older people tend to fare worse in all natural disasters; HelpAge International reported that older people had disproportionately high death rates in the 2004 Asian tsunami and their needs were overlooked in chaotic relief operations. Hurricane Katrina forced the evacuation of 1.7 million people in 2005 and led to deaths and long-term health problems for 200,000 New Orleans residents. The true toll of the October floods in Pakistan 2010 will not be known for years as the poverty resulting from destroyed livelihoods continues to claim lives. 2010 was the hottest summer on record in Russia with Moscow temperatures topping 38 °C; the death rate from respiratory problems triggered by air pollution from widespread forest fires increased dramatically.

Global poverty

Whilst the developed world struggles with diseases of affluence, most of the world struggles with poverty. Global poverty is falling, but this is mainly due to China – poverty in Sub-Saharan Africa is increasing.

There is a marked positive correlation between the per capita income in a country and life expectancy (see Figure 1.5), but there is a wide range at the lower end. Individual countries can be looked at dynamically on Gapminder. However, there may be marked variation within countries (see the discussion on effect of social class in the UK in Chapter 2).

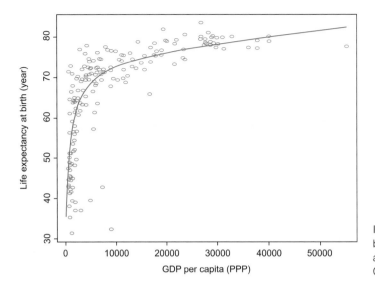

Figure 1.5 The relationship between Gross Domestic Product and life expectancy. Courtesy of Gapminder.

Inter-generational strife

This is a potential problem in both developed and under-developed countries. Strains and conflict could arise due to the falling dependency ratio (i.e. fewer working people to support those in need of care). There is the prospect of poverty in old age for the current young due to increased life expectancy but a decline in provision for pension payments (compared with current retirees). There is also an increased expectation of those growing old in the next two decades, e.g. aspiring to early retirement with decreased disability levels but still expecting enhanced care services.

The inverse of the dependency ratio is the support ratio. The number of working-age adults per older adult will decrease in all regions between 2010 and 2050 (see Figure 1.6).

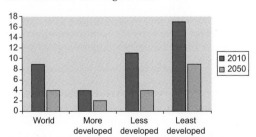

Figure 1.6 The number of adults aged 15–64 per adult aged 65 or older in different development regions in 2010 and projections for 2050 (Population Reference Bureau 2010).

Social aspects of ageing

Old age is unfortunately often a time of loss. The potential losses are varied, often interrelated, and include:

- Health and eventually life, due to increasing pathology.
- Wealth due to termination of employment (in the UK, the default retirement age of 65 was removed in April 2011, making compulsory retirement at any age unlawful unless justified).
- Companionship following bereavement (spouse, siblings and friends).
- Independence due to acquired disabilities.
- Homoeostasis due to impairments of the autonomic nervous system and renal function.
- Status following retirement and loss of independence.

The above changes and losses may expose people to the following consequences:

- Unhappiness, grief, depression, suicide (see Chapters 4 and 16).
- Increased incidence of illness.
- Increased risk of accident.
- Poverty; though the proportion of pensioner households with low incomes has fallen.
- Dependence and abuse.
- Malnutrition and subnutrition (see Chapter 11).
- Hypothermia (see Chapter 12).

Loss of wealth

Income falls on giving up paid employment. Pensions are not normally equivalent to wages and the average pension is about half of the average working wage for a couple. Disabilities themselves may result in additional costs, e.g. for help, aids and adaptations.

Retirement

Retirement is a mixed blessing: 20% of workers fear retirement but 50% look forward to it. Retirement is a potential period of loss – of income, status, companionship and self-confidence.

To counteract the disadvantages, there are positive aspects of retirement:

- It may occupy one-third of life.
- Many remain fit and healthy for most of this time.
- It is an opportunity to redesign lifestyle and to promote good health.
- Time is available for new or renewed interests, activities and relationships.

But retirement may bring social problems and it is a time when some difficult decisions will have to be made. Dilemmas encountered may include:

- Becoming a carer, e.g. of parents or grandchildren early in retirement or of spouse or siblings later on.
- Where to live – it is probably best to stay put where comfortable and well known. If a move is contemplated, earlier is better than later, as the retiree is likely to be fitter and one of a pair.
- What sort of accommodation? Somewhere enabling independence, despite acquired disabilities.
- Driving – may need to be given up at some stage, so beware of geographical isolation (see Chapters 4 and 16).
- Sex – it is 'allowed' even in the very old so long as it gives pleasure to both partners (see Chapter 13).
- Boredom affects 10% of the retired – another 20% (although not bored) would prefer still to be working. People who are poor, disabled, poorly educated and isolated are most likely to be dissatisfied with retirement.
- The economic consequences of an expanding population of retired persons dependent on pensions are causing widespread concern within the developed world. As a consequence, the retirement age may be gradually increased to 70+ years. There will be a need to review the nature of paid employment in later years with consideration of plans to make partial or gradual retirement easier without loss of status, pay or pension rights. Preparation for retirement is vital.
- The increasing vulnerability and unpredictability of the global financial markets also pose threats to pension provision. The pension aspirations of many current workers may not be met and may be considered a potential threat to world finance.

> **Recommended physical activity in retirement**
>
> - Regular moderate-intensity activity for 30 min on most days.
> - Short bursts of exertion may have a cumulative effect.
> - Start slow and gradually build up intensity and duration.
> - Work on strength, flexibility and balance.
> - If an activity is not provoking symptoms, it is unlikely to be doing harm.
> - Generally benefits of activity outweigh risks.
> - When activity requires special equipment or clothing, make sure it is appropriate and in good condition.

Some myths of ageing

- **It is a new problem** No – there have always been elderly people; there are now more. In the past, most people were denied the opportunity of old age by dying young. Now, most babies born in developed countries can expect to survive into their 80s.
- **All elderly people are decrepit and senile** No – most live independent lives and mainly in their own homes (96% in the UK).
- **The chronic conditions of old age are untreatable** No – medical treatment at all ages is primarily the management of chronic conditions. The courses of disease can be slowed or modified, e.g. Parkinson's disease or Alzheimer's

disease, symptoms can be alleviated, e.g. pain, breathlessness, and in deficiency diseases (pernicious anaemia, osteomalacia and myxoedema) normal function can be restored.

- **Natural decline cannot be prevented** No – regular physical activity can rejuvenate and physical capacity can be improved by 10–15 years. Also, adopting a 'healthy lifestyle' in middle age (no smoking, avoidance of obesity and taking regular exercise) can delay the onset and decrease the eventual severity and duration of disability towards the end of life.
- **Treating elderly patients is a waste of money** No – not to treat is not only inhumane (see Human Rights Act 1998) but also often expensive, and neglected problems may lead to longer-term, higher expenditure (i.e. 'care' can be more expensive than 'cure').
- **Care of the elderly is bankrupting the NHS** No – it is true that elderly people account for more costs within the NHS than the young (except for the management of children). However, most people make few demands on the NHS until the 15 years prior to their death. Costs for this terminal period are similar if death occurs at any age, i.e. 40, 50, 60 years, and so on. In fact, death in very old age may be gentle and not incur the high cost of unrealistic heroics.
- **All elderly people are depressed and lonely, and are better off dead** No – the majority of elderly people are not depressed. Well-being and contentment may feature in later life more than during the ambitious and frustrated productive years. Although the general population thinks that 90% of elderly people are lonely, only 10% of the elderly consider themselves to be so.
- **The elderly are of no use** No – they are a valuable resource with experience and, sometimes, wisdom. The majority of carers are elderly and these include grandparents assisting in the rearing of their grandchildren because of absent or working parents. The old are the backbone of the voluntary services.
- **Old patients have a limited future and poor prognosis** No – life expectancy at 65 years is in excess of 17 years for a man and 20 years for a woman. Survival for 5 years after many surgical and oncological treatments is recorded as a success.

 REFERENCES

All websites accessed September 2011.

Bloom DE, Mahal A, Rosenberg L, Sevilla J (2010) *Economic Security Arrangements in the Context of Population Ageing in India*. http://onlinelibrary.wiley.com/doi/10.1111/j.1468-246X.2010.01370.x/full#b17.

HelpAge India (undated) *Economic and Health Survey on India's Oldest Old (80+) – Needs, Care and Access*. http://www.helpageindia.org/pdf/Economic-&-Health-Survey-on-India%27s-Oldest-Old-%2880+%29.pdf.

Kovats RS, Haines A. (2005) Global climate change and health: recent findings and future steps. *CMAJ* 172(4): 501–502, doi: 10.1503/cmaj.1050123.

Population Reference Bureau (2010) *World Population Highlights 2010*. http://www.prb.org/Publications/PopulationBulletins/2010/world-populationhighlights2010.aspx.

United Nations (2009) *World Population Ageing 2009*. Department of Economic and Social Affairs. http://www.un.org/esa/population/publications/WPA2009/WPA2009_WorkingPaper.pdf.

WHO (1999) *Ageing in India*. IJ Prakash. http://whqlibdoc.who.int/hq/1999/WHO_HSC_AHE_99.2.pdf.

 FURTHER INFORMATION

Lancet and UCL Institute for Global Health Commission (2009) *Managing the Health Effects of Climate Change*. http://www.ucl.ac.uk/global-health/ucl-lancet-climate-change.pdf.

National Academy of Sciences (2006) *Aging in Sub-Saharan Africa: Recommendations for Furthering Research*. http://www.ncbi.nlm.nih.gov/bookshelf/picrender.fcgi?book=nap11708&blobtype=pdf. http://www.ncbi.nlm.nih.gov/books/NBK20296/.

2

Health and social care for elderly people in the UK

How many older people are there?

The UK population topped 60 million for the first time in 2005. As well as increasing, the population is ageing, with the biggest percentage changes at extreme old age. The 2001 census was the first where the number of pensioners was greater than the number of children. The proportion of people aged 65 and over is projected to increase from 16% in 2009 to 23% by 2034. Different sources give figures for different age bands and areas, i.e. UK/Great Britain/England and Wales, and since the last census in 2001 figures are estimates, you will find different numbers quoted. However, all agree that the proportion of the population aged 75+ and 85+ is increasing markedly and, in line with this, the most dramatic change is seen in centenarians (11,600 in 2009 increasing over seven-fold to an estimated 87,900 in 2034). This can be explored in detail on the dynamic map on the ONS website (ONS 2010).

Is life expectancy still increasing?

Life expectancy at birth has continued to increase steadily from the 1970s (Figure 2.3). However, despite all the government's attempts, the difference between social class groups (here grouped into manual and non-manual) has persisted and even widened slightly. This is the main explanation for the regional differences in life expectancy; people living in the north of England live around 2 years less than those in the south.

What is your life expectancy when you are old?

Life expectancy at extreme old age has always been longer than people think; if a woman born in 1850 lived to 80 years her life expectancy at 80 was another 4 years. For a women born in 1950 this is estimated to be 8.5 years. This is important for clinical management – an 80-year-old newly diagnosed diabetic will have time to develop complications! Currently, in the UK, a man of 65 can expect another 17.6 years of life and a woman another 20.2 years. Unfortunately the gain in healthy life expectancy is not keeping pace with the overall gain in life expectancy, so women in particular spend more time in late life in poor health.

Does living longer mean more suffering in old age?

The answer to this question is 'it depends'. In England in the 21st century, social class – as defined by the Registrar General's Socio-economic Class (RGSC) – still has a marked effect on life expectancy and disability-free life expectancy. Table 2.1 shows

Lecture Notes Elderly Care Medicine, Eighth Edition. Claire G. Nicholl and K. Jane Wilson.
© 2012 John Wiley & Sons, Ltd. Published 2012 by John Wiley & Sons, Ltd.

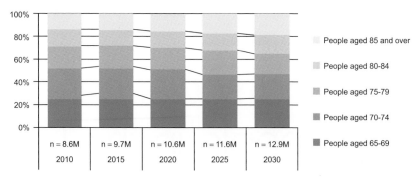

Figure 2.1 Percentage composition of the population aged 65+ in England and estimated changes to 2030, with the total number of those aged 65+. *Source:* Office for National Statistics licensed under the Open Government Licence v.1.0.

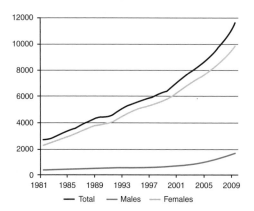

Figure 2.2 Population (number of people) aged 100 years and over in the UK, 1981–2009.

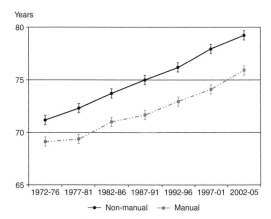

Figure 2.3 Male life expectancy at birth by social class in England and Wales, 1972–2005.

Table 2.1 Life expectancy and disability-free life expectancy by Registrar General Socio-economic Class in England, 2001–2003 (ONS 2010)

Sex and age	RGSC	LE (years)	DFLE (years)	HLE as a proportion of LE (%)
Men at birth	I	80.2	70.2	88
	V	73.5	56.9	77
Women at birth	I	85.5	71.6	84
	V	78.7	60.4	77
Men at 65	I	18.3	11.6	64
	V	13.9	6.3	45
Women at 65	I	22.7	12.8	56
	V	17.6	8.1	46

RGSC, Registrar General's Social Class; LE, life expectancy; DFLE, disability-free life expectancy; HLE, healthy life expectancy.

that in each class women live longer than men, but the advantage especially for disability-free life expectancy, of being a member of RGSC I as opposed to V whether calculated at birth or 65 for both men and women is staggering. In social class I, men spend a greater proportion of their lives than women without limiting illness.

What are the characteristics of the older population?

Gender

In the population aged 65+, women outnumber men because of their longer life expectancy and the death of young men in World War II, but this ratio is falling. In 1984 there were 156 women aged 65 and over for every 100 men of the same age, compared with the current sex ratio of 129 women for every 100 men, as the war generation dies. By 2034 it is projected that the 65 and over sex ratio will have fallen still further to 118 women for every 100 men. In 2003, there were 40 men per 100 women aged 85+; for 2031 the estimate is 65 per 100 (Figure 2.4).

Ethnicity

There is less ethnic mix in old age than in the general population, where 7.9% were described as non-white in 2001. Whereas 12% of people under 16 are from an ethnic minority group, this is 2.5% at 65+ and only 1% at 85+. However, 10% of Black Caribbean and 7% of Indian people were over 65 years in 2001 (reflecting the earlier migration of these groups to the UK). The London borough of Brent, for example, has a very significant number of older people from ethnic minorities, so local planning is essential.

Geographic variation

Older people migrate from towns to the country and seaside so the distribution of people above state pension age (currently women of 60+ and men of 65+) is uneven. London is a young city. In 2010, 30% of the population was 65+ in Christchurch, Dorset. By 2033, it is projected that over 40% of the population will be aged 65+ in areas such as West Somerset, Berwick-upon-Tweed, South Shropshire, West Dorset and North Norfolk, compared with the UK average of 22.9%.

Health status

In the General Lifestyle Survey (GB) 2010 (ONS 2009), 1/3 adults aged 65–74 and 1/2 adults aged 75 and over report a limiting longstanding sickness or disability. Both proportions are similar to a decade ago. Some conditions have a very high prevalence: 16% of women and 10% of men aged 65–74 have diabetes.

For those aged 65–74, the proportion with a disability increases as income decreases. The effect

Thousands

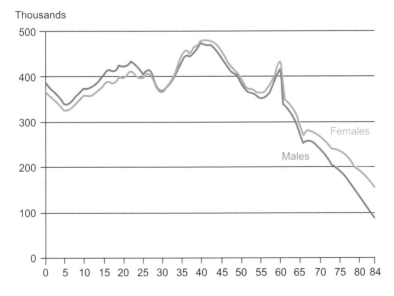

Figure 2.4 Population (in thousands) by age in the UK, 2007. *Source*: Office for National Statistics licensed under the Open Government Licence v.1.0.

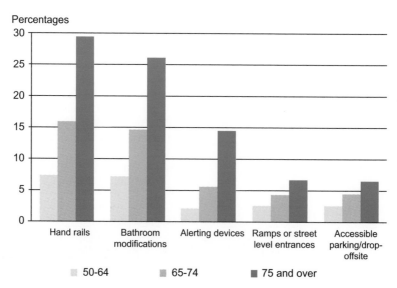

Figure 2.5 House adaptations by age of the household reference person in England, 2006.

of income is less marked for those aged 75 and over. Figure 2.5 shows the relationship between increasing age and common adaptations for disability.

Sensory impairment

In 2008, 64% of the 153,000 on the register of blind people and 66% of the 156,300 people on the register of those with partial sight were aged 75 or over. Twelve percent of the over 75s have visual impairment. Seventy percent of the over 70-year-olds in the UK have some hearing loss, mild in 27%, moderate in 36% and severe in 7%.

Living companions

In 2007, in Great Britain, 30% of women and 20% of men aged 65–74 lived alone. Aged 75+ this rose to 61% and 33%. White people are more likely to live alone than those from ethnic minority groups. Overall, one-third of pensioners live alone (Figure 2.6); half of them live with their spouses and only one-fifth live with children, siblings or friends. The extended family is rare in the UK and probably always has been.

Income

In 2008/09, 1.8 million pensioners lived in poverty (defined as below 60% of contemporary median income), fewer than in 2007/08 when there were 2 million pensioners in poverty (Figure 2.7).

The largest source of income for pensioners is state 'benefit income', which includes state pension income and benefits (Figure 2.8). Older pensioners tend to be poorer and spend a higher percentage of their total expenditure on essentials, e.g. heating, food and housing. In the UK, the safety net provided by the social security system is complex and this acts as a deterrent to taking up benefits. Occupational pensions and investment income are increasing in importance.

Where do elderly people live?

Ninety-five percent of people over 65 in the UK live in their own home (including sheltered flats). This is termed living in 'the community', in contrast to institutional care, although care homes should be part of the local community too! Owner-occupiers account for about 70%. A higher percentage of elderly people than middle-aged live in rented accommodation (Figure 2.9). Results from the English House Condition Survey 2004 (Department for Communities and Local Government 2004)

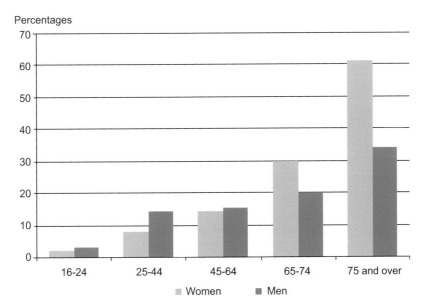

Figure 2.6 People living alone by sex and age in Great Britain, 2007.

showed that housing is steadily improving, al-though 33% of people aged 75+ still lived in a 'non-decent' home (versus 28% of all households) and are more likely to be in an energy-inefficient home (12% versus 8%), or a home in serious disre-pair (11% versus 10%). Eight percent of over 65-year-olds live in sheltered housing.

Sheltered housing

This usually comprises the following:

• A group of small flats (typically one bedroom, living room, kitchenette, bathroom and toilet)

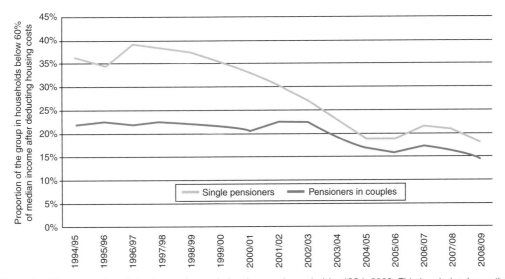

Figure 2.7 The proportion of single pensioners in low-income households, 1994–2009. This has halved over the last decade, with smaller falls for pensioner couples. *Source*: Households Below Average Income. DWP UK. Updated September 2010.

Percentages

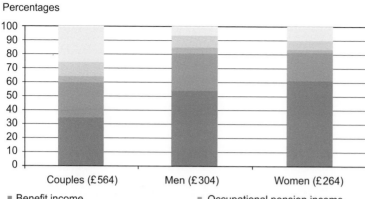

Couples (£564)   Men (£304)   Women (£264)

- Benefit income
- Personal pension income
- Earnings
- Occupational pension income
- Investment income
- Other income

Figure 2.8 Average gross weekly income of pensioners, 2008–09.

often around communal facilities for meals or social activity.
- Provided by the local authority, housing associations, voluntary sector and increasingly the private sector.
- Scheme manager or 'warden' who may work office hours only.
- Buzzer system allows residents to summon help.
- Residents are usually able to wash, dress, transfer and mobilize independently (including wheelchair users) and prepare their own food.
- They may have the usual help from social services.
- Benefits those with physical disability.
- Newer schemes are being set up with staff on site 24 h to provide 'extra care' (for washing, dressing, meals, etc.), enabling much frailer residents to live there. There were around 20,000 places in 2005.
- Purpose-built developments may include components of 'assistive technology'.

Institutional care

In 2010 it was estimated that only 3.7% of people over 65 lived in institutions, but this rate rose rapidly with increasing age to 12% aged over 75 years and 20% over 85 years. The rate in the UK was higher than in many continental European countries, but is now similar (number of people 65+ in care: 319,937; total of 65+: 8,585,000 = 3.7%).

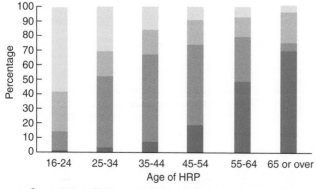

Own outright   Buying with mortgage   Social renters   Private renters

Figure 2.9 Age of household reference person by housing tenure, 2008. *Source*: English Housing Survey (2010). Full household sample. Crown copyright.

Institutionalization occurs when the person can no longer be supported at home *within the resources available* because of:

- severe physical disabilities;
- immobility;
- severe mental disability requiring constant supervision;
- unpredictable and frequent care needs.

This point is reached sooner if the person has a passive personality and there is no family support or even hostility to the person remaining at home.

Complications of institutionalization include:

- depersonalization;
- marked restriction of choices;
- accelerated dependence.

NB: All of these can be minimized by persistent effort by staff, visitors and sometimes the residents.

What types of institutions are there?

Long-stay hospitals

These have almost disappeared but have left a difficult legacy regarding who pays for care of this frailest group. Successive governments struggle with the NHS being 'free at the point of delivery', whereas care provided by social services is means-tested in England (free in Scotland). Thirty years ago, many elderly people spent their last months in a geriatric long-stay hospital. This care had its limitations, but was free to the patient. Long-stay hospitals were shut to save money; patients were placed in nursing homes, transferring some of the costs to the individuals. Geographical variation in the availability of long-stay NHS beds resulted in inequity.

NHS continuing care (NHS CC)

This was introduced to try to restore equity; individuals are assessed against criteria to determine whether they are entitled to free care for the remainder of their days. To qualify, an individual must have a 'primary health need', and the nature, complexity and unpredictability of their conditions are considered. A patient granted NHS CC is usually bed-bound with multiple problems needing regular skilled nursing, e.g. for pressure sores or tube feeding, unpredictable medical needs and a very short prognosis.

The assessment is in two stages: if the initial checklist is positive, a full assessment is done assessing 12 domains (behaviour, cognition, psychological needs, communication, mobility, nutrition, continence, skin integrity, breathing, medication and symptom control, altered consciousness and special factors). Geographical variation persists. The right of appeal is used quite often, as if you have to pay for a nursing home, you may have to sell your house rather than leaving it to your family. If the patient is granted NHS CC, the care can be provided at home, a nursing home or, occasionally, a hospital. A patient who is dying and wishes to die at home may be 'fast tracked' home with NHS CC. Scotland takes a fairer view, where the 'personal care' element is not separated from nursing care and is not means-tested.

Care homes providing nursing care

These are often still referred to as nursing homes. Most new residents are over 80, suffer from multiple disabilities (both physical, usually being chair/bed-bound, and mental) and need 'hotel services', help with personal hygiene *and* nursing care. Medical cover is provided by the resident's general practitioner (GP). They may keep their GP if the home is local, but the move often results in a change of GP at a very vulnerable time. A registered nurse must be on duty 24 h a day. The weekly fee for a private nursing home bed is around £650.

Care homes providing personal care

These are often still referred to as residential homes. Residents need hotel services and help with personal hygiene and also have their own GP. Most of the staff are care assistants. On admission, a new client would usually be able to move from bed to chair and walk (with help as needed) to the communal dining and sitting areas. Nursing care, if needed for a short period, is usually provided by a district nurse. The average weekly fee for a private

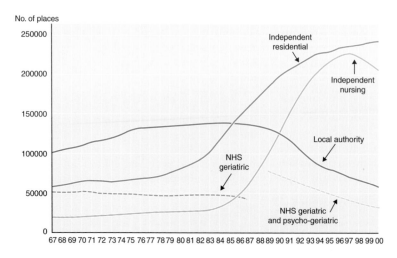

No. of places

Independent residential

Independent nursing

Local authority

NHS geriatiric

NHS geriatric and psycho-geriatric

67 68 69 70 71 72 73 74 75 76 77 78 79 80 81 82 83 84 85 86 87 88 89 90 91 92 93 94 95 96 97 98 99 00

Figure 2.10 Long-term trends from 1967–2000 in the long-term care sector. (Adapted from Laing and Buisson.)

residential care home bed is around £500 (more for people with dementia, in London, etc.).

Residential homes and nursing homes are now all regulated by one authority, but the beds are registered for a specific client group. If a residential home resident becomes ill and is admitted to hospital, the home can refuse to take the resident back 'as it can no longer meet their needs', forcing the unfortunate individual to move again to a care home with nursing. This causes frustration as the resident may have been deteriorating for some time prior to admission; the wait for nursing home care increases length of hospital stay and the individual may deteriorate further or even die from nosocomial infection. This situation is better if the home has both nursing and personal care beds ('dual registered'). There is a lot of variation in the flexibility of both homes and local authorities.

Specialist homes for people with dementia

It is relatively easy to maintain a physically disabled but cognitively intact person at home – if problems arise between care visits they can summon help. Whilst extra-care sheltered flats with assistive technology (see above) can provide a good care setting, the commonest reason for people to need 24-h care is dementia on top of physical problems. Therefore, most care homes will cope with a degree of dementia but have to be registered for this. If dementia is the main problem, in the form of wandering or disruptive behaviour, a specialist Dementia (elderly) or DE unit will be needed.

Who provides institutional care?

Care homes with nursing are mainly in the private sector. Care homes providing personal care were traditionally run by local authorities, but over 90% of beds are now provided by the private sector. There is some voluntary sector provision. The care home market is a difficult one. An initial rapid expansion in private beds has been followed by contraction. In England, since 2003 there has been a steady decline in the number of council-supported residents. In 2009, councils purchased just under half of all the registered places in care homes in England for older people (171,207 places), 43% of the beds with nursing for older people and 52% of the beds for older people needing personal care.

As more people are supported at home, patients entering institutional care are frailer and the costs outstrip the available funding. The major trends in bed provision are shown in Figure 2.10.

How is institutional care paid for?

In England and Wales, if an older person has enough savings, they can enter a private or voluntary sector home of their choice if they meet its admission criteria. If a person needs state financial support, an assessment is carried out to see if they meet the criteria for care home admission and whether personal care or nursing care is appropriate. Then their financial situation is assessed. The individual has to contribute to the cost, ranging from forfeiting their allowances to paying the full amount for residential care if they have > £23,250 capital (2012–13). Residents must be left with a weekly personal allowance of £22.30. Owner-occupiers often have to sell to finance care unless a dependent relative continues to live in the house or insurance arrangements have been made; there is a '12 week disregard' which gives a brief window when the council must ignore the value of a house to allow the property to be sold. In a nursing home, the 'board and lodging' and 'personal care' components are means-tested but the state contributes to the cost of nursing care regardless of means – the rate in 2012–13 is £108.70. An assessment for this must be done by an NHS employed registered nurse prior to placement.

In a locality, the commissioners (social services/Primary Care Trusts) have a benchmark price for a nursing bed and a residential bed and a list of 'approved homes'. They may block purchase beds in a home. Approval is designed to improve standards but reduces choice, as does block-booking. Homes may be able to charge more in the private market so a social services client may only get a bed in the home of their choice if they or their family 'top-up' to pay the gap between the benchmark cost and the price the home wishes to charge. A NOP survey (Partnership 2010) showed that most people are aware that they are likely to live into their 80s and that many people will go into care (roughly 40%) but are over-optimistic in their expectation of how long for (5 years). The overall average is 2 years, but it is 4 years plus for self-funders and 1 in 10 will live 8 years in care. However, the majority have no realistic idea of how much it will cost.

In 2009, the annual average cost of residential care in the UK was estimated at nearly £25,000, with the cost for a nursing home at around £35,000. Care at home is also expensive; at an average of £17.30 per hour, 3 h of daily home care would amount to more than £18,000 per year (Laing and Buisson 2009).

In Scotland, people aged 65 or over who live in care homes and are assessed as self-funders receive a weekly payment of £149 (2008) for personal care and a further payment of £67 if they require nursing care; self-funders still pay for 'hotel costs'.

> **Challenges for the UK care sector**
>
> - Increasing numbers of very old (i.e. > 85 years).
> - Increasing frailty of residents – especially dementia with behavioural problems.
> - Staff recruitment and retention problems.
> - Financial consequences of increasing staff numbers, training and pay.
> - Rising public expectations.
> - Demands of recent legislation regarding space.
> - Inadequate benchmark funds (self-funders subsidize state-funded clients)

How is care for older people organized?

Traditionally, health care was the responsibility of the NHS and social care of the social services department of the local authority; over the decades, the government departments responsible have been aggregated and disaggregated. All agencies providing services have a responsibility to older people – law and order, town planning, housing, transport, even education, as all impact on the quality of life and opportunities for older people.

Health care for older people

The organization of the NHS

The Department of Health (DH) controls the NHS. The Secretary of State for Health is the head of the DH and reports to the Prime Minister. The structure of the NHS is immensely complex and is always being reorganized. Until September 2010, the DH supervised England's 10 Strategic Health Authorities (SHAs), which oversaw all NHS activities in England, supervising the NHS trusts in its area. The devolved administrations of Scotland, Wales and Northern Ireland run their local NHS services.

In England, each SHA contained around 15 organizations called Primary Care Trusts (PCTs). PCTs assess local need and **commission** care for their population. This means buying care, according to contracts that specify the type, volume and quality parameters for different clinical problems, e.g. emergency admissions or elective cataract surgery. Many PCTs provide services themselves and were encouraged to separate these 'provider services' from their main business of commissioning. PCTs had to work with their councils on a local delivery plan to try to ensure that services are 'joined up'. In a few areas they actually merged with social services to form 'care trusts'.

The NHS services to be commissioned included primary care (provided by GPs and their teams); a range of community services, e.g. community hospitals, specialist nurses; secondary care – traditionally provided in the District General Hospital (DGH) – and tertiary care (specialist hospital care in regional or national centres, usually teaching hospitals). To complicate things, groups of GP practices (which are of course providing primary care) could be given funding to commission the other care their patients needed – this is called **practice-based commissioning**. For patients with psychiatric problems, GPs provide primary care, but community, secondary and the rare tertiary mental health services are run by separate organizations, Mental Health Trusts.

NHS hospitals have been encouraged to gain more independence from government by becoming Foundation NHS Trusts (FTs) which are financially accountable to an agency called Monitor. Once, a hospital had a budget to treat its local population. Now, FTs have moved to **payment by results** (PBRs) – really payment by numbers as the outcome is not considered. FTs then compete with their neighbours and any community services offering the same 'product line' (e.g. endoscopy) for business from local or more distant PCTs and GP commissioning groups.

In the last decade, the government wished to increase **patient choice**. Private and voluntary sector health care providers were encouraged to compete with NHS providers. Thus a PCT may choose to buy knee replacement surgery from the local DGH, an established private hospital, an Independent Sector Treatment Centre (set up to process patients needing a narrow range of short-stay surgical single procedures) or an NHS national centre, e.g. the Royal National Orthopaedic Hospital. As the 'market' develops, there is some evidence that, as predicted, easy elective surgery is creamed off into the private sector leaving the NHS with complex cases and emergencies – both of which include a disproportionate number of older people.

In 2010, a further reorganization was announced. The principles are not contentious and include:

- a commitment to putting the needs of patients and the public first;
- use of improved health outcomes as the driver and measure of success;
- empowerment and engagement of clinical health care professionals.

However, the way in which these aims are to be achieved is causing considerable debate. As a first step, SHAs in England have merged to form four SHA-clusters. They will remain in place until March 2013, when the SHA-clusters will become the 'local' organizations of a new NHS Commissioning Board. PCTs will be phased out and clinical commissioning consortia (GPs, consultants and nurses) will become responsible for commissioning, under direction from the Commissioning Board. How this round of changes will evolve and the implications for maintaining a similar system across the four nations (this plan only covers England), public health, strategic planning and the care of frail older people remains to be seen. Above all, elderly people want a dependable local service.

General practitioners

In the UK every person is registered with a GP. The GP was the first point of contact for all NHS services, but some services can now be accessed directly, e.g. self-referral to physiotherapy, walk-in centres, calling the NHS Direct phoneline for advice. This increases patient choice but may fragment care. If multidisciplinary care is to succeed in the community setting, it is essential that the GP becomes the effective leader of the team. A good GP needs:

- wide knowledge of medicine and the skills of other team members;
- comprehensive past records and current information about the patient's problems and treatment;
- an approachable manner so that neither elderly patients nor their carers (formal or informal) are deterred from seeking help;
- ready access to hospital-based specialists' help and advice.

During any consultation, there is an opportunity to pick up other health or social problems and look ahead. The GP contract ensures that the practice is paid for a number of specific QOF points (quality and outcomes framework). GP practices usually have very well-developed IT systems and the opportunities for paid prevention are flagged to GPs on screen. Some practices are developing registers of 'Vulnerable Older People'.

Potentially preventable diseases in old age

- Seasonal influenza – annual vaccination.
- Pneumococcal pneumonia – 5-yearly vaccination.
- Multi-infarct dementia and stroke by treatment of high BP and anticoagulation for atrial fibrillation.
- Osteoporosis by achieving good peak bone mass in adult life and continuing to exercise.
- Ischaemic heart disease by avoidance of tobacco and promotion of exercise and 'Mediterranean' diet.
- Alcoholic dementia, heart failure, pancreatitis and cirrhosis, by safe drinking.
- Obesity, with its effect on osteoarthritis and carbohydrate metabolism.
- Type 2 diabetes, by maintaining ideal body weight and regular walking.
- Diverticular disease by increasing dietary fibre.
- COPD and bronchogenic carcinoma; risks reduced by avoiding tobacco.
- Dietary deficiency states.
- Iatrogenic disease.

GPs who wish to demonstrate their special expertise with older patients can take the Diploma of Geriatric Medicine examination of the Royal College of Physicians. They can take on extra responsibilities as a GP with a special interest in older people.

Community nursing staff

An increasing number of nurses work in the community, outside hospitals and GP surgeries. They are employed by the PCT, GP practices or the voluntary sector. Examples include district nurses, disease or system-specific specialist nurses, e.g. for heart failure, COPD/asthma, Parkinson's disease, continence, stoma specialists, palliative care symptom control (Macmillan) and hands on help (Marie Curie). Many have prescribing rights. The concept of the community matron was based on an American model; in that different health care economy, it was an effective way of case managing older complex patients. As is often the case when

government dictates health policy, the system was rolled out before evidence that it worked here and it probably does not!

Much of the total time of these nurses is devoted to the care of elderly people. They provide:

- treatment, e.g. injections, enemas and dressings;
- specialist care, e.g. stoma management and continence advice;
- liaison with other services;
- hands-on nursing (mainly supervising health care assistants).

Community psychiatric nurses (CPNs) are registered mental health nurses based in community mental health teams of the Old Age Psychiatry service. They work mainly with patients with depression and dementia to:

- support the patient and carers;
- monitor progress;
- liaise with other services.

Hospital care of older patients

This can take the following forms:

- Ambulatory care, i.e. accident and emergency attendance and outpatient clinics.
- Acute inpatient care.
- Intermediate care (IC)/rehabilitation (see below).
- Long-term care (see above).

Emergency department (ED)

Because of their liability to accidents and the sudden onset of illness, older people are frequent users of the emergency department (ED). Their management may be sub-optimal for several reasons:

- Inability to give an account of themselves owing to impaired consciousness, confusion or dementia, communication difficulties (speech, hearing impairment), anxiety or fear.
- Their problems are frequently multiple and complex.
- They are often unaccompanied.
- Their accident or illness is often a consequence of long-term neglect or lack of support.
- They are more likely than most patients to require transport back home.

An overnight stay may allow sufficient time for an older person to regain their equilibrium and be assessed and discharged the next day with increased support. The Department of Medicine for the Elderly should have sufficient staff to provide an immediate 24 h per day expert advisory service to their local ED.

Outpatient department

Irrespective of age, all appropriate patients have a right to be referred to any specialist clinic.

- Frail elderly patients are more likely to require assistance with transport to, and within, the hospital.
- All clinics should be user-friendly for elderly patients; e.g. appropriate seating (chairs with arms enable older people to get up independently), effective arrangements for deaf or partially sighted patients and wheelchair-users in the waiting area, a working communicator in the clinic room and variable height couches. Help with dressing and undressing is likely to be needed.
- Complex patients with multiple pathologies are best managed in specialist geriatric clinics, supported where necessary by organ-specific specialists.
- Follow-up clinics where necessary should be held near to the patient's home, e.g. GP surgery or community hospital and not necessarily at the DGH.

During the last 20 years, the acute bed numbers in British hospitals have been reduced by 2% annually. At the same time, admissions have risen by 3.5–5% each year. Elderly people are the greatest users of hospital beds (65% of inpatients are over 65 years of age). Occupancy rates have always been high and often reach 97%. The system has only continued to function by the steady reduction in the length of stay for each patient including the elderly.

Most admissions are considered appropriate, but inappropriate admissions may be higher among older patients, up to 20%, especially in the very old. However, the rates of inappropriate admissions are very variable and depend on the quality of local general practice and the availability of alternative forms of care. Reasons why elderly people have higher admission rates are:

- Pathology, both acute and chronic.
- Living alone and social disadvantage.
- Polypharmacy.
- High accident/fall rates.

Intensive case management of older patients with chronic disease is designed to reduce admissions (e.g. by identifying deteriorating cardiac failure before admission is necessary), and if admission is needed, faster discharge should be expedited by better, flexible care in the community.

The acute hospital is a dangerous place for frail elderly people, which should act as a stimulus to improving the safety of patients through better hospital design, improved staffing levels and mix, and improving standards of cleanliness and catering.

- Up to 50% of deaths of elderly patients in hospital may be precipitated by poor prescribing.
- Ten percent of all hospital inpatients suffer from cross-infections, especially MRSA. This rate is highest in frail elderly people.
- Broad-spectrum antibiotics may precipitate bowel overgrowth by *Clostridium difficile* and the resulting diarrhoea may be fatal.
- Falls are common because of impaired physical and cognitive function of the patient, hospital design and inadequate staff supervision. The situation is often made worse by the inappropriate use of various forms of restraint (both physical and pharmacological).
- The nutrition of malnourished patients may deteriorate further owing to poor catering and feeding arrangements.
- Dependency may be encouraged by poor staff attitudes and practices.
- Elderly patients are not always given appropriate priority when investigations are needed. Delays can be detrimental. Sophisticated techniques may be needed as elderly patients are less able to cope with demanding and invasive investigations than younger patients.
- Surgery is more dangerous, especially if delegated to junior surgeons and anaesthetists.
- Malnutrition hampers surgical recovery.
- Ignoring pre- and post-operative medical conditions compromises the success of essential surgery.
- Post-operative complications are more common and more serious.
- Lack of appropriate community services and/or accommodation may delay discharge. Up to 70,000 patients are trapped in this way in UK hospitals at any one time. Six percent of acute hospital beds are occupied by 'delayed discharges' who continue to be exposed to the above dangers.

As the NHS moves to a more financially driven model, delays in hospital at all ages are being measured in a new way. For each category of diagnosis, there is a predicted length of time needed in hospital. This is known as the 'trim point'. If the patient stays in longer, these extra days are termed 'outlier' bed days.

The department of medicine for the elderly

This is the ideal setting for the medical and nursing management of frail elderly patients with multiple and complex problems. Ideally it is based within the DGH, but has out-reach facilities in community hospitals, the community itself and care homes. It should also provide advice and support for other hospital departments caring for elderly patients, especially the ED, orthopaedic surgery, general surgery and old age psychiatry.

Admission to a department of geriatric medicine should hasten and not limit access to other specialist opinions, such as cardiology, neurology, etc.

Roles of IC

- Supporting people at home and avoiding admission by intensifying care provision at times of need (e.g. an acute minor illness).
- Aiding recovery by the provision by rehabilitation services.
- Enabling discharge of elderly patients through active rehabilitation programmes.
- Rehabilitation in a community hospital.
- 'Step down care' in the community hospital, i.e. less intense, more user-friendly, less clinical, more domestic provision of inpatient services.
- Enhance the domiciliary support at the time of discharge.
- Thus is in danger of being all things to everyone.

Some of the provision may be nurse-led, moving away from the doctor-led medical model. However, patients receiving IC are likely to be very frail and vulnerable to repeated episodes of deterioration in their health, and the input of geriatricians is essential.

Mental health services for older people

Departments of old age psychiatry are usually based in secondary care but do much of their work in the community. Psychiatry operates an age cut-off; a patient with a psychiatric problem reaching 65 'graduates' from the adult service to the old age service and new patients aged 65+ go straight to old age psychiatry. The multidisciplinary team comprises specialist nurses, therapists, psychologists and social workers or case managers in addition to the psychiatrist. Patients are usually assessed at home by one of the team, and are usually managed at home with ongoing support, not least because so many beds have been cut in this sector.

Intermediate care

Intermediate care (IC) incorporates services that sit between primary care and the DGH which are designed to be therapeutic, rather than provide care. See Standard 3 of the National Service Framework.

Day hospitals

These are units that provide day treatment. Physically frail people attend units run by Medicine for the Elderly services, whereas people with mental health problems attend services run by Old Age Psychiatry. Transport has always been problematic. Day hospitals provide many of the services available to inpatients, i.e. diagnosis, investigation, procedures, e.g. blood transfusion, multidisciplinary assessment and rehabilitation. Many day hospitals were shut because they provided 'social day-care'. Some survived by rebadging themselves as 'rehabilitation day units'. If money is ever really diverted back into the community, the day hospital may be due for a renaissance as it was successful in providing 'intermediate care' before the term was invented – a method of avoiding admission, shortening hospital stay and providing post-discharge support.

Social care for older people

Most elderly people wish to continue to live in their own homes. This aspiration is supported by the

Table 2.2 Estimated number of clients aged 65 and over receiving services in England, 2008–2009.

Domiciliary care	No. of recipients
Day care	106,000
Meals	95,000
Professional support	204,000
Equipment and adaptations	394,000
Home care	453,000

www.ic.nhs.uk/webfiles/publications/009_Social_Care/car-estats0910asrfinal/Community_Care_Statistics_200910_Social_Services_Activity_Report_England.pdf.

government, but good community services are not a cheap option, and the services are often fragmented, inadequate and underfunded or inefficient, depending on your viewpoint.

The local authority was responsible for assessing and purchasing domiciliary and community social care for residents, but in many areas social care and health care have merged. Over 95% of the elderly population lives independently, but about 10% need formal community services in order to remain at home (Table 2.2). In 2008–09, 1.78 million clients received services, of whom 1.22 million clients are aged 65+, mainly requiring help because of physical disability. Over the last decade fewer clients have received home care as resources are focused on those most at need.

When the person stays in their own home what types of care can be provided?

Twenty-four-hour care

This is extremely expensive. At least two carers are needed to cover shifts and holidays. Individuals may pay for this privately or it is occasionally paid for as NHS CC.

Regular visits for care

Frail people are enabled to stay at home by domiciliary care.

- Private care via care agencies or advertisements. All agencies must carry out Criminal Records Bureau checks because the clientele are vulnerable. Private care is limited only by the financial means of the individual and the local availability of suitable carers.
- Statutory care involves assessment by a care manager and a care package is drawn up. The care may be commissioned from in-house staff (social services or PCT), or the private sector through agencies.
- Care is now generally provided by generic care assistants who will perform a range of tasks, e.g. a morning visit (30 min) to get the client up, washed, dressed and breakfasted, a lunchtime visit (15 min) to heat the pre-delivered frozen meal, and an evening visit (20 min) to get the client back to bed.
- Once the client can no longer use the toilet independently between visits, or make themselves a hot drink, the situation become precarious, but many such individuals prefer to remain at home.
- If the client cannot transfer with the help of one person, 'double-up' care may be needed (two carers) and such patients will usually be padded up (incontinence) and sit in their chairs until the next visit (risk of pressure sores).
- In England and Wales this type of care is means tested.
- Personal care is free in Scotland.
- Domestic tasks, e.g. shopping and cleaning, have to be paid for privately, so good-value services such as those run by Age UK are much in demand.

The Community Care Survey (2008 data published in 2009) documented that the average number of contact hours per household was 11.7 h a week, up from 8.1 in 2002. More intensive services are being provided for a smaller number of service users, continuing the trend seen over the last 10 years. Statutory services have had to focus on frailer clients as funding has not kept pace with the increasing numbers of old people.

Meals-on-wheels/frozen meals service

This provides clients with hot meals in their own home at mid-day. There are practical problems in providing meals that remain appetizing and nutritious after delays caused by storage and delivery; some clients love them, others throw them away or are too muddled to eat them. Special meals, e.g. vegetarian, diabetic, kosher and halal, may be available. Some areas have moved to a system of delivering frozen ready meals. The client needs a freezer and a microwave and reasonable cognitive function to learn what may be an entirely new method of heating food.

Luncheon clubs

These are centres where meals are provided, usually at subsidized prices, run by either the local authority or voluntary organizations. Luncheon clubs usually run just once or twice weekly, but also offer companionship. Transport is often a limiting factor.

Day centres

These are very varied and may be run by the local authority or voluntary groups, but must not be confused with day hospitals. Staff may be trained (social workers, therapists) or untrained or a combination of both. A charge for attendance is usually made and transport may be provided. About 5% of elderly people attend day centres.

> **Day centre aims**
>
> - To combat loneliness.
> - To provide diversional activity and recreation.
> - To provide a meal and other comforts.
> - To relieve carers.
> - To disseminate health education, e.g. about falls risk.
> - To encourage activity, e.g. regular exercise and balance groups.
> - To introduce clients to other forms of care.

Respite care

This is the temporary provision of a bed, usually in a care home, for frail patients with chronic irremediable diseases, to give the informal carers a well-earned break. The service is organized by social services/PCT and is means-tested. It may smooth the path to eventual permanent placement, e.g. for a person with dementia. However, periods of respite care often have an adverse effect on the recipients – especially if they are unable to comprehend the reasons for such respite care. Respite care should not be confused with crisis intervention, i.e. when a supporting system suddenly collapses, nor should it be considered as top-up rehabilitation. However, because of the bed

shortages and pressures if a frail person suddenly deteriorates in a non-specific way (see Chapter 3), they may be put in a respite bed only to be admitted to the DGH 3 days later with severe pneumonia.

Specialist equipment

A range of traditional equipment can be provided, e.g. a pressure relieving mattress, toilet frame, bath board, grab rails, handling belts, a commode and even a hospital bed, hoist and wheelchair. Lifeline pendant alarms enable the wearer to summon help. More expensive equipment such as stair lifts can be fitted and modifications made to the house, e.g. doorways widened for wheelchairs, a level access shower; there are often delays and wrangling over who pays.

Telecare is the use of electronic technology to monitor and assist people to maintain independence in their own environment. A telecare service can monitor three components: safety and security, physiological parameters and activity. Devices include video-monitoring, fall detectors, sensors to monitor activity (a pressure mat activated as the person gets out of bed can turn on the light, detectors monitoring the fridge and front door can be used to monitor feeding and wandering, etc.), wet bed alerts can summon a night carer, automatic taps prevent floods, etc. Everyone should have smoke alarms.

Roving warden schemes

These are area-based and support a number of older people living in their original accommodation.

Regulation of health and social care

In England a new health and social care regulator, the Care Quality Commission (CQC) was set up in 2009. It is responsible for ensuring that all providers (state, charitable and for-profit) meet essential standards of quality and safety, monitors compliance with the standards, inspects all types of provision (including hospitals, mental health services, nursing and residential homes) and uses enforcement powers when needed. It remains to be seen how effective this system will be. Details for the Regulatory bodies for the devolved nations are given below:

- Scottish Commission for the Regulation of Care: www.carecommission.com/.
- Health Inspectorate Wales: www.hiw.org.uk.
- Northern Ireland Regulatory and Quality Improvement Authority: www.rqia.org.uk.

Who cares?

Paid carers provide the care described above, but 'informal carers' provide the majority of care. These are the most important members of the caring workforce. They are unpaid, untrained, but devoted and effective. Although the generations tend to live apart, there continues to be frequent contact within a family and almost 50% of elderly people living alone have regular daily contact with a family member. The bulk of community support is provided by family and friends – the following points are relevant to the situation within the UK:

- The proportion of dependants, i.e. children under 16 years, men over 65 years and women over 60 years of age in the community, is around 40% and has not increased during this century. There are now more dependent elderly people in the community than dependent children.
- However, consider how much support goes into helping people look after children in comparison with older dependants.
- It is calculated that in the UK there are 6 million informal carers.
- Most carers are women (60%) and over half of 'housewives' can expect to be called upon at some time to help an elderly and infirm person.
- Many carers are elderly (24% are 65+). The mean age of carers of confused elderly people is 61 years.
- There is a high social cost to informal carers in England (2009).
- Forty-eight percent of carers were providing care for 20 h or more per week, 30% for 35 + h and 22% for 50 + h.
- Carers have the right to an assessment. Of the 398,000 carers assessed (2009), an estimated 355,000 carers (89%) received a service following a carer's assessment or review. Of these, 58% received 'carer specific' services and 42% received information and advice.

Needs of carers

Recognition

- By family and friends.
- By professionals.
- By the state.

Support

- Financial.
- Social.
- Psychological.
- Professional.
- Self-help groups.

Respite

- Short periods (e.g. day care).
- Long periods – intermittent admission to care.
- Sitting services (e.g. Crossroads).
- Immediate in emergencies.

Information

- About the patient's illness.
- About available services.

Strategies to improve care of older people

Although it is 10 years old, the National Service Framework for Older People (NSF OP) 2001 is still relevant. It is one of a series of 'frameworks' developed by a multidisciplinary committee set up by the government and the aim was to improve standards of care for older people.

Recommendations of the NSF OP

- Standard 1 – routing out age discrimination. NHS services will be provided regardless of age on the basis of clinical need alone. Social care services will not use age in their eligibility criteria or policies to restrict access to available services. Ageism is, however, often covert rather than explicit.
- Standard 2 – person-centred care. NHS and social care services will treat older people as individuals and enable them to make choices about their own care. This is achieved through the single

assessment process, integrated commissioning and provision of services including community equipment and continence services.

- Standard 3 – intermediate care (IC). Older people will have access to a new range of IC at home to promote independence, prevent unnecessary hospital admission, enable early discharge from hospital and to prevent premature admission to long-term care.
- Standard 4 – general hospital care. Older people's care in hospital is delivered through appropriate specialist care and by staff who have the right set of skills to meet their needs.
- Standard 5 – stroke. The NHS will take action to prevent stroke, working in partnership with other agencies where appropriate.
- Standard 6 – falls. The NHS, in partnership with councils, will take action to prevent falls and reduce resultant fractures or other injuries.
- Standard 7 – mental health. Older people who have mental health problems will have access to integrated mental health services provided by the NHS and councils to ensure effective diagnosis, treatment and support for them and their carers.
- Standard 8 – the promotion of health and active life in older age. The health and wellbeing of older people is promoted through a coordinated pro-gramme of action led by the NHS with support from councils.
- An appendix on medicines management.

A New Ambition for Old Age (2006) was the second phase of the NSF and focused on dignity, joined-up care and healthy ageing.

Financial allowances that can be claimed by some UK pensioners

Pensions are very complicated and always chang-ing. Know the basics, look on the Age UK website for details and always suggest that patients get advice from the Citizens Advice Bureau. Benefits may differ between England, Scotland, Wales and Northern Ireland. Attendance Allowance is a very important benefit.

Basic state pension

The basic state pension is paid to men at 65. It was paid to women at 60, but since April 2010, a process of rapid equalization has begun so a woman's state pension age (SPA) will reach 65 by November 2018. Then, both men and women will see their SPA rise to 66 by October 2020.

The basic state pension is provided if you have paid sufficient National Insurance contributions (NICs). From April 2010, you need 30 'qualifying years' for the full rate, but if you have not worked, your contribution record may be protected by National Insurance Credits. In 2012–13, a single person's pension is £107.45 a week, £171.85 for a couple. From April 2011 the basic state pension rises each year in line with average earnings, the Consumer Price Index or 2.5%, whichever is greater.

Over 80 pension

People aged 80 and over, in England, Scotland and Wales, are eligible for the Over 80 pension of £64.40 a week if they do not get the basic State Pension at all, or if it pays them less than this.

Pension credit

This is a benefit with two parts, Guarantee credit and Savings credit. It replaces Income Support for those of SPA. If you live in Great Britain, have reached the SPA (for women this is rising) and have savings below £10,000 you may be entitled to **Pension Guarantee Credit**. This guarantees a minimum income by topping up your weekly in-come to £142.70 if you are single, £217.90 if you have a partner. These amounts may be more if you are disabled, have caring responsibilities or certain housing costs, such as mortgage interest pay-ments. **Pensions Savings Credit** is paid to people aged 65 and over. It depends on the level of retire-ment provision you have made. It may be paid as well as Guarantee Credit.

Council tax benefit

Council tax helps pay for local services like policing and refuse collection. This benefit is means-tested and paid if you have less than £16,000 in savings. Council tax is also reduced if you have severe dementia or receive an Attendance Allowance.

Housing benefit

This is a means-tested benefit to help with paying rent.

Attendance allowance (AA)

This is a non-means-tested benefit paid to a person who needs help with personal care; there is a qualifying period of 6 months, unless there is a prognosis of < 6 months when the payment can be made at once and even if the claimant does not currently need help. In 2012–13, the higher rate (day and night) is £77.45 a week, the lower rate is £51.58 (day or night).

Extra money for carers

The Carer's Allowance is paid to a carer who earns less than £100 a week (2012–13) and provides more than 35 h of care per week to a person in receipt of a qualifying benefit, e.g. AA (£58.45 a week). NICs are paid to protect pension rights of working age carers. Carers receiving state pension should apply for Carer's Allowance, but it is paid as a Carer Premium in Pension Credit.

Prescription charges, sight tests and dental care

If you are 60+, you are entitled to free prescriptions and sight tests. You get free sight tests at 40 years if there is glaucoma in the family. Free dentistry is available if you receive Pension Guarantee Credit.

Health care travel costs

Costs of getting to hospital may be paid if a person gets Pension Guarantee Credit.

Blind person's allowance

For 2011–12 this is £1,980 – there are no age or income restrictions.

Keeping warm

- Winter fuel payment is an annual non-means-tested benefit: in 2011–12, above the SPA you get £100–300 depending on your circumstances.
- The Warm Front Scheme, for those on a qualifying benefit, e.g. AA, provides a package of insulation and heating improvements up to the value of £3,500 (or £6,000 for oil, low carbon or renewable energy).
- Cold weather payments are a means-tested payment made for each 7-day period of very cold weather between 1 November and 31 March.

Concessions

Older people get concessions for bus and rail travel and entry to places of entertainment, but there are local variations in generosity and age

qualifications; eligibility for free national bus passes in England will rise with SPA. All pensioners over the age of 75 are entitled to a free television licence.

Christmas bonus

An annual £10 is available if you get a state pension.

Social fund (community care grants)

Means-tested discretionary loans may be made for replacement of clothing, home repairs, redecoration, bedding and furniture, etc.

Funeral expense payment

This must be requested before the funeral is carried out (fees plus up to £700).

 REFERENCES

Department for Communities and Local Government (2004) *English House Condition Survey 2004.* http://www.communities.gov.uk/documents/housing/pdf/151924.pdf.

English Housing Survey (2010). http://www.communities.gov.uk/documents/statistics/pdf/1479789.pdf.

Health and Social Care Information Centre (2009) Community Care Statistics 2008. Home care services for adults, England. http://www.ic.nhs.uk/webfiles/publications/Home%20Care%20%28HH1%29%202008/HH1%20Final%20v1.pdf.

Laing and Buisson,Care of Elderly People UK Market Survey 2009. www.statistics.gov.uk/hub/population/ageing/older-people.

ONS (2009) *General Lifestyle Survey.* See Appendices for data. http://www.ons.gov.uk/ons/search/index.html?newquery=General+Lifestyle+Survey.

ONS (2011) *Bulletin Focus on Older People.* http://www.ons.gov.uk/ons/rel/mortality-ageing/focus-on-older-people/older-people-s-day-2011/index.html http://www.ons.gov.uk/ons/rel/mortality-ageing/focus-on-older-people/older-people-s-day-2011/index.html.

Partnership (2010) *Financial Advisers Left Out in the Cold on Long Term Care Advice, Warns Retirement Specialist Partnership.* NOP survey.

http://www.partnership.co.uk/press/2010/June/Press-Release-7-June-20101/.

UK National Statistics (2009) *Older People: UK National Statistics Publication Hub.*

➜ FURTHER INFORMATION

Age UK: http://www.adviceguide.org.uk/index.htm.

Citizens Advice Bureau: http://www.adviceguide.org.uk/index.htm.

Communities and Local Government (2010) *English Housing Survey Headline Report 2008–09.* http://www.communities.gov.uk/documents/statistics/pdf/1479789.pdf.

Department of Health: http://www.dh.gov.uk/en/Home.

DH (2006) *A New Ambition for Old Age: Next Steps in Implementing the National Service Framework for Older People.* http://www.dh.gov.uk/en/Publicationsandstatistics/Publications/PublicationsPolicyAndGuidance/DH_4133941.

Health Inspectorate Wales: www.hiw.org.uk.

NHS (2011) The health and social service information centre. *Community Care Statistics 2009–10*: Social Services Activity, England 2009-10. http://www.ic.nhs.uk/webfiles/publications/009_Social_Care/carestats0910asrfinal/Community_Care_Statistics_200910_Social_services_Activity_Report_England_Tables_and_Charts.xls.

NHS (2011) *Quality and Outcomes Framework.* http://www.qof.ic.nhs.uk/

Northern Ireland Regulatory and Quality Improvement Authority: www.rqia.org.uk.

ONS (2010) *Pensioner Income and Expenditure.* http://www.ons.gov.uk/ons/search/index.html?newquery=Pensioner+income+and+expenditure.

Putting People First (2011) *People Who Pay for Care: Quantitative and Qualitative Analysis of Self-funders in the Social Care Market.* www.puttingpeoplefirst.org.uk/_library/Resources/Personalisation/Localmilestones/People_who_ pay_for_care_-_report_12_1_11_final.pdf.

Scottish Commission for the Regulation of Care: www.carecommission.com/.

Scottish Government (2010) *Free Personal and Nursing Care, Scotland, 2008–09.* http://www.scotland.gov.uk/Resource/Doc/317110/0100996.pdf.

3

Special features of medicine in the elderly

The ageing of populations

We have seen that the proportion of elderly citizens increased in developed countries during the 20th century and similar changes are happening even faster in less developed countries. Reasons for this include falling fertility rates and falling death rates at all ages but particularly in infancy and early childhood, owing to improved living standards. The increasing number of very elderly people is, however, partly due to the improvements in medicine in adult life.

Blessing or curse?

Increasing longevity sounds like a blessing, but only if the extra years are healthy and active. Figure 3.1 shows the possible outcomes (after Tallis 2003). Scenario A is the current situation; people tend to be relatively healthy until their late 60s when chronic disabilities start to accumulate until death. Scenario B shows a situation in which both morbidity and death are postponed. However, the added years may be associated with 'compression of morbidity' into the final months of life, the desirable outcome shown in scenario C, or, the worst case scenario, to a prolonged period of disability and dependency, shown in scenario D. One recent estimate gave a 65-year-old English man an average of 10.2 further years of active life followed by 7.3 years of significant disability, and a woman 11.4 years and 8.8 years, respectively (ONS 2010).

The ageing process

Cells, tissues and organs all change with age and eventually function begins to deteriorate. Ageing is very complex and poorly understood. There are two major groups of theories:

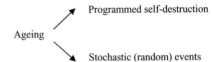

Wyllie and colleagues have worked on cell death since the 1970s. Whereas an injured cell will swell, burst and release its contents, causing an inflammatory and immune cascade, when a cell dies a normal death, it shrivels up and is consumed by nearby cells so fast it never gets a chance to spill its contents. They named their discovery apoptosis (pronounced apotosis), from the Greek for 'falling off', as in leaves from a tree. An array of intracellular and extracellular signals can trigger the cell to enter the process of programmed cell death. Apoptosis occurs from the earliest stages of development (e.g. leading to the separation of fingers), is very active during growth and continues throughout life. Aberrant regulation of apoptosis contributes to cancer, autoimmune disorders, neurodegenerative diseases and systemic viral infection.

It is clear that individual cells can undergo programmed death. There has been debate as to whether multicellular organisms carry programmes to self-destruct ('a ticking clock'). Ageing

Lecture Notes Elderly Care Medicine, Eighth Edition. Claire G. Nicholl and K. Jane Wilson.
© 2012 John Wiley & Sons, Ltd. Published 2012 by John Wiley & Sons, Ltd.

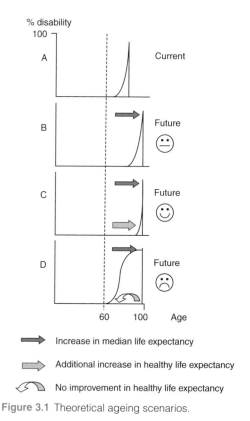

% disability

Increase in median life expectancy

Additional increase in healthy life expectancy

No improvement in healthy life expectancy

Figure 3.1 Theoretical ageing scenarios.

as a predetermined, genetically controlled process would be supported by the characteristic lifespans of different organisms. A single gene mutation in the roundworm *Caenorhabditis elegans* doubles its life expectancy to around 6 weeks. This gene, *daf-2*, codes for a primitive insulin receptor and regulates an array of other genes which influence longevity. This is part of the mechanism that allows the worm to suspend its development when the environment is harsh. The situation is more complex in man, but the insulin pathway is important in diabetes and cancer which has links with ageing.

Sirtuins are nicotinamide adenine dinucleotide (NAD+)-dependent protein deacetylases that extend the lifespan of yeast, worms and flies and may be involved in the mechanism by which calorie restriction increases lifespan in animals. There are seven mammalian sirtuins, SIRT1 to SIRT7, which have complex roles in metabolism, homeostasis and the stress response. Different sirtuins are found in the nucleus, mitochondria and cytosol. Major research effort is being targeted at

developing sirtuin activators aiming to treat obesity, diabetes and neurodegeneration and even extend lifespan. Resveratrol (a natural compound found in the skin of red grapes and in wine) was thought to be a SIRT-1 activator but the results may have been an artifact. Nevertheless, there is a huge range of Resveratrol supplements for sale on the internet; anti-ageing is big business (see the website of Sirtris Pharma).

Although no genes have been found that double lifespan in man, a study of the genomes of more than 1,000 centenarians, scouring about 300,000 sequence variations for possible links to longevity, has identified around 150 variations in DNA sequence that can predict (with 77% accuracy) whether a person has the genetic wherewithal to live to 100.

Single genetic disorders causing premature ageing (progeria) do occur. These are 'segmental ageing' syndromes as they do not result in all the typical features of ageing, but it seems likely that some of the mechanisms involved will be relevant to normal ageing.

- Hutchinson–Gilford syndrome: very rare, sporadic, autosomal dominant causing death around 13 years from MI or stroke. Usually a silent substitution from glycine GGC (*A*, *C*, *G* and *T* represent the four nucleotide bases of a DNA strand – adenine, cytosine, guanine, thymine) to glycine GGT in codon 608 of the lamin A (LMNA) gene on 1q, which activates a cryptic splice donor site to produce abnormal lamin A. The nuclear fragility of lamin A-deficient cells increases apoptosis and may exhaust stem cell-driven regeneration.
- Werner's syndrome: rare, autosomal recessive progeria of adulthood caused by mutations in a gene on 8p coding for a member of the RecQ helicase family. Characteristic features include premature greying, skeletal changes and death around 50 years. The Werner protein unwinds, separates and repairs damaged DNA and may be important in maintaining telomeres.

In *C. elegans*, although genotype determines the mean lifespan of a population, individual longevity has a large stochastic component, with several-fold differences observed even with an isogenic population in a uniform environment.

Wear and tear theories claim that ageing is caused by random accumulated injuries from ultraviolet light, physical damage, toxic by-products of metabolism, etc.

The ageing cell

Neurons, renal and myocardial cells do not divide and have to last a lifetime, although the numbers fall. Normal human embryonic fibroblasts have a fixed capacity to divide around 50 times, but those from mature subjects have a reduced capacity for reduplication.

One factor contributing to this may be telomerase inactivation in somatic cells (unlike the germline). Telomerase maintains telomeres, regions of repetitive non-coding DNA at the tips of chromosomes that protect them from destruction.

When cells divide, the enzymes that replicate DNA cannot continue all the way to the end of the chromosome so telomeres are gradually used up, becoming shorter every time a cell divides. Eventually they reach a critically short length, the cell cannot divide any more and apoptosis may be triggered. The Nobel Prize for medicine 2009 was awarded for the discovery of how chromosomes are protected by telomeres. Telomerase-deficient mice appear prematurely aged and telomerase reactivation resulted in rejuvenation of some tissues. However, this may carry a cancer risk as telomerase reactivation is a possible explanation for the immortality of malignant cells in culture. A commercial blood test is already available to get your telomere length tested and compared to an age-matched sample to 'assess your biological age'. This is fascinating, but more work is needed, particularly with regard to the relationship to cancer.

Many other features of cells from aged individuals reflect stochastic events. The biochemistry of the cell is noisy. All cellular processes – transcription, translation, protein folding, every enzymic reaction and all the inbuilt regulatory mechanisms – are subject to random errors. The workings of cells get noisier as they get older, and this might contribute to increasing cellular dysfunction with age. Features of cells from aged individuals include:
- Aneuploidy (variable chromosome numbers).
- Accumulation of somatic mutations of DNA in the cell nucleus and mitochondria.
- Dysregulation of gene expression.
- Misfolded proteins tend to aggregate and 'gum up the works', e.g. amyloid. Cells deploy 'chaperones' to refold misshapen proteins, but this mechanism may be overwhelmed.
- Lipofuscin pigment granules accumulate in cytoplasm in liver, kidney and muscle (from damaged red cells).
- Oxidative stress and damage as reactive oxygen species are not mopped up by antioxidants and damage key molecules including DNA.
- Less effective cellular pumps (a family of proteins called multidrug resistance proteins) fail to remove toxic products from cells.
- Adducts on macromolecules, e.g. glycation may reflect failure of processes for repair and turnover of macromolecules.

Ageing tissues

- Loss or dormancy of stem cells: ageing could in part be due to the inability of stem cells to replenish the tissues of an organism with functional differentiated cells needed to maintain them.
- Cross linkages (e.g. disulphide bonds) in collagen and elastin cause increased stiffness in connective tissue especially in skin, elastic laminae of blood vessels, tendons and lens of eye.
- Mitochondrial respiratory-chain function (energy release) is less efficient in skeletal muscle.

Immunity and ageing

- Thymic involution and attenuated T-cell-mediated immunity lead to reactivation of quiescent infections, such as TB and varicella. There seems to be a decline in delayed-type skin-hypersensitivity reactions to injected antigens (anergy) in many frail aged subjects.
- Autoantibodies occur more frequently (e.g. antiphospholipid antibodies) and are associated with vascular disease, but their significance in older people is uncertain.
- Proliferative disorders of the lymphocyte are very common.
- Malnutrition and diabetes compound these problems.

Unifying hypothesis

Many of the stochastic cellular events described appear to lead to telomere shortening and many drugs with which we are all familiar lengthen telomeres. Whilst this is too simplistic it is increasingly likely that ageing will eventually be understood in terms of interacting genetic, programmed and random events.

Declining function

Many physiological parameters decline with age, but the magnitude of the decline is hard to estimate. These figures are almost always based on cross-sectional rather than longitudinal studies, which will include individuals within the elderly cohort who have acquired diseases that may affect function, e.g. renal function will suffer as a result of hypertension or diabetes, or whose sedentary lifestyle in retirement has caused cardiorespiratory fitness to decline through disuse. To be attributable to ageing per se, a phenomenon must be universal, intrinsic and progressive. Watching the London Marathon will reveal many 70 or even 80+ year olds fitter than most people in their 30s and 40s.

Special features of illness in older patients

Illness in older people is usually a continuum of conditions found in middle age, but the impact of the illness will be modified by the context of ageing and loss of fitness, and the social situation the person is in (Figure 3.2).

Background of ageing

Ageing changes are seen in *most organs* (go through the body in your mind), including the brain, special senses and peripheral nerves.

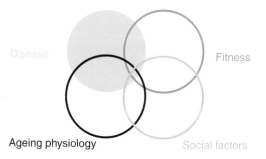

Figure 3.2 Interaction between disease, ageing physiology and the individual's fitness and social situation.

Why do ageing changes matter?

- There is increased variability between individuals.
- Okay at rest, significant when stressed (e.g. fasting glucose minimally higher in the elderly, but glucose levels higher after meals).
- Impaired homeostasis results in problems when the environment becomes more challenging. In extreme old age the challenge may be minimal, such as maintaining BP on standing. Some physical signs have different significance, e.g. small pupils, poor upgaze and wasting of small muscles of the hand.

Multiple pathology and aetiology

Why do elderly people often have several diseases?

The prevalence of many diseases increases with age (e.g. stroke, PD, AD) so the fact that older people have several diseases may simply reflect this. Some chronic diseases have complications affecting several systems (e.g. diabetes may lead to heart, eye, kidney and nerve problems) or may predispose to other disorders (e.g. infections). Also, a risk factor may predispose the individual to several diseases (e.g. smokers are more likely to have chronic bronchitis, lung cancer, heart disease, strokes, gangrene, macular degeneration and osteoporosis). One problem may also have several causes; e.g. falls are usually multifactorial (previous stroke + cognitive impairment + poor vision + osteoarthritis of the knees, etc.). As discussed later, multiple diseases mean multiple drugs, so the common situation in an older person presents multiple interactions, as shown in Figure 3.3.

Different risk factors

It must not be assumed that parameters (e.g. high lipid levels) that constitute a risk factor in the young carry the same risk in the elderly in the absence of positive evidence. An 85-year-old with a cholesterol level of 8 mmol/L presumably has 'protective' genes and so the significance of this finding is not the same as in a 40-year-old.

Different susceptibility to disease

This is more of a theoretical possibility than a practical consideration. The expected increase in TB as the cohort of people who had survived TB in

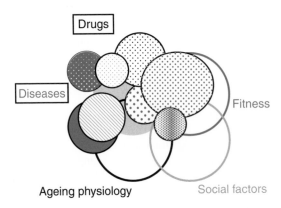

Figure 3.3 Multiple interactions.

the pre-drug era became old and frail with poor nutrition and reduced immunity is limited.

Different differential diagnoses

Although the range of possible diagnoses may be similar at any age, age is important in determining what is most likely. For example the commonest cause of fits, jaundice and anaemia will be different in the neonate, child, young adult and elderly person.

Altered response to disease

Many older people present in exactly the same way as middle-aged people, e.g. crushing central chest pain in an MI. However, this is not always the case, making diagnoses in the frail older person a challenge. There may be:

- Missing symptoms, e.g. lack of pleuritic pain, fever and thirst in pneumonia.
- Missing signs, e.g. lack of neck stiffness in meningitis.

Finally, non-specific presentation is common. The 'geriatric giants' – the big 'I's – are common features of illness in old age:

- Intellectual failure (acute or chronic confusion).
- Incontinence (if this is new, why?).
- Immobility ('off her feet').
- Instability (falls).
- Iatrogenic disease (see pharmacological treatment).
- Inability to look after oneself (functional decline or, in an analogy to paediatrics, 'failure to thrive').

All of these vague and dull-sounding clinical pictures, often labelled 'social problem' in the medical records, are almost never due to social problems and could be because of a huge range of serious and treatable conditions – if you look – such as MI, stroke, PD, etc.

Low expectations

Why do older people sometimes present so late in their illness?

Older people may have poor expectations of the health care system, fuelled by friends and family and sometimes, sadly, by previous experience of health care professionals. 'What do you expect at your age?' is a remark familiar to many. The problem may be compounded by lack of medical understanding, so that urinary incontinence and swollen ankles are assumed to be normal in old age.

Social problems

Old age is a time of loss (family, friends, income, housing, mobility, independence and life itself). There may be practical solutions. However, often what are most appreciated are support and a little of your time to hear about how things were.

Advantages and disadvantages of 'labels'

Be circumspect before labelling people. It is part of the doctor's job; the label usually helps the patient to understand what is causing their symptoms and helps the clinicians to manage the condition. For example, the Alzheimer's Society campaigns to get people with dementia recognized and given a diagnosis, as without this they cannot access the help that is available. However, sometimes labels are unhelpful: a 93-year-old woman with impaired glucose tolerance labelled 'diabetic' may be refused Christmas cake in her residential home. It is very difficult to shake off an incorrect label and so, if in doubt, remain descriptive, e.g. 'breathless with shadow on CXR', pending further investigation.

The importance of functional assessment and rehabilitation

Expensive and technically successful intervention is of limited value if the patient does not recover the ability to enjoy a worthwhile quality of life. Overall assessment should include a comprehensive list of medical problems and their prioritization in terms of threat to quality and quantity of life (an assessment of cognitive function, evaluation of functional abilities, some idea of the social background ['ecological niche'] and who is there to do tasks for the patient when they are unable to do them for themselves). It will take an older person longer to recover strength and function after a severe systemic illness – this may be obvious to the reader, but is not always obvious to the patient, family and medical attendant.

Rehabilitation

Rehabilitation is defined as the restoration of the individual to their fullest physical, mental and social capability. It takes several forms:

- Restoration to full activity after a severe illness (e.g. abdominal surgery or MI).
- Restoration of maximum achievable function following a specific impairment (e.g. stroke and fractured hip).
- Facilitating the achievement of as much independence as possible despite continuing impairment (e.g. PD, amputation, stroke and hip disease).

Rehabilitation can take place in a variety of settings (see box below). It is an active process and it is important that the multidisciplinary team, including the patient and carer, share common goals and objectives. If the patient is not progressing as well as anticipated, it is important to look for barriers that may be interfering with the process. These include depression, uncontrolled pain and hidden agendas, e.g. 'If I improve, I will be a burden to them'.

Rehabilitation from acute illness

Hospital admission is often required, not for specific investigations or medication that cannot be administered at home, but because the weakness associated with a chest infection or heart disease

---

The rehabilitation team

Patient.
Family and friends.
Nurses.
Rehabilitation professions (physiotherapists, occupational therapists, speech therapists).
Doctor.
Clinical psychologist.
Dietician.
Podiatrist.
Orthotist.
Social worker.
Voluntary workers.

Rehabilitation settings

Acute hospital ward (includes orthopaedic wards).
Rehabilitation ward in acute hospital.
Intermediate care ward in community hospital.
Stroke units, wherever situated.
Outpatient therapy departments.
Geriatric day hospital or rehabilitation and falls unit.
Psychiatric counterparts of the above.
Primary-care premises.
Care homes.
Sheltered flats.
Community groups, e.g. stroke clubs, keep-fit classes.
Patient's own home (e.g. home-based exercise programme).

---

renders patients unable to attend to their bodily needs (nutrition, fluid intake, bowel, bladder, hygiene, etc.) unassisted. They may feel too unwell to get out of bed. Unless there is adequate support at home, early admission is essential to prevent pressure sores, contractures, constipation, incontinence and loss of confidence, which would necessitate protracted rehabilitation.

Remobilization is achieved by suitable exercises (passive, assisted, resisted), combined with functional exercise, such as transfers, sitting to standing and walking. Activities of daily living (ADL) abilities are assessed and various items of equipment may be deployed to facilitate independence. An attempt at quantitative measurement of function is provided by the Barthel scale (see Appendix 2). Following discharge, the able-bodied may consider positive measures to promote physical fitness. In some health care settings a new term 'reablement' has been coined; this applies to the lower level rehabilitation process that is needed to get an elderly person back to their previous level of function following an illness or spell in hospital.

Even if there is irremediable impairment, it may be possible to reduce disability or handicap.

- **Impairment**: loss or abnormality of structure or function, e.g. weak leg and arm following stroke.
- **Disability**: the resulting loss of ability to perform an activity in the normal manner, e.g. a diminished ability to walk.
- **Handicap**: the ensuing disadvantage in terms of fulfillment of the individual's role, e.g. unable to cook and do the housework or participate in leisure activities, and so on.

Principles of rehabilitation

1 Rehabilitation is needed after all illnesses not just after stroke or fracture, etc.
2 A multi-disciplinary activity including the patient and the patient's informal carers.
3 Essential to know what the patient could do before the current illness.
4 Full assessment of the patient's problems is required before the process starts.
5 Goals must be realistic with defined end points.
6 Logical step-by-step approach to achieve the set goals.
7 A continuous process – 'every activity is a therapeutic opportunity', i.e. rehabilitation does not just occur when face to face with a therapist.
8 Maintenance is required if the achieved improvements are to be retained.
9 Rehabilitation can take place in a variety of settings depending on circumstances.

Rehabilitation is not always the most appropriate way to manage severe disability. Palliation is sometimes the best and kindest option.

Barriers to successful rehabilitation

- Global impairment of higher cerebral function.
- Poor motivation (patient or carers).
- Depression.
- Unrealistic expectations.
- Communication difficulties.
- Sensory deprivation.

- Loss of body image, sensory ataxia, disordered visuospatial perception.
- Co-morbidities (arthritis, heart failure).
- Sub-optimally treated pain.
- Pressure sores, contractures.
- Swallowing problems.
- Poor nutritional state.

Ethical problems

The whole area of denial of access to high-class care versus overaggressive and futile intervention – discriminating ageism versus compassionate ageism – is a major minefield and one of the fascinations of geriatric medicine. See Chapter 16.

Examination of the aged patient – things to look out for

Gait

- Aided or unaided?
- Foot drop?
- Shuffling or striding? Stable or unstable?
- Difficulty up/down from chair?
- Parkinsonian or multi-infarct?

Face

- Parkinsonian (lack of expression).
- Depression.
- Hypothyroidism, anaemia, vitiligo.
- Angular stomatitis (often due to ill-fitting dentures).
- Orofacial dyskinesia.
- Ptosis – symmetrical ('age-related') or unilateral (eye surgery or Horner's).
- Basal-cell carcinoma.
- Facial palsy.

Joint disease

- Stiff neck.
- Tentative handshake of rotator-cuff atrophy, difficulty getting in/out of sleeves.
- Stiff hips/knees.
- Kyphosis and protuberant abdomen suggestive of osteoporosis.

Self-neglect

- Dirty hands/face/body.
- Dirty clothing, evidence of incontinence.
- Unshaven, hair unkempt.
- Neglected nails.

Nutrition

- Obesity.
- Protein–energy undernutrition – compare weight with previous records; signs of recent weight loss or extreme cachexia.
- Hydration.

Conversation

- Dyspnoea?
- Good account of circumstances?
- Plausible, with obvious lacunae?
- Mood?
- Speech – dysphasia, dysarthria, dysphonia?
- Emotional lability.

Formal examination

- Extrasystoles – common and seldom significant.
- Neglected breast cancer.
- Displaced apex beat – due to chest deformity which also affects typical radiation of murmurs.
- Peripheral pulses – palpate and auscultate.
- Abdomen – ribs tend to sit over pelvis, so hard to ballot kidneys, distended bladder and faecal impaction.
- Defective up-gaze – common, dubious significance.
- Ankle jerks – usually present, plantar strike often the best technique.

Pharmacological treatment: special considerations

- Polypharmacy refers to the use of multiple medications by a patient; there is no standard definition, but ≥ four drugs is commonly used.
- Polypharmacy is increasing. In the past decade, the average number of items prescribed to people aged 60 or over has almost doubled from 22.3 to 42.4 items for each person per year.
- Elderly patients consume most drugs (prescribed or over-the-counter). The oldest 15% of the population receive 45% of all drug prescriptions.
- Asymptomatic people are treated to reduce risk from chronic disease. The risk of adverse events has to be traded against the theoretical benefits.
- The prevalence of chronic disease increases with age. Treatment to national guidelines for each condition can lead to a complicated cocktail of drugs.
- ADR-related hospital admissions are increasing (see Figure 3.4), account for 5–12% of all hospital admissions in older patients, and have a high in-hospital mortality rate of 2–10%.
- One-third to half of all medicines for long-term conditions are not taken. If the prescription is appropriate this is a loss to the patient, the health care system and the country. Full, blame-free discussion is needed and if the person does not intend to take the drugs, do not prescribe them.

Older people are:

- More sensitive to drugs (weight, renal function, etc.). The estimated glomerular filtration rate (eGFR) can be looked up easily on the internet.
- More susceptible to side-effects and adverse effects.
- More likely to have side-effects that have serious sequelae.

Pharmacokinetics and pharmacodynamics

Pharmacokinetics (what the body does to the drug) and pharmacodynamics (what the drug does to the body) are both affected by ageing. Examples include:

- Slower gastric emptying.
- Increased ratio of adipose to lean tissue (increased volume of distribution for fat-soluble drugs, e.g. diazepam).
- Reduced plasma albumin.
- Altered liver metabolism – affects first pass (chlormethiazole and paracetamol).
- Reduced renal clearance (very important when a drug excreted by the kidney has a narrow therapeutic index, e.g. digoxin).
- Increased receptor sensitivity (psychoactive drugs and warfarin).

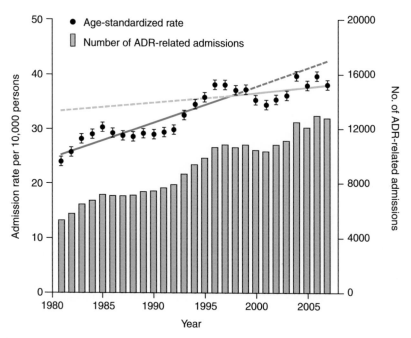

Figure 3.4 Adverse drug reactions (ADRs) – annual number and age-standardized rates per 10,000 persons aged ≥ 60 years in the Netherlands, 1981–2007. Separate regression lines are fitted to the period 1981–96 (blue) and the period 1997–2007 (red). Solid lines indicate regression lines fitted to data. Reproduced from Hartholt et al. (2010).

When problems arise there are often many causes

Example

Nellie Smith does not get out much because of her arthritic knees. She is prescribed a non-steroidal anti-inflammatory drug (NSAID):

- She decides indigestion is normal at her age (expectations).
- She has a haematemesis (more prone to side-effects).
- She collapses (impaired homeostasis, exacerbated by her furosemide).
- She fractures her hip (co-existing osteoporosis).
- She is not found until the next day (social factors – lives alone).
- She is admitted but has complications (need for speed to avoid complications of immobility).
- Antibiotics are prescribed (iatrogenic – third-generation cephalosporins should be avoided unless essential).
- She develops *Clostridium difficile* diarrhoea from which she may die.

Was the NSAID indicated initially?

Multiple pathologies means multiple drugs

Older people on several drugs are:

- More likely to experience side-effects, drug interactions and adverse drug reactions.
- Likely to have problems with concordance, especially if confused.
- Often on one drug to treat the side-effects of another!

Previous criteria to support drug prescription were not widely used in Europe as they reflected American prescribing. The STOPP/START (Screening Tool of Older Person's Prescriptions/Screening Tool to Alert Doctor's to the Right Treatment) evidence-based criteria have shown benefit when used for individuals in hospital and the community and for prescription reviews.

START identified prescribing omissions in 60% of elderly hospital admissions:

- Statins in atherosclerotic disease (26%).
- Warfarin in chronic AF (9.5%).
- Antiplatelet therapy in arterial disease (7.3%).
- Calcium/vitamin D supplementation in symptomatic osteoporosis (6%).

STOPP identified that 9% of the drug budget for $\geq$ 70 years in Ireland in 2007 could potentially be saved by stopping:

- Proton pump inhibitors at maximum therapeutic dose after > 8 weeks.
- NSAIDs after > 3 months.
- Long-acting benzodiazepines after > 1 month.
- Duplicate drugs.

Reviewing the drugs – repeat prescriptions

Review your patient's problem list and prioritize the treatable. The patient is usually on many drugs already. For each drug consider:

- Does the likely benefit outweigh the risk? (E.g. 74-year-old man on warfarin for stroke risk reduction secondary to AF, has dementia, is prone to falls and is found to have an unexpected INR of 7.2: stop the warfarin and you may save his life.)
- Still indicated? (Oxybutinin, sulphonylureas, etc. are often continued with little evidence of efficacy.)
- 'Nicest' drug for the job? (E.g. clarithromycin has fewer gastric side-effects than erythromycin.)
- Is the drug causing the symptoms? (E.g. nausea or confusion due to codeine; furosemide and fludrocortisone are an illogical combination.)
- Could a single agent replace two? (E.g. ACE inhibitor for hypertension with CCF.)
- Is the formulation/route of administration the best? (Syrups and patches may help.)
- Timings appropriate? (Once or twice-a-day options aid adherence for the patient or carers.)
- Aids to administration? [E.g. spacer for inhalers, no childproof tops, Medicines administration record (MAR) chart.]
- Aids to adherence? (E.g. Dosette box.)
- Regular or 'as required'? (Analgesics are best given on a regular basis.)
- Does the patient understand the medications and any precautions? (Supply written information and record advice in the notes.)
- Cheapest, if there are equivalents? (E.g. proton pump inhibitors.)
- Check against STOPP criteria.

Should a new drug be started?

- Aim for cure or disease modification, symptom control, or primary or secondary prevention.
- Start low; go slow, but increase dose until in the therapeutic range or side-effects develop.

- Give a drug for long enough time before deciding it is ineffective, e.g. antidepressants.
- Where the aim is prevention, consider the overall burden of pathology and drugs, but avoid therapeutic nihilism.
- Check against START criteria.

How many drugs are reasonable?

Cardiac guidelines in many countries, including NICE Guidelines for treatment after MI, recommend multiple drugs:

- Beta-blocker.
- Aspirin.
- Clopidogrel (a thienopyridine antiplatelet agent which acts by inhibiting the P2Y12 receptor) for a year after non-ST elevation myocardial infarct (NSTEMI) or percutaneous coronary intervention (PCI), commonly known as coronary angioplasty.
- ACE inhibitor and perhaps ARB too [according to the Candesartan in Heart Failure Assessment of Reduction in Morbidity and Mortality (CHARM) programme (McMurray et al. 2003)].
- Statin.
- With heart failure – loop diuretic and spironolactone.
- With diabetes – insulin in the acute phase, usual treatment later.
- With AF – warfarin or aspirin and dipyridamole.
- With angina – nicorandil.

Summary: the overall picture

- If there are multiple drugs, are they all essential?
- Avoid drugs treating the side-effects of another drug.
- Look for potential interactions.
- If the patient has renal/hepatic failure, do not rely on memory; check every drug in the British National Formulary (BNF).
- The patient will change. Always review medication. Is secondary prevention still appropriate?

Surgery in elderly patients

The outcome of surgery depends on the patient (current diagnosis, co-morbidities, fitness and social support), the surgery and the urgency of the situation.

Currently, 40% of all surgical inpatients are over 65 years old; this figure will increase as the population ages. Some operations are essential if the patient is to have a chance of survival and reasonable function, e.g. repair of a fractured hip or resection of a colonic cancer. The fracture is repaired as an emergency. The cancer will be removed as an emergency if there is perforation of the bowel or obstruction, but semi-electively otherwise. If the risk of surgery is too high, non-operative management is used. The balance depends on the situation and to some extent custom and practice. It is deemed so painful to die with a broken hip that surgery is usual, even when death is likely in the next few days (both non-operative management and deaths are recorded). An obstructing bowel cancer may be treated palliatively even though death from obstruction can be a challenge to manage; surgeons have to publish individual figures for death rates and non-operated cases are not recorded.

These indications for surgery contrast with operations that may be desirable to improve quality of life, e.g. knee replacement, which are always elective and for which the patient will need to be fitter.

The type of surgery is a major factor. Very frail patients can have cataract surgery under local anaesthetic. Less invasive options have been devised as alternatives to very major procedures, e.g. endovascular aneurysm repair (EVAR) for aortic aneurysm, endoscopic stapling of pharyngeal pouches, laparoscopic parathyroidectomy and percutaneous endoscopic colopexy (PEC) for recurrent sigmoid volvulus.

Emergency versus elective

Over 75 years, the 30-day mortality for emergency surgery is 10–30% (Figure 3.5). The main risk factors for elective surgical patients are:

- Cardiac: infarction during preceding 3 months or failure.
- Respiratory: COPD, current smoking.
- CNS: stroke during preceding 3 months, dementia.
- Metabolic: diabetes, steroids, renal failure.
- Significantly overweight or underweight.
- Frailty and poor mobility.

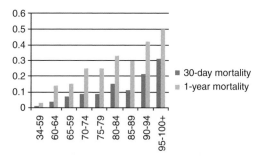

Figure 3.5 Age and post-operative mortality. Thirty-day and 1-year mortality rates related to age at operation in patients who had non-elective general or

Pre-operative care

The amount that can be achieved pre-operatively depends on the urgency of surgery. For elective surgery aims should include:

- Stop smoking – reduces post-operative chest infection.
- Improve fitness – often not achievable if the surgery is for chronic pain, e.g. knee replacement.
- Improve nutrition – by nasogastric tube if necessary.
- Optimize management of co-morbidities, e.g. is an ECHO needed?
- Optimize drugs:
  o Anticoagulant and antiplatelet agents: depends on the indication and procedure, but usually stop warfarin a week before and swap to enoxaparin, stop clopidogrel a week before.
  o Stop non-essential drugs particularly if they will add to delirium.
  o Diabetics may need insulin on a sliding scale.
  o Plan which drugs should be taken on the morning of surgery with a little water (long-term beta-blocker, drugs for PD).
- Delirium – predictable in patients with cognitive impairment; forewarn the patient and family as this reduces distress and possibly complaints and enables the family to help with reorientation after surgery. Written information may help.
- Swab for MRSA and eliminate if present.
- Pre-op therapy input – plan aids and appliances.
- Pre-op social work input if a package of care will be needed.
- Special considerations, e.g. stoma nurse.

Even for emergency surgery it is essential to correct heart failure, salt and water depletion, respiratory infection and severe anaemia as rapidly as possible. The volume depletion associated with fractured hip is easy to underestimate and more aggressive fluid replacement prior to surgery improves outcome.

Anaesthetic care

The skill of the anesthetist is as important as the surgeon in ensuring good operative outcome; frail elderly people are usually assessed pre-operatively by a senior anaesthetist who will decide whether general or regional anaesthesia is appropriate. Ageing affects the pharmacokinetics and pharmacodynamics of many anaesthetic drugs. Pre-medication is often avoided in the very old and reduced doses are needed for many drugs. During surgery the aim is to avoid episodes of excessive hypotension after induction of anaesthesia or large blood loss, or the combination of hypertension and tachycardia after noxious stimulation. Patients also need good care of their pressure areas and maintenance of body temperature.

Post-operative care

Post-operative analgesia requires careful control to maximize pain relief with minimal sedation or respiratory depression. Other measures include support and encouragement, early mobilization, careful fluid and electrolyte balance, remove catheter as soon as possible, maximize nutrition with dietetic support, avoid constipation, minimize sleep deprivation and use non-drug measures as first line for confusion.

Post-operative complications

1 Respiratory infection – resulting from atelectasis due to suppression of full inspiration by pain (abdominal surgery) or sedation.
2 Confusion – commonest on day 3 or 4 and following orthopaedic rather than general surgery possibly related to cerebral fat embolism. See Chapter 4 for other causes of acute confusional states; drugs and alcohol or their abrupt withdrawal are particularly important. Another predictable cause is hyponatraemia caused by bladder irrigation during prostatectomy. Risk factors include sensory deprivation, pain, bladder distension and constipation.
3 Cardiac failure (in 5–10% of surgical patients over 65) – sometimes due to overenthusiastic fluid replacement; surgery and pain increase ADH secretion.
4 MI (1–4% of cases); half are painless, 'failure to thrive' post-operatively. Compare new and pre-operative ECG.
5 Stroke (3% of patients over 80 undergoing surgery).
6 DVT affects 25–33% of patients. Follow prophylactic guidelines.
7 Pressure sores (see Chapter 15).

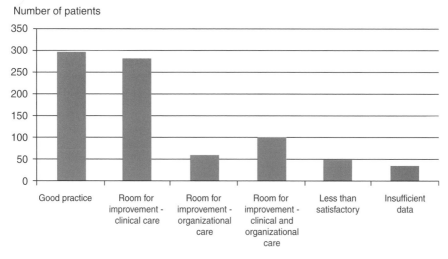

Figure 3.6 Overall assessment of care. Reproduced with permission of NCEPOD 2010.

Changes in the organization of surgical care

The development of an orthogeriatric service improves outcomes for hip fractures in some hospitals. A similar multidisciplinary approach to management in elective general surgery has been pioneered in London. The 2010 National Confidential Enquiry into Patient Outcome and Death (NCEPOD 2010) examined the care of people over 80 years old who died within 30 days of an operation in a 3-month period in 2008. Data for all aspects of care, from admission to death, were gathered by review of case notes and questionnaires. The report describes its findings as 'depressing' and 'unfortunate'. As Figure 3.6 shows, only 37% (295/786) were considered to have received 'good' care.

If good care is to be provided, there will need to be more emphasis on older people in undergraduate and postgraduate training in all specialties and an expansion in the number of geriatricians.

📖 REFERENCES

Hartholt KA, van der Velde N, Looman CWN, et al. (2010) Adverse drug reactions related hospital admissions in persons aged 60 years and over, The Netherlands, 1981–2007: less rapid Increase, different drugs. *PLoS One* 5: e13977. doi: 10.1371/journal.pone.0013977.

McMurray JJV, Pfeffer MA, Swedberg K, Granger CB, Yusuf S (2003) The CHARM programme. *Lancet* 362: 1678–1679.

NCEPOD (2010) *Elective & Emergency Surgery in the Elderly: An Age Old Problem*. www.ncepod.org.uk/2010eese.htm.

Neary WD, Foy C, Heather BP, Earnshaw JJ (2006) Identifying high-risk patients undergoing urgent and emergency surgery. *Annals of the Royal College of Surgeons England* 88: 151–156, doi: 10.1308/003588406X94896.

ONS (2010) *Health Expectancies at Birth and at Age 65, United Kingdom, 2006–08*. http://www.ons.gov.uk/ons/taxonomy/index.html?nscl=National+Health+Expectancies.

Tallis R (2003) *Is the Ageing Population a Threat to Sustainable Health Care?* http://www.cardi.ie/userfiles/ageing_and_health_care.pdf.

➡ FURTHER INFORMATION

Adams J (2008) Genetic control of ageing and life span. *Nature Education* 1(1), www.nature.com/scitable/topicpage/genetic-control-of-ageing-and-life-span-847.

Aubert G, Lansdorp PM (2007) Telomeres and ageing. *Physiology Review* 88: 557–579, doi: 10.1152/physrev.00026.2007.

Barry PJ, Gallagher PF, Ryan C, O'Mahony D (2007) START (Screening Tool to Alert doctors to the Right Treatment) – an evidence-based screening tool to detect prescribing omissions in elderly patients. *Age and Ageing* 36: 632–638, ageing.oxfordjournals.org/content/36/6/632.abstract.

Cahir C, Fahey T, Teeling M, et al. (2010) Potentially inappropriate prescribing and cost outcomes for older people: a national population study. *British Journal of Clinical Pharmacology* 69: 543–552, www.ncbi.nlm.nih.gov/pubmed/20573091.

Gallagher P, Ryan C, Byrne S, et al. (2008) STOPP (Screening Tool of Older Person's Prescriptions) and START (Screening Tool to Alert doctors to Right Treatment). Consensus validation. *International Journal of Clinical Pharmacology Therapy and Toxicology* 46: 72–83.

Haigis MC, Sinclair DA (2010) Mammalian sirtuins: biological insights and disease relevance. *Annual Review of Pathology* 5: 253–295. www.ncbi.nlm.nih.gov/pmc/articles/PMC2866163/?tool=pubmed.

Harari D, Hopper A, Dhesi J, et al. (2007) Proactive care of older people undergoing surgery ('POPS'): designing, embedding, evaluating and funding a comprehensive geriatric assessment service for older elective surgical patients. *Age and Ageing* 36: 190–196, www.gsttcharity.org.uk/pdfs/POPSpaper.pdf.

Kudlow BA, Brian K, Kennedy BK, et al. (2007) Hutchinson–Gilford progeria syndromes: mechanistic basis of human progeroid diseases. *Nature Reviews Molecular Cell Biology* 8: 394–404, doi: 10.1038/nrm2161, www.nature.com/nrm/journal/v8/n5/full/nrm2161.html.

Ledford H (2010) Genetic variations offer longer life. *Nature News* doi: 10.1038/news.2010.328.

Merideth MA, Gordon LB, Claus S, et al. (2008) Phenotype and course of Hutchinson–Gilford progeria syndrome. *New England Journal of Medicine* 358: 592–604, www.nejm.org/doi/full/10.1056/NEJMoa0706898.

NICE Clinical Guideline 76 – Medicines adherence: www.nice.org.uk/nicemedia/live/11766/43042/43042.pdf.

O'Neill D (2011) Respect and care for the older person. *Lancet* 377(9766): 640, www.thelancet.com/journals/lancet/article/PIIS0140-6736(11)60234-1/fulltext.

Pearson H (2008) The cellular hullabaloo. *Nature* 453: 150–153, doi:10.1038/453150a.

Sirtris Pharma: www.sirtrispharma.com/about.html.

Stefan M, Lino LI, Fernandez G (2011) Medical consultation and best practices for preoperative evaluation of elderly patients. *Hospital Practice* 39, doi: 10.3810/hp.2011.02.373.

Summary of the STOPP criteria: ageing.oxfordjournals.org/content/suppl/2008/10/01/afn197.DC1/afn197_suppl_data.pdf.

Willyard C (2010) Ageing cells lose protein pumps. *Nature News* doi: 10.1038/news.2010.373.

Zhu H, Belcher M, van der Harst P (2011) Healthy ageing and disease: role for telomere biology? *Clinical Science* 120: 427–440, doi: 10.1042/CS20100385, www.clinsci.org/cs/ev/120/0427/cs1200427_ev.htm.

4

Old age psychiatry

Age changes

- Brain weight decreases by 20% from its young adult weight by the age of 90.
- Selective neuronal loss of 5–50%, and cells tend to shrink.
- Fifteen to twenty percent reduction in synapses in the frontal lobes.
- Lipofuscin accumulates in some cells (significance uncertain).
- Plaques and tangles are found in aged brains, but seldom in middle-aged ones.
- Granulovacuolar degeneration can often be found in the hippocampus and occasional vascular amyloid deposits are seen in cortical blood vessels.
- All these changes are more pronounced in Alzheimer's disease (AD), but AD is not just exaggerated ageing.
- Performance in intelligence testing, learning ability, short-term memory and reaction time tend to decline with age (see age-associated memory impairment, p. 53) but often not significantly until about the age of 75.

Sleep

Sixty percent of older people complain about insomnia; sleep quality worsens with ageing. Studies indicate that the overall duration of sleep is the same, but sleep is more disturbed with more arousals. Periods of rapid eye movement sleep change little but there is less slow-wave sleep. Apnoeic episodes are more common. The worst sleep patterns are found in patients with dementia.

Simple advice for poor sleepers

- Have realistic expectations.
- Rise at a regular and early hour.
- Maintain activity during the day, avoid daytime napping.
- Avoid caffeine in the evening.
- Keep the bedroom for sleeping, not watching TV, etc.
- Wind down before trying to get to sleep.
- Do not go to bed hungry.
- Take a warm milky drink in the evening.
- Do not go to bed too early.

Factors that disturb sleep patterns

- Anxiety.
- Depression.
- Pain.
- Discomfort due to constipation.
- Urgency, frequency, nocturia.
- Restless legs (pramipexole and ropinirole are licensed treatments).
- Cramps.
- Nocturnal cough or breathlessness.
- Drugs (theophylline, sympathomimetics, high dose steroids; alcohol initially sedates but alerts later).
- Drug withdrawal (sedatives, hypnotics).

If simple corrective measures do not help, look for and treat any factors listed in the above list. Avoid hypnotics if possible as elderly persons are more likely to fall, e.g. if they have to get up to go to the

Lecture Notes Elderly Care Medicine, Eighth Edition. Claire G. Nicholl and K. Jane Wilson.
© 2012 John Wiley & Sons, Ltd. Published 2012 by John Wiley & Sons, Ltd.

toilet, and there may be a hangover effect the next day. If the situation is causing distress to the patient or carer, a short course of a hypnotic may be justified. Melatonin, the pineal hormone involved in circadian rhythms, is licensed for insomnia, but evidence that this is preferable to hypnotics is scant.

Obstructive sleep apnoea/hyponoea syndrome (OSAHS) increases with age; the jaw tends to shorten especially if edentulous and the airways tend to be narrower and less well supported as muscles and connective tissues age and become fatty. Extreme daytime sleepiness with poor concentration and reports of night-time 'choking' or extreme snoring should trigger referral for a sleep study. Continuous positive airways pressure (CPAP) with a modern mask is well tolerated, improves sleep, mood and cognition and reduces the associated high blood pressure.

REM sleep behavioural disorder is more common in old age, often associated with neurological disease, and is characterized by purposeful sometimes violent movements reflecting dream activity. It responds to low dose clonazepam or melatonin.

Problem drinking

Older people are less tolerant of alcohol due to:

- a lower ratio of body fat to water;
- a lower hepatic blood flow and reduced metabolism;
- increased brain sensitivity.

At any age, repeated excessive ingestion leads to dependency, physical disease or harm. Consumption peaks at age 55 and declines thereafter, but this may change as the middle aged who are used to drinking more than earlier generations grow old. Older people may benefit from low to moderate alcohol intake, for example cardiovascular benefits and improved quality of life. However, the Royal College of Psychiatrists (2008) estimates that 1 in 6 older men and 1 in 15 older women are drinking enough to harm themselves.

There are three patterns of drinking, described below.

Early-onset drinkers or survivors

- Males = Females, i.e. there is no gender preponderance.

- Two-thirds of elderly drinkers have a continuing alcohol problem that began when younger.
- Likely to be resistant to help.

Late-onset drinkers or reactors

- F > M.
- Use alcohol in an attempt to assuage loneliness and sadness.
- Depression common.

Intermittent or binge drinkers

- A less common pattern.

Problems linked to alcohol

- Falls, with increased risk of osteoporosis and therefore fractures, accidents, bruising.
- Self-neglect.
- Acute confusion, anxiety, depression, neuropathy, hallucinations, Wernicke's encephalopathy, dementia, fits.
- Gastrointestinal and liver disease.
- Heart problems including cardiomyopathy and atrial fibrillation.
- Haemorrhagic stroke.
- Bone marrow suppression.
- Many cancers.
- Hypothermia.
- Interaction with medications.

The usual problem is daily dosing rather than bingeing, so the alcohol problem may not be apparent. Consider a simple screening tool like CAGE (see Appendix 3), but this may be less valid in older drinkers.

Treatment entails total withdrawal: delirium tremens is managed with chlordiazepoxide (use lower doses). In problem drinking, it may be possible to reduce intake: check who is buying the alcohol. The Institute of Alcohol Studies produces a useful fact sheet, and Alcoholics Anonymous (AA) offers helpful support for those who find their methods acceptable.

Anxiety

Anxiety is very common in older people. It may accompany depression, dementia and physical illness or may cause physical symptoms (palpitations, breathlessness, giddiness, abdominal discomfort, bowel fixation). Always consider anxiety or depression in recurrent attenders and in rehabilitation patients who fail to make progress. When severe (Generalized Anxiety Disorder) it decreases social functioning and has a marked impact on health-related quality of life. Treatments include reassurance or cognitive therapy, but if associated with panic attacks, try duloxetine (a serotonin and noradrenaline reuptake inhibitor, SNRI), escitalopram (a selective serotonin reuptake inhibitor, SSRI), or pregabalin (antiepileptic GABA agonist).

Late-onset delusional disorder

This is a schizophreniform paranoid psychosis in which personality, affect and self-care skills are well preserved and there is no thought disorder. It most often affects single women who live alone, especially those who suffer from deafness. Isolation is thought to be a significant factor in its development. There is often a highly structured system of delusions and hallucinations, which may centre on a conspiracy involving the neighbours or have a sexual content. The response to antipsychotic drugs is good if concordance can be achieved. Newer agents, such as low-dose risperidone, were thought to cause fewer long-term side-effects but were more expensive. However, now they are cheaper, but it is recognized that they have a range of serious side-effects.

Causes of hallucinations

- Bereavement.
- Depression.
- Acute brain syndrome (including drugs, e.g. dopaminergic treatment for PD).
- Dementia.
- Late onset schizophrenia.
- Poor vision (Charles Bonnet syndrome – no other features of psychiatric illness – patients need explanation and reassurance that this is not a harbinger of mental illness).

Depression

Prevalence

Depression occurs in around 10–15% of people aged over 65 years and is severe in 3%. Unipolar depression is most common, but bipolar disorders make up 5–10% of more severe cases and the hypomanic

phase is often missed. The key is to consider the possibility of a mood disorder. Ask the patient – most will tell you and there is a surprisingly good correlation between a Yes/No answer to the question 'Are you depressed?' and the result of a full psychiatric assessment. Screening tools such as the Geriatric Depression Score (see Appendix 5) may be helpful. Many old, ill people in hospital are anxious, lose their appetite and cannot sleep or concentrate. In the list of features that follows, physical aspects are least helpful in discriminating between physical and psychiatric disease and anhedonia perhaps the most.

Features

- Association with physical illness especially chronic disease. Growing evidence for a subtype of depression in later life associated with cerebrovascular disease.
- Somatization of symptoms, hypochondriasis.
- Pervasive anhedonia ('when did you last enjoy anything?').
- Guilt, worthlessness, low self-esteem.
- Hopelessness and helplessness.
- Apathy or agitation, anxiety, delusions.
- Sleep disturbance.
- Withdrawal, poor concentration and memory ('pseudodementia').
- Self-neglect, malnutrition, dehydration.
- Suicide risk.

In almost all industrialized countries, men aged 75 years and older used to have the highest suicide rates. Suicide attempts in older people are often long planned, involve high-lethality methods and, as the elderly are more fragile and frequently live alone, often lead to fatal outcome. In later life, in both sexes, major depression is the most common diagnosis in those who attempt or complete suicide. In the UK, the greatest reductions in male suicide rates have been seen in men over 75 years, from 25 per 100,000 population in 1991 to 14 per 100,000 population in 2009 ($n = 262$). The trend in older women is similar but with rates of about one-third. This is strong evidence that recognition and treatment of depression in old age has improved (Figure 4.1). However, a previous serious attempt, bereavement and isolation all point to high risk.

Management

Supportive

- Mild depression is managed in primary care.
- Counselling.

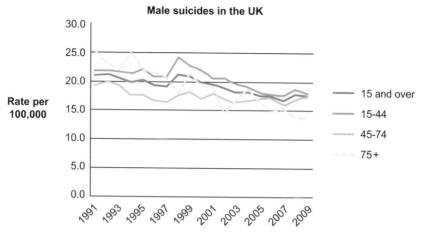

Figure 4.1 Age-standardized suicide rates in the UK, 1991–2009. *Source*: ONS 2011, Crown copyright.

- Relieving loneliness.
- Practical measures, e.g. benefits check.
- More severe depression is often best managed with help of the local Old Age Psychiatry service, involving community psychiatric nurses (CPNs), social workers and a consultant. The team usually assesses the patient in their own home and will support them to continue with medication or cognitive behavioural therapy.
- Old Age Psychiatry service may offer day hospital care, which might include exercise, cognitive behavioural therapy (CBT) and art therapy, with different days for clients with depression or psychosis and dementia.
- Referral to Cruse Bereavement Care if relevant.
- Remember to support the carers; depression is extremely common and it is essential to offer support, e.g. respite care or a sitting service such as Crossroads for the patient, before deterioration in the carer's mental health precipitates a crisis.

Drugs

- SSRIs are the drugs of choice, because of fewer sedating and anticholinergic effects than the tricyclic antidepressants. Watch for hyponatraemia.
- They are relatively safe in overdose.
- Nausea, diarrhoea and restlessness can occur.
- To minimize nausea, start at a very low dose for the first week and increase gradually. Explain to the patient that any nausea will wear off.
- Give a simple explanation of the chemical basis of depression and explain that depression cannot just be shaken off by 'counting your blessings' or having a bit more moral fibre!
- Explain to patients that SSRIs are different from benzodiazepines, do not usually cause dopiness, and will be stopped gradually when no longer needed.
- Strongly reinforce the need to stick with the tablets for at least 6 weeks before expecting the cloud to lift. Information sheets can be useful. Treatment should be continued for a year, or possibly even for life in severe cases.
- Our current practice is:
  o Citalopram (SSRI) starting with 10 mg for most patients.
  o Mirtazapine (a presynaptic α_2-antagonist, which increases noradrenergic and serotinergic transmission) stimulates appetite and aids sleep.
  o Trazodone (tricyclic with few antimuscarinic effects) if sedation is needed.
  o Venlafaxine (SNRI) for resistant depression.
- Lithium is helpful as a mood stabilizer in bipolar disorder, but it has a narrow therapeutic index and levels must be checked if toxicity is suspected (tremor, ataxia, impaired renal function).
- Fluoxetine, fluvoxamine and paroxetine (all SSRIs) are more likely to be involved in significant drug–drug interactions than citalopram or sertraline.
- If SSRIs cause nausea and the patient is sleepy try lofepramine (a tricyclic with few antimuscarinic side-effects), building up from 70 mg.

Electroconvulsive therapy

Electroconvulsive therapy (ECT) is comparatively quick, safe and effective in severe depression, but most psychiatrists are now very reluctant to consider ECT because of the bad press it has received. The Mental Health Act 2007 states that ECT may not be given to a patient with capacity who refuses it, and may only be given to an incapacitated patient where it does not conflict with any advance directive, the decision of a donee (the person who is given the power of attorney) or deputy, or the decision of the Court of Protection.

Acute and chronic confusion

Many old people are described as confused. Anyone can become delirious when they are ill, but this is common in frail older people. Simplistically, delirium is the term used for acute confusion and dementia describes chronic confusion. The interrelationship between the two is complex.

- Dementia is the biggest risk factor for delirium; a person with dementia typically gets much more muddled when ill and improves to some extent (but not always back to baseline) if they recover.
- Delirium may persist for months (or years according to some) – when does this become 'dementia'?
- Some causes of dementia are reversible.
- Long-term cognitive decline is common after an episode of delirium.
- Dementia with Lewy bodies (see later) has features more typical of delirium.

Delirium

Delirium is a transient, reversible syndrome that is acute and fluctuating, and occurs in the setting of a medical condition. Delirium is common and occurs in up to half of frail older patients admitted to hospital. It can be a key component in the cascade of events leading to a downward spiral of functional decline, institutionalization and eventually death.

Susceptibility factors

- Age.
- Cognitive impairment.
- Previous episode of delirium.
- Depression.
- Multiple comorbidities.
- Multiple drugs.
- Falls (a marker of frailty).
- Sensory impairment.

Precipitating factors

Intracranial

- Infarction – any stroke, especially right parietal and most confusing for the doctor if no physical signs; often frontal.
- Infection – meningoencephalitis.
- Injury – head injury with contusion or intracranial blood, fat embolism.
- Post-ictal – (if the fit is missed the patient is just found on the floor).
- Iatrogenic – drugs acting on the CNS (including abrupt withdrawal, e.g. benzodiazepines not charted).

Extracranial

- Infection – commonly chest, urine and cellulitis.
- Metabolic and nutritional – fluid and electrolyte imbalance, hypoglycaemia, hypo-/hyperthermia, refeeding syndrome, Wernicke's encephalopathy.
- Anoxia – cardiac or respiratory failure, 'silent' myocardial infarction, anaemia.
- Toxic – drugs and alcohol.
- Stress response.
- Anaesthesia and surgery.

Consequences of illness and hospitalization

- Pain.
- Emotional distress.
- Sleep deprivation.
- Unfamiliar environment exacerbated by loss of glasses, hearing aids.
- Catheters, drips, etc.
- Urinary retention, constipation.

The pathophysiology is poorly understood (see Figure 4.2); susceptibility factors all impair neurotransmission. The precipitating events cause further acute breakdown of network connectivity, by increasing inhibitory tone within the brain

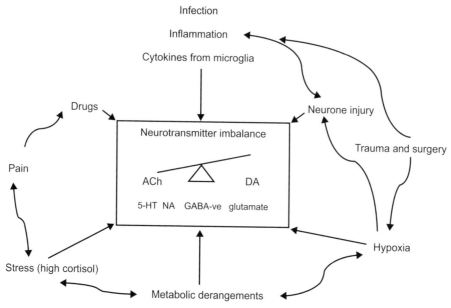

Figure 4.2 Pathogenesis of delirium.

(GABAergic neurotransmission). All transmitters may be affected, but a frequent pattern is cholinergic hypofunction and dopaminergic excess. The form of delirium that results, hypoactive, hyperactive or mixed, depends on which networks are affected. A small study with single-photon emission computerized tomography (SPECT) has shown hypoperfusion in the frontal, parietal and pontine regions.

Clinical features of delirium (acute confusion)

- Onset typically rapid over hours to days.
- Marked fluctuation: lucid intervals.
- Reversal of sleep–wake cycle is common.
- Altered consciousness often described as 'clouding'.
- Inability to sustain, focus or shift attention.
- Disturbed cognition, e.g. disorganized thinking, disorientation.
- Illusions, misinterpretation, e.g. thinking an IV line is a snake.
- Hallucinations, perception in the absence of a stimulus.
- Delusions, false beliefs; the patient may deny they are ill and escape from the hospital.
- Fear, bewilderment, restlessness or hypoactivity.
- Possibly signs of underlying cause.

Management

- **Prevention**: attention to orientation, food and fluids, sleep and sensory inattention has been shown to reduce the incidence of delirium. Avoid suddenly stopping sedatives and antidepressants unless essential, and use caution with new drugs that cross the blood–brain barrier.
- **Identification** of high-risk patients and educating the family reduces distress.
- **Recognition** of delirium is the key. An algorithm such as the CAM (see box) may help. Agitated delirium is obvious, but apathetic delirium with withdrawal and drowsiness is easy to overlook.
- Treat underlying cause/s.
- Look for exacerbating factors, e.g. faecal impaction, urinary retention, pain.
- Correct additional factors: fluid and electrolyte imbalance, nutritional deficiencies.
- Reassurance and explanation: avoid confrontation; ask the family to sit with patient.
- Optimize environment and sensory input: glasses, hearing aid, quiet familiar music, dim light at night, but avoid overstimulation.
- Minimize moves around the hospital and ward.
- Avoid complications: nurse sitting with the patient, 1 to 1 'specialling', mattress on floor to reduce risk of hip fracture, pressure mattress.

- Serious restlessness or agitation not responding to above measures: haloperidol or risperidone, start with 0.5 mg, increasing if necessary in increments after 2 h; if neuroleptics are to be avoided (concern about DLB – see later) try lorazepam. Give drugs orally if possible (will take 30–60 min to start to have effect) or IM if essential to sedate rapidly for the person's safety.

The Confusion Assessment Method (CAM) Diagnostic Algorithm

Four features are assessed:

1 Acute onset and fluctuating course – need information from a family member or carer
  Is there an acute change in mental status from the patient's baseline? Does the (abnormal) behaviour fluctuate?

2 Inattention
  Does the patient have trouble keeping track of what is said, are they easily distractible or do they have difficulty focusing attention?

3 Disorganized thinking
  Is the patient's thinking disorganized, rambling, irrelevant or illogical?

4 Altered level of consciousness
  Is the patient's level of consciousness alert (the only normal answer), vigilant (hyperalert), lethargic (drowsy but easily roused), stuporose (difficult to arouse) or comatose (unrousable)?

The diagnosis of delirium by CAM requires the presence of features 1 and 2 and either 3 or 4. (With training, sensitivity is around 94% and specificity 89%.)

Dementia

Dementia is a clinical and public health problem of enormous magnitude.

What is dementia?

Dementia is a *syndrome* (lots of causes) of *acquired* (not learning difficulties), *chronic* (lasts months to years), *global* (not just memory or just language problems) impairment of higher brain function, in an *alert patient* (not drowsy), which *interferes with* *the ability to cope* with daily living (it does not usually matter if an old person does not know 'it's Tuesday', but if he or she does not know 'it's winter', he or she might freeze).

Remember:

My	**m**emory – short-term memory loss predominates in early dementia
Old	**o**rientation
Grandmother	**g**rasp and other executive functions such as planning
Converses	**c**ommunication
Pretty	**p**ersonality change
Badly	**b**ehavioural changes including dyspraxia – difficulty with complex motor tasks, e.g. dressing oneself and agnosia – problems recognizing people and objects, leading to a variety of behaviour that is difficult to manage.

After Brice Pitt (Emeritus Professor of Old Age Psychiatry at St Mary's, London)

Causes of the dementia syndrome

Primary dementias, where the disease mainly affects the neurons in the brain, are categorized as:

- Alzheimer's disease (AD), the commonest cause.
- Dementia with Lewy bodies (DLB).
- Frontotemporal lobar dementias (FTD).

Rarer causes are:

- Prion diseases such as familial, sporadic and variant Creutzfeldt–Jakob disease.
- Huntington's disease: autosomal dominant trinucleotide repeat disorder in which an excessive number of CAG repeats results in a polyglutamine sequence in the huntingtin protein, which leads to neurone death. It causes dementia with abnormal movements, usually presenting in middle age.
- Normal pressure hydrocephalus (NPH) presents with a triad of incontinence, gait dyspraxia and dementia (while the dementia is still mild), probably due to abnormal CSF flow, although by the time CSF pressure is measured it is in the 'normal' range. It may respond to shunting.

Secondary dementias occur in which the neuronal damage is due to other pathology:

- Vascular dementia (which includes multiple small infarcts and white matter ischaemia).
- Potentially reversible conditions which can present as dementia.
- Rule out any major metabolic problem especially hypo- or hyperthyroidism, hypercalcaemia, hyponatraemia, recurrent nocturnal hypoglycaemia, major organ failure (usually obvious), vitamin deficiencies, especially thiamine, folate and B_{12}, toxicity from centrally acting drugs and alcohol, head trauma (either repetitive, e.g. punchdrunk syndrome in boxers) or the sub-acute confusion of a subdural haemorrhage following a fall and head injury, an expanding brain tumour and, very rarely in the UK now, neurosyphilis, or the dementia occurring with HIV.

Remember:

Drugs and alcohol.
Eyes and ears.
Metabolic.
Emotional (really, psychiatric problems).
Nutritional.
Trauma and tumours.
Infections.
Atheroma – vascular dementia.

How common is dementia?

Dementia is rare below 55 years, but the prevalence increases dramatically with age to about 2% in the over 65s and rises to about 20% in the over 80s. There is a slight female preponderance. In elderly people, AD probably accounts for half to two-thirds of cases of dementia. About 800,000 people in the UK have dementia. The lifetime risk for any individual developing AD is around 10%.

What happens in dementia?

The onset is insidious with gradual changes in memory and concentration, thinking processes, language use, personality, behaviour and orientation. Short-term memory is impaired early, long-term recall is often much better. Thinking becomes rigid and concrete. The condition progresses to obvious problems with short-term memory and managing basic activities of daily living, increasing disorientation and sometimes difficult or distressing behaviour such as night-time wandering,

aggression or apathy. These behavioural and psychological symptoms of dementia (BPSD) cause a lot of distress for carers. A tendency to lose things easily turns into paranoia and even delusions. Constant repetition of the same questions can be very trying for carers. Eventually, the patient is completely disorientated, no longer recognizes close family members, ceases to communicate and becomes doubly incontinent, bed-bound and totally dependent. The typical duration is 8–10 years.

Why does dementia matter?

Dementia is a devastating condition for the patient while insight is preserved and for their family, who witness the progressive deterioration. For the spouse this has been likened to 'being bereaved without being widowed'. Dementia also has major economic consequences. Owing to increasing life-span, there are more of the 'oldest old', one in five of whom may have dementia, a major cause of dependency and need for institutional care. Politicians and society are beginning to grapple with the issues and the costs of health and social care. In the UK the national cost of dementia (2007) is about £17 billion per year (direct costs to health and social care £8.2 billion) and in 30 years the cost will treble to over £50 billion per year. The costs of dementia are greater than the costs of stroke, heart disease and cancer. The impact of dementia on other health outcomes is dramatic. A person with a fractured hip and dementia is over 2.5 times as likely to die and 18 times more likely to be discharged to a care home than a person with normal cognition.

In addition to the considerable morbidity, it is believed that AD is the sixth leading cause of death in the West. However, 'bronchopneumonia' usually appears on the death certificate. Despite this burden, dementia is only just beginning to command the attention it deserves.

How is a diagnosis of dementia made?

The GP is usually the first port of call, but a survey performed by the Alzheimer's Society (AS) suggests that it is often difficult to get a diagnosis. In 2006, at age 65–69, 5 people per 1,000 had a diagnosis of dementia whereas the estimated actual prevalence is 13 per 1,000. At 80+ the figures were 60 and 122 per 1,000 respectively. There are many reasons for this, discussed below.

Difficulties getting a diagnosis of dementia

Doctor factors

- Lack of confidence/training in this area.
- Lack of awareness that a simple cognitive screen may be essential to identify a problem masked by 'a good social front'. Quick screening tests include Hodkinson's Abbreviated Mental Test Score (see Appendix 4).
- Reluctance to diagnose an 'untreatable illness' (but much can be done; see management below).

Patient/carer factors

- Need to know previous level of function to identify decline.
- Patients with dementia do not give the best medical histories – they get muddled or may focus on previous problems (e.g. 'It's the doctor … what did I want to say? … Ah, doctor, it's my back').
- Patients are elderly and often live alone; family may be distant, so corroborative information may be limited. However, if family members are concerned, there is usually a problem, whereas if only the patient is complaining, the diagnosis is often anxiety, depression or 'worried well'.

Environmental factors (Figure 4.3)

- The point at which the person has difficulty coping depends on their environment and support network as well as their cognitive abilities.

It is important to understand that dementia does not equate with a number on a cognitive function score such as the MMSE, Folstein's Mini Mental State Examination (scored out of 30). A barrister with a complex brief may present with difficulty managing at work and is still able to score 30, but there may be a strong clinical suspicion, confirmed by the passage of time, that this is AD. An elderly resident in a care home who has not been noted to be confused may have an MMSE of 16, as coping with the daily routine does not require a high degree of cognitive function.

Dementia often presents acutely because of a social crisis (e.g. death of caring spouse) or physical crisis (any illness, often a chest or urine infection, which worsens the confusion).

Cognition changes with age – what is normal and what is pathological?

- Many old people are slightly forgetful and it is difficult to distinguish ageing changes from the earliest stages of dementia.

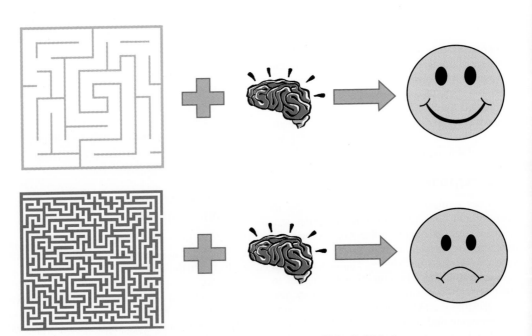

Figure 4.3 The interplay between the brain and the environment. © Claire G. Nicholl.

Age-Associated Memory Impairment is a subjective complaint of forgetfulness in those over 50 years, with a performance on memory testing one standard deviation below the normal for a young adult. Almost 20% of people over 50 years meet these criteria and the significance is uncertain. Older people often compensate well for memory changes using pattern recognition from experience.

Mild Cognitive Impairment (MCI) has been coined for people who have evidence of memory loss in comparison with those of the same age, confirmed by testing and noticeable to other people. There is no single accepted definition; the Mayo Clinic criteria include impairment of language, attention, reasoning, judgement, reading and writing as well as memory problems. Other definitions restrict MCI to memory impairment. However, all definitions agree that the problems are not severe enough to affect activities of daily living. Even this is not objective; different lifestyles place different demands on the individual (see above). The American College of Physicians suggests that 20% of the population over 70 may have MCI. Some people with MCI are in the early stages of Alzheimer's or another dementia, others have stress, anxiety, depression or physical illness and others may have always had a poor memory. Some people with MCI eventually develop dementia. Others remain stable and some return to normal. In memory clinic series, depending on the population, definitions and protocols adopted, around 10% of people with MCI progress to dementia per year (compared to around 1% in the normal population).

Figure 4.4 shows cognitive change with ageing in three normal individuals with different baselines: an individual with two episodes of acute illness and two individuals who develop dementia. At the single point in time shown by the arrow, it will be difficult to be certain about what a given level of cognitive function means for an individual.

Disease factors

- Most dementias develop slowly over many years, so there is not a single time point when the disease becomes apparent.

Having identified possible dementia, the GP may manage the patient or refer on to a neurologist (younger people), a geriatrician (frail older people), an old age psychiatrist (older people with behavioural problems) or, increasingly, a multidisciplinary memory clinic.

The aims of a clinical assessment

Is it dementia?

A full history, with more detailed cognitive function testing, including assessment of language, visuospatial skills and reasoning, e.g. MMSE, or in the more able a more detailed instrument such as the Addenbrooke's Cognitive Examination (ACE-R), usually answers this question. However, even in expert hands there is often uncertainty which is only resolved by the passage of time. Cognitive scores are affected by education, language fluency, impaired hearing and vision, acute illness, dysphasia and low mood. These conditions must be ruled out, as must psychiatric problems like schizophrenia and mania.

What type of dementia is it?

The next step is to identify the cause. The dementia may be reversible (e.g. hypothyroidism), treatment may slow disease progression (e.g. treating hypertension in vascular dementia), specific treatment may be available (e.g. AD), genetic counselling may be required (e.g. familial AD) or it may be important to avoid certain medication (e.g. neuroleptics in DLB). The major causes are discussed in more detail below.

There is no diagnostic test for most of the primary dementias until a post-mortem examination, so the *likely* cause is determined by the *clinical features* and the results of *investigations*. Common conditions such as vascular dementia (VaD) and AD may co-exist and are probably additive.

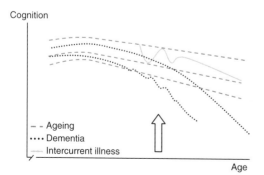

Cognition

– – Ageing
···· Dementia
— Intercurrent illness

Age

Figure 4.4 Cognitive change with ageing.

History

Progressive deterioration is usual in AD. Where it occurs, step-wise deterioration suggests vascular dementia. Hallucinations and delusions are features of DLB. Parkinsonian features would suggest vascular dementia or DLB. Most patients with dementia show some fluctuation, known as 'sun-downing' because the confusion worsens in the evening, but marked fluctuation affecting conscious level can occur in DLB. Weighted scores, such as the Hachinski ischaemia score, may improve diagnostic accuracy, and work is in progress to determine whether patterns of change found on neuropsychological and language testing add to diagnosis. Younger patients are more likely to have a frontotemporal dementia.

Examination

- Ill or well and clues from general appearance (self care or neglect).
- Cardiovascular system; BP, cardiac rhythm, burden of atheroma.
- Neurological system (walk and turn, undress, get onto couch swiftly, follow commands):
  o stroke disease or other focal problems;
  o other neurological conditions, e.g. PD.
- Psychiatric state, mood, hallucinations.

Investigations

- Blood tests to exclude reversible causes or other major pathology (blood count, biochemical profile, ESR, thyroid function, B_{12} and folate (syphilis serology and HIV testing are rarely relevant).
- CXR and ECG.
- Head CT early on is likely to be normal but is useful to exclude space-occupying lesions or a subdural haematoma. Disproportionately large ventricles with little sulcal atrophy raise the possibility of NPH.
- In the late stages, a CT scan usually shows cerebral atrophy.
- MRI is more sensitive than CT in documenting volume loss (particularly in the medial temporal lobe in AD) and the amount of vascular damage.
- CIT SPECT labels presynaptic dopamine transporters and helps distinguish between AD and DLB. $[^{123}I]$-β-CIT is $[^{123}I]$-2β-carbomethoxy-3β-(4-iodophenyl)tropane, a radiotracer with high affinity to monoamine transporters.
- Genetic tests, e.g. apolipoprotein E alleles that predispose to AD, are not routine.

- At present, older people with dementia rarely have a lumbar puncture, functional scanning or serial morphometric scans to document progressive atrophy, but this is likely to change over the next 5 years.

How is dementia managed?

Management depends on the severity of the dementia and whether the patient lives alone and comprises a multidisciplinary, multi-agency package of care. Much of the management is similar regardless of the aetiology. The package needs to be well coordinated and to evolve as the needs of the patient and carer change. The many options include:

- Coping strategies (diaries, reminder alarms), psychological techniques (CBT), reminiscence work (life-story book) and validation therapy (approach where care staff accept the reality of the dementia sufferer's world to them, but there is no evidence for benefit).
- Optimize hearing, vision and improve general health.
- Treat other conditions that may impair cognition (e.g. anaemia, heart failure).
- Treat risk factors (e.g. hypertension in vascular dementia).
- Treat specific symptoms and behaviours (major tranquillizers, unfortunately, are often the only option).
- Education and support for patients and carers: the AS deals with all types of dementia, produces excellent leaflets and Caring with Confidence training packages; Carers UK.
- Genetic counselling (only in rare early-onset dementias).
- Legal advice (e.g. a Lasting Power of Attorney may obviate the need for the Court of Protection at a later date, advice about driving, advance decisions, etc.).
- Advice on driving (excellent information sheet from AS, patients can pay for a driving assessment at a special centre).
- Therapy assessments: occupational therapy, speech and language therapy (for swallowing and communication) and physiotherapy; usually aimed at arranging appropriate care and advising carers, rather than treating the patient.
- Assistive 'smart' technology: includes pressure mats to turn on lights, fridge and door monitors to detect movement, automatic fall detectors if the person cannot press the buzzer, automatic tap cut-off.

- Assessment for benefits and care by social services (see Chapter 2).
- Regular district nurse/community psychiatric nurse support.
- Continence services.
- Sitting services (Crossroads), day hospitals, respite care.
- Admiral nurses (support carers).
- Optimum provision of long-term care.
- Encourage training for staff in care homes.
- Palliative care in the terminal stages.
- Drugs may be used:
  - for secondary prevention, e.g. aspirin, statins and antihypertensives may delay vascular dementia, but there is no clear evidence base;
  - to treat specific symptoms (see debate on antipsychotics in BPSD);
  - to enhance cholinergic transmission in AD.

The Mental Capacity Act

In England, when your patient may lack capacity, if you propose to act on their behalf you must respect the MCA in the following situations:

- Decisions regarding serious medical treatment, e.g. investigations, cancer treatment, feeding tubes.
- Moving from home to a care setting.
- Drug trials.
- The Act will affect how you consult the patient's family and friends; patients with no-one to support them need an Independent Mental Capacity Advocate (IMCA).

Management of BPSD

The best approach is to try to understand the basis of the particular behaviour from the individual's perspective and rectify the cause:

- Physical: delirium, thirst, constipation, pain (see delirium).
- Psychological: anxiety, depression, boredom.
- Environment: poor facilities (no space to wander, lack of views, no aids to orientation), over- and understimulation, disturbed behaviour of others, inadequate numbers or training of staff.

Drug treatment

- Unfortunately, these behaviours often persist.
- No drugs are licensed for long-term management of BPSD but antipsychotics are widely used.
- Doses are lower than those in schizophrenia but parkinsonian side-effects were common with first-generation drugs like haloperidol.
- Newer atypicals, e.g. risperidone, olanzapine, quetiapine, were thought to have fewer side-effects.
- However, meta-analysis of 17 trials (modal duration of 10 weeks) demonstrated that the risk of death (variety of causes including cardiovascular) associated with the drugs was 1.7 times that of placebo.
- 180,000 people with dementia in England are treated with antipsychotics per year. Of these, 20% may benefit, but around 1% will die and 1% will have a stroke.
- Use the lowest dose possible, for the shortest time possible; once the patient has settled, aim to reduce and then stop the drug.
- Risperidone has a licence for up to 6 weeks use.
- If you use these drugs, explain the rationale and risks to the family and document this.

Recognition that dementia is a terminal illness

- In early dementia, patients should be supported to live a full life.
- However, clinicians must recognize when the patient is entering the terminal phase.
- In a study of 323 nursing home residents with advanced dementia, 6-month mortality was high (nearly 25%), complications such as pneumonia, febrile episodes and eating problems were common and distressing symptoms were frequent.
- In the last 3 months of life 40% of residents had a burdensome intervention such as hospital admission or tube feeding.
- One-third of patients in nursing homes with end-stage dementia and aspiration are tube-fed in the USA.
- This is more likely where the family and carers had not appreciated the clinical course; therefore it is essential to educate relatives regarding poor prognosis and change to a palliative approach.
- There is no evidence of benefit in terms of nutritional state, pressure sores or mortality.

- Involving a speech therapist and dietician may enable adequate oral intake for longer during the patient's decline.
- Avoid keeping people 'nil by mouth', offer food and fluid as patient can manage.
- Considerable resources would be released by allowing people to die with comfort and dignity.
- Asking for a second opinion is often advisable.

Alzheimer's disease

Alzheimer's disease is the commonest dementia. It is named after Alzheimer who looked after Auguste D, a 51-year-old inmate of an asylum with memory impairment and behavioural problems. After her death Alzheimer studied her brain and in 1906 presented his findings of brain atrophy, plaques and with a new stain, neurofibrillary tangles.

Pathologically AD is characterized by:

- amyloid-containing extracellular plaques;
- intraneuronal neurofibrillary tangles containing tau protein.

It was divided into early-onset and late-onset, but the pathology is identical so this distinction is used less. However, younger patients present different management challenges because they are often still at work and have younger families. In AD, beta amyloid (Aβ) is clipped from a normal transmembrane protein, amyloid precursor protein (APP), by two enzymes – beta-secretase and gamma-secretase. Aβ is produced in the AD brain at a normal rate but is not cleared from the brain efficiently and sticks together to form amyloid plaques. According to the amyloid hypothesis, accumulation of Aβ drives the rest of the disease process, including formation of neurofibrillary tangles and cell death. Figure 4.5 shows a simplified scheme for APP metabolism.

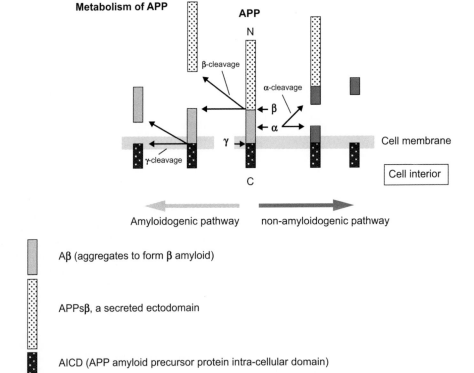

Figure 4.5 The metabolism of APP. N and C, the N and C terminus of a polypeptide. Simplified from Cole and Vassar (2007), doi: 10.1186/1750-1326-2-22. © 2007 Cole and Vassar; licensee BioMed Central Ltd.

Risk factors for Alzheimer's disease

- Down's syndrome.
- Age.
- Female sex.
- APOE ε4.
- Obesity in middle age.
- Head injury.
- Elevated homocysteine levels (can be decreased by folate, so may be counterbalanced by fruit and vegetables).

Protective factors for Alzheimer's disease

- Education (partly a threshold effect, but confounding with other associations with social class, e.g. diet high in antioxidants).
- Continued brain activity (keep reading!).
- Social activity.
- Exercise.
- Wine, coffee and turmeric in curry (so it is not all bad news!).
- Diet rich in foods containing vitamin E (but not vitamin E supplements).
- Tobacco (may be the nicotinic effect on cholinergic transmission, but the possible benefit does not outweigh the harm done by smoking).
- NSAIDs and aspirin (trials to date have been disappointing).
- Hormone replacement therapy (fitter population and not reproduced in trials).
- Statins (could be reduction in vascular damage; evidence to date disappointing).

Genetics and AD

There are rare autosomal dominant forms of AD with mutations in three genes, all of which probably increase brain levels of amyloid, the APP gene on chromosome 21, presenilin 1 on 14q and presenilin 2 on 1q. People with trisomy 21 (Down's syndrome) almost all develop AD in their 40s because of the gene dose effect of APP. Most cases of AD appear sporadic but there is evidence of a polygenic genetic predisposition in these cases too. The best established association is with the Apolipoprotein E4 gene on chromosome 12. There are three common alleles, APOE ε2, APOE ε3 and APOE ε4.

- APOE ε2 is less common and may provide some protection against AD.

- APOE ε3, the most common allele, appears neutral with regard to AD.
- APOE ε4 increases the risk of getting AD and getting symptoms at a younger age (40% of people who develop AD v 25–30% of the population) but the mechanism is unknown. APOE ε4 is a risk-factor gene; it increases the risk of AD, but some with the e4/e4 genotype never get the disease.

Phases of AD

The National Institute on Ageing and the Alzheimer's Association (NIA–AA) workgroup (2011) has produced new guidelines for the diagnosis of AD in three phases:

1. Asymptomatic preclinical phase (for research)

The pathophysiological process of AD (and brain shrinkage) is thought to begin many years before AD becomes clinically apparent. If interventions that delay or arrest progression of the pathology become available, identifying pre-symptomatic people will be very important.

2. The symptomatic, pre-dementia phase (MCI due to AD)

People in this stage may be slower, less efficient and make errors completing complex functional tasks such as paying bills, preparing a meal or shopping. However, they still function independently. Prominent impairment in episodic memory is a strong predictor of progression to AD, but other patterns of cognitive impairment, e.g. visiospatial impairment, can also progress. A number of biomarkers may indicate that the underlying pathology is AD. These are currently used in research but may become part of clinical diagnosis. In this stage, encourage patients to remain as engaged as possible in three domains: physical activity (improves mood as well as fitness), cognitive activities, e.g. crosswords, and social engagement.

Possible biomarkers for MCI-AD

Aβ deposition:

- CSF Aβ42 (lower than normals).
- Positron-emission tomography (PET) amyloid imaging.

Neuronal injury:

- CSF tau/phosphorylated-tau (increased).

- Hippocampal volume or medial temporal atrophy by volumetric measures.
- Rate of brain atrophy.
- FDG-PET imaging: ^{18}F-fluorodeoxyglucose is a radioactive analogue of glucose so the concentrations of tracer imaged reflect tissue metabolic activity
- SPECT perfusion imaging.

Associated biochemical change:

- Inflammatory biomarkers (cytokines).
- Oxidative stress (isoprostanes).

3. The dementia phase

At this point the cognitive deficits start to impact on functional independence. How long the patient remains in their own home depends on the robustness of the available family support and the pattern their dementia takes. Behavioural problems and urinary and particularly faecal incontinence are factors predicting institutionalization.

A number of therapeutic approaches relating to amyloid are being developed, from small-scale trials of vaccines (one early study had severe side-effects in man), to Phase III trials of agents that alter aspects of amyloid biology, e.g. formation, deposition, metabolism – gamma-secretase inhibitors and alpha-secretase enhancers and binding. IV Ig (normal human immunoglobulin) contains naturally occurring antibodies against Aβ and is being tested but is scarce and costly, so monoclonals such as bapineuzumab and solanezumab may be a better way forward.

The metabolism of acetylcholine

The rationale for the current drugs used for AD is based on earlier work showing that most neuronal death occurs in cholinergic projections. Cholinergic transmission could be enhanced by increasing the availability of the precursor, via direct stimulation of the receptors or by preventing the breakdown of endogenous acetylcholine (see

Figure 4.6). Three drugs, which are all acetylcholinesterase (AChE) inhibitors, are available:

- Donepezil: reversible inhibitor of AChE.
- Galantamine: reversible inhibitor of AChE with nicotinic receptor agonist properties.
- Rivastigmine: reversible non-competitive inhibitor of AChE and butyryl cholinesterase (available as a patch).

All have cholinergic side-effects especially nausea, vomiting and diarrhoea. To minimize these, the drugs are started at a low dose and gradually increased. Care must be taken in sick sinus syndrome, peptic ulcer disease, COPD and urinary retention, and there may be interactions with muscle relaxants in anaesthesia. The drugs have limited efficacy and do not seem to benefit all patients, but many get a useful response in terms of memory or behaviour, with another 6 months of better function. AChE inhibitors are widely available in most countries. Restrictive guidelines in the UK were relaxed to some extent in 2011 (NICE 2011).

Use of acetylcholinesterase inhibitors

- AD is diagnosed in a specialist clinic.
- Indicated for mild and moderate AD (typically mild equates to MMSE 21–26 and moderate to 10–20, but clinical judgement is needed to assess severity).
- The carer's views should be considered and it needs to be feasible to expect compliance with taking the tablets.
- Drug should be continued if there is cognitive or behavioural benefit (stable MMSE indicates benefit, as decline is expected).
- Carry out 6-monthly specialist review or shared care protocols.
- Stop drug if benefit is no longer apparent or MMSE falls below 10 (though if the patient is still at home many would not withdraw treatment).

Although the licensed indication is AD, trials have shown benefit in DLB and vascular

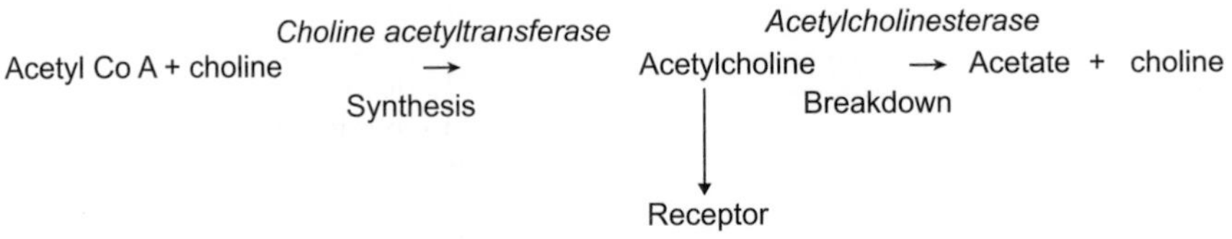

Acetyl Co A + choline → Synthesis (Choline acetyltransferase)

Acetylcholine → Acetate + choline Breakdown (Acetylcholinesterase)

Receptor

Figure 4.6 The metabolism of acetylcholine.

dementia, and so the lack of diagnostic precision is not a danger.

Although the cholinergic system is primarily affected, other neurotransmitter systems are involved in AD. Memantine is an *N*-methyl D-aspartate receptor antagonist which reduces glutamate-induced neurotoxicity. NICE only recommends memantine in moderate AD if there is intolerance or a contraindication to AChE inhibitors, but it is the only drug licensed for severe AD.

In addition to anti-amyloid approaches and new cholinergic agents, ongoing drug trials in AD include nerve growth factor, statins, high-dose folate/B_6/B_{12} supplements, a combination of omega-3 fatty acids, uridine and choline (needed by neurons to make phospholipids) and lithium and valproate for agitation. Over-the-counter preparations include: epigallocatechin, the major polyphenol in green tea which enhances non-amyloidogenic breakdown of APP; huperzine, an alkaloid from moss, a cholinesterase inhibitor; caprylidene, an FDA-approved foodstuff, a triglyceride which is metabolized to ketones and may increase brain energy; and resveratrol, the natural phenol in red grape skins which may be neuroprotective.

Dementia with Lewy bodies

Think of DLB if your patient seems to have a combination of symptoms of AD, PD, neuropsychiatric phenomena, particularly visual hallucinations, and postural instability, with wide fluctuations that can even involve conscious level. Lewy bodies, intracytoplasmic deposits of misfolded alpha-synuclein, are found throughout the cerebral cortex, whereas in PD they are restricted to the *substantia nigra*. DLB closely resembles the dementia typically associated with Parkinson's. Pragmatically, if cognitive symptoms precede physical symptoms by one year, the patient is considered to have DLB. Extreme care must be taken with all antipsychotic drugs as the patient may become drowsy, rigid and die. The course tends to be more rapid than AD. The hallucinations can be very troublesome but may respond to rivastigmine and low-dose levodopa preparations may improve mobility.

Frontotemporal dementias (Figure 4.7)

Six patients with a frontal dementia were first described by Pick in 1892. It is now recognized that frontal dementia is not a single entity but a

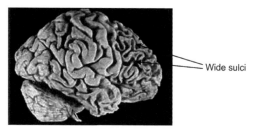

Figure 4.7 Brain showing frontal degeneration.

family of disorders with frontotemporal lobar degeneration in the brain (FTLD). Frontotemporal dementias (FTD) cause around 15% of dementia with onset below 65 years (mean age of onset 58 years) but can present later, accounting for about 8% of all dementias. They tend to be more rapidly progressive than AD (mean life expectancy 8 years).

Pathologically they are characterized by loss of neurons, frontotemporal atrophy, gliosis and intraneuronal inclusion bodies consisting of abnormal amounts or forms of protein. The first protein to be identified was tau. Until around 2006 (Forman et al. 2006), all FTLDs were thought to be 'tauopathies', but tau abnormalities account for around 45% of cases (FTLD-tau). Another protein, transactive response DNA-binding protein TDP-43 has been identified in 50% of cases, the TDP-43 'proteinopathies' (FTLD-TDP). In the remaining 5%, the protein that aggregates is an RNA binding protein, fused in sarcoma protein (FTLD-FUS). Ubiquitin may also be found in the inclusion bodies, but this is non-specific as ubiquitin is attached to damaged or misshapen proteins as the cell's way of marking them for disposal. Whatever the nature of the inclusion bodies, serotinergic systems are more affected than dopaminergic systems, with cholinergic and noradrenergic pathways being relatively normal.

Fifteen percent of cases are familial. The remainder appear sporadic, but there may be a genetic predisposition. Six genes (2011) have been associated with familial cases. In these, genetic mutations result in abnormal proteins.

Typical symptoms of frontotemporal dementias include:

- **Impaired executive functioning** – problems with planning and sequencing, prioritizing, multitasking, self-monitoring and correcting behaviour.

- **Perseveration** – repeating the same word or activity when it no longer makes sense.
- **Social disinhibition** - 'private behaviour in public' with no regard for social norms or legal limits, acting impulsively with no regard for the impact on others, e.g. flirting with teenage children's friends, laughing or swearing at a funeral.
- **Compulsive eating** – gorging on food, may take food from other people's plates.
- **Utilization behaviour** - difficulty resisting impulses to use or touch objects, e.g. will pick up a phone receiver when the phone is not ringing and the person does not intend to make a call.
- **Aphasia**.
- **Dysarthria**.
- **Apathy and abulia** – loss of interest and motivation to perform a task.
- **Loss of empathy** – loss of ability to appreciate how others will feel.
- **Dystonia** – abnormal postures of the hands or feet.
- **Gait disorder** – shuffling, frequent falls.
- **Tremor** – usually of the hands.
- **Clumsiness** – dropping or difficulty manipulating small objects.

In comparison with AD, memory and orientation tend to be well preserved. There is considerable overlap between the clinical pictures and, as the disease progresses, more symptoms emerge.

Management

This is supportive as for other dementias. SSRIs may be helpful for disinhibition, repetition and compulsive behaviours, trazodone for disruptive behaviours and methylphenidate for apathy. AChE inhibitors worsen symptoms.

Vascular dementia

Vascular dementia (VaD) is caused by brain damage secondary to impairment of the blood supply to parts of the brain. This can happen in several ways:

- Multiple strokes (usually thrombotic or embolic but can be haemorrhagic) 'multi-infarct dementia' – the individual strokes may be clinically silent.
- Single stroke in a critical part of the brain, e.g. angular gyrus or thalamus especially left brain.
- Subcortical ischaemic vascular disease (SIVD):
  - o Lacunar disease: small, spherical strokes in the deep parts of the brain.
  - o Binswanger's disease: damage to small blood vessels in the white matter (myelinated fibre tracts).
  - o CADASIL: **c**erebral **a**utosomal **d**ominant **a**rteriopathy with **s**ubcortical **i**nfarcts and **l**eukoencephalopathy. CADASIL is linked to abnormalities of a specific gene, Notch3, on chromosome 19p. It causes multi-infarct dementia, stroke, migraine and mood disorders. Individuals usually develop symptoms in their 30s and often die by age 65, but older individuals may not be identified.
  - o Cerebral amyloid angiopathy (CAA) amyloid is deposited in the media and adventitia of small and mid-sized arteries. Some cases are sporadic and some familial, and six types of protein have been described in the aggregates. Beta-amyloid is the commonest and may be associated with AD but also occurs in elderly brains without typical AD pathology. Gradient echo MRI (T2*) sequences may demonstrate multiple small, chronic haemorrhagic lesions in patients with CAA which often present with lobar intracranial haemorrhage. PET with a carbon 11-labelled Pittsburgh compound B (^{11}C–PiB) ligand, which binds to beta-amyloid, can be used to quantify amyloid deposition within the cerebral cortex.

The textbook description is of stepwise deterioration temporally related to series of small infarcts, but many cases show slowly progressive cognitive and motor decline. The number of pure VaD cases is small, and many cases thought to be AD have mixed pathology (see Figure 4.8). Studies using ^{11}C-PiB to image amyloid and MRI to quantitate vascular damage suggest that the effects of the two pathologies are additive. White matter changes can be seen in many people who appear to have no cognitive complaints, but as the total volume of these changes increases, cognitive difficulties are more likely.

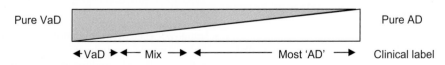

Figure 4.8 Overlap between AD and vascular pathology.

Risk factors for VaD are similar to those for stroke and include hypertension, smoking, obesity, high cholesterol, diabetes, atrial fibrillation and a South Asian or African-Caribbean ethnic background.

Symptoms of VaD can be very similar to AD. There are often physical signs of vascular damage. Frequent features include:

- Cognition: executive function is often affected more than memory, encoding is more of a problem than retrieval, inattention and poor concentration.
- Psychological symptoms: apathy and depression, emotional lability, hallucinations and delusions. Insight may be better preserved.
- Motor: focal neurological signs and findings such as parkinsonian features, pseudobulbar palsy, marche à petits pas, incontinence and epilepsy.

Treating vascular risk factors is recommended but the evidence base is poor. Blood pressure lowering trials have given inconsistent results, perhaps as few trials have had cognition as an endpoint. The apparent beneficial effect of statins seen in observational trials has not been replicated in RCTs. See McGuiness et al. (2009a,b).

Transient global amnesia

This curious episodic disorder which predominantly affects older people is not predictive of stroke or dementia. In an episode the person remains alert and capable of high-level intellectual activity (e.g. driving), but if questioned may be perplexed and has impaired memory for past and present events. Several new hypotheses for the pathogenesis of TGA have been proposed, including psychological disturbances, personality traits and hypoxia associated with venous congestion in memory relevant structures (e.g. hippocampus) or small vessel changes – there is no consensus about the cause.

Features

- Sudden-onset amnesia – retrograde for recent events, anterograde preventing new memories being laid down.
- Bemusement, perplexity, disorientation, repetitive questioning.
- Preservation of alertness, verbal fluency, motor activity.

- Duration mostly 2–12 h, although complete recovery may take a few days; very low recurrence rate.

Self-neglect

Old people are not infrequently encountered living in conditions of extreme degradation with total disregard for hygiene and self-care: the 'senile squalor syndrome'. Some will be found to have mental illness (dementia, alcoholism, schizophrenia, obsessive compulsive disorder) but others appear normal despite hoarding vast quantities of rubbish. This has been termed the Diogenes syndrome after Diogenes of Sinope, the ancient Greek philosopher who showed his contempt for material things by living in a barrel. He believed that happiness is attained by satisfying one's natural needs in the simplest way possible. In this context, the perpetrator is seen to have made a bizarre lifestyle choice, rather than having an illness, but the condition may lead to hypothermia, malnutrition and infections, as well as vigorous protests from the neighbours!

Risk factors associated with self-neglect

- Dementia.
- Depression.
- Bereavement and isolation.
- Disability.
- Alcohol.
- Previous psychiatric disorder.
- Learning difficulties.
- Obsessive compulsive disorder.
- Lifelong difficult personality/eccentricity.

📖 REFERENCES

Cole SL, Vassar R (2007) The Alzheimer's disease β-secretase enzyme, BACE1. *Molecular Neurodegeneration* 22, doi: 10.1186/1750-1326-2-22.

Forman MS, Farmer J, Johnson JK, et al. (2006) Frontotemporal dementia: clinicopathological correlations. *Annals of Neurology* 59: 952–962, doi: 10.1002/ana.20873.

McGuinness B, Todd S, Passmore P, Bullock R (2009a) Blood pressure lowering in patients without prior cerebrovascular disease for prevention of cognitive impairment and dementia. *Cochrane Database of Systematic Reviews* 4, CD004034, doi: 10.1002/14651858.CD004034.pub3.

McGuinness B, Craig D, Bullock R, Passmore P (2009b) Statins for the prevention of dementia. *Cochrane Database of Systematic Reviews* 2, CD003160, doi: 10.1002/14651858.CD003160.pub2.

NIA–AA (2011) *The Diagnosis of Dementia Due to Alzheimer's Disease: Recommendations from the National Institute on Ageing – Alzheimer's Association Workgroups on Diagnostic Guidelines for Alzheimer's Disease 2011.* http://www.alzheimersanddementia.com/article/S1552-5260%2811%2900101-4/fulltext. The same website will direct you to the criteria for MCI and other up-to-date literature.

NICE (2011) *Donepezil, Galantamine, Rivastigmine and Memantine for the Treatment of Alzheimer's Disease (TA217).* http://egap.evidence.nhs.uk/ta217.

ONS (2011) *National Statistics Online.* http://www.statistics.gov.uk/downloads/theme_health/suicide-rates-in-the-uk-1991-2009.xls.

Royal College of Psychiatrists (2008) *Alcohol and Older People – A Public Health Perspective. Report for the Vintage Project.* http://www.epicentro.iss.it/vintage/pdf/VINTAGE%20Report%20Alcohol%20and%20older%20people_final.pdf.

Royal College of Psychiatrists (2010) *Information on Older People's Mental Health.* http://www.rcpsych.ac.uk/mentalhealthinfoforall/problems/depression/depressioninolderadults.aspx.

→ FURTHER INFORMATION

Alcohol and the Elderly 2010: http://www.ias.org.uk/resources/factsheets/elderly.pdf.

Alzheimer's Disease Education and Referral (ADEAR) Centre's National Institute of Ageing websites for AD and FTLD: http://www.nia.nih.gov/alzheimers., http://alzheimers.about.com/od/typesofdementia/a/What-Is-Frontotemporal-Dementia.htm.

Alzheimer Research Forum trials in progress: http://www.alzforum.org/dis/tre/drc/default.asp.

Alzheimer's Society: http://alzheimers.org.uk/.

Association for Frontotemporal Degeneration (AFTD): http://www.theaftd.org/frontotemporal-degeneration/disorders.

Banerjee S (2010) *The Use of Antipsychotic Medication for People with Dementia: Time for Action.* http://www.dh.gov.uk/prod_consum_dh/groups/dh_digitalassets/documents/digitalasset/dh_108302.pdf.

Carers UK:. http://www.carersuk.org/.

Davis UC (2010) *Update on vascular dementia. Prof Charles DeCarli, Head of AD Center.* http://www.uctv.tv/search-details.aspx?showID=18366.

Fong TG, TulebaevSR, Inouye SK (2009) Delirium in elderly adults: diagnosis, prevention and treatment. *Nature Reviews Neurology* 5: 210–220, doi: 10.1038/nrneurol.2009.24.

Inouye S, van Dyck C, Alessi C, Balkin S, Siegal A, Horwitz R (1990) Clarifying confusion: the confusion assessment method. *Annals of Internal Medicine* 113: 941–948.

Ittner LM, Götz J (2011). Amyloid-β and tau – a toxic pas de deux in Alzheimer's disease. *Nature Reviews Neuroscience* 12: 65–72, doi: 10.1038/nrn2967. A good review on latest thoughts about pathophysiology of AD.

The Lewy body Society: http://www.lewybody.co.uk/.

Mind – information on many mental health problems: http://www.mind.org.uk/.

Mitchell SL, Teno JM, Kiely DK, et al. (2009) The clinical course of advanced dementia. *New England Journal of Medicine* 361: 1529–1538 or http://www.nejm.org/doi/full/10.1056/NEJMoa0902234.

National Dementia Strategy (2009) *The Main Policy Documents for England and the Devolved Nations.* http://www.dh.gov.uk/en/SocialCare/NationalDementiaStrategy/index.htm.

Sampson EL, Candy B, Jones L (2009) Enteral tube feeding for older people with advanced dementia. *Cochrane Database System Review* 2, CD007209.

University of California, San Francisco – frontotemporal dementia: http://memory.ucsf.edu/ftd/overview/ftd.

UNT (2011) A different way of learning – watch American experts giving a grand round. The spectrum of FTD Mario Mendez Prof of Neurology and Psychiatry, UCLA. http://www.hsc.unt.edu/education/PACE/ArchivedGrandRounds.cfm.

US National Institutes of Health clinical trials: http://www.clinicaltrials.gov/.

5

Falls and immobility

Falls

Age changes

- Reduced visual acuity, reduced contrast sensitivity and slower dark adaptation.
- Balance impairment secondary to loss of labyrinthine hair cells reducing vestibular input.
- Sarcopenia: loss of muscle mass and strength, and increased fatigability.
- Slower reaction time.
- Increased prevalence of osteoporosis (kyphotic posture).
- Increased body sway.
- Reduced walking speed with shorter broad-based or more irregular gait pattern, less effective heel strike and more time spent in double support (i.e. both feet on the ground at the same time).
- Cerebrovascular changes, contributing to cognitive impairment.

Introduction

- Falls are common: one-third of over 65s and half of over 80s living in the community fall per year; 50% of these are multiple falls.
- Women fall more frequently; they tend to be frailer than age-matched men and have increased body sway.
- Older people in care homes fall most – most frail.
- Falls are multifactorial, due to interplay between internal and external risk factors. An older person slipping on a wet floor cannot compensate quickly enough to save themselves, lands heavily and is likely to sustain a fracture.
- Falls are not an inevitable part of ageing, but the risks increase with age.
- Only 15% of falls are caused by circumstances that would cause anyone to fall, i.e. a true mechanical fall.
- Falls have important sequelae.
- Falls are a symptom, not a diagnosis.
- The NSF for Older People Standard 6 addresses assessment and prevention of falls and osteoporosis.
- There are multiple guidelines, e.g. NICE (2004) and the Royal College of Physicians (2011).

A simple mnemonic for falls

DAME (reminds you that women fall more frequently than men):

- **D**rugs (polypharmacy, alcohol).
- **A**ge-related changes (as above: gait, balance, sarcopaenia, sensory impairment).
- **M**edical (stroke disease, heart disease, PD).
- **E**nvironmental (obstacles, trailing wires, poor lighting, etc.).

Intrinsic risk factors

History

An accurate history is an essential part of the detective work to determine all the risk factors leading to falls. It is also important to obtain a witness report.

Lecture Notes Elderly Care Medicine, Eighth Edition. Claire G. Nicholl and K. Jane Wilson.
© 2012 John Wiley & Sons, Ltd. Published 2012 by John Wiley & Sons, Ltd.

> **Aid to remembering what to ask: SPLATT!**
>
> - Symptoms: dizziness, light-headedness, chest pain, palpitations?
> - Previous falls: is this the first fall? (acute event) or one of many? (frailty/dementia)
> - Location: falls occurring outdoors have a better prognosis than those in the home.
> - Activity: walking, hanging out washing, extending neck, standing on chair?
> - Time: getting out of bed, after taking tablets, after a meal, when coughing/straining/passing urine?
> - Trauma sustained?

Symptoms

- Do you ever feel dizzy or light headed?

    Dizziness is usually multifactorial. See Table 5.1.
- Do you get the sensation of the world spinning around you?

    This suggests vertigo. Vertigo lasting only a few minutes after changing position is suggestive of benign positional paroxysmal vertigo (BPPV). This is diagnosed using the Hallpike manoeuvre. See Examination below. A longer history of vertigo suggests vestibular neuronitis.
- Did you get palpitations? Were they regular/irregular, fast or slow?

    This would suggest an arrhythmia.
- Did you get any chest pain?
- Do you think you blacked out? How long for? How did you feel afterwards?

    Syncope/transient loss of consciousness (TLOC) is transient global hypoperfusion which resolves completely with no neurological deficit. Exposure to an emotional or unpleasant stimulus, e.g. a funeral or phlebotomy, leading to a brief blackout with rapid and complete recovery is very suggestive of vasovagal syncope/simple faint. Recurrent blackouts merit investigations including tilt table, carotid sinus massage and heart rate monitoring. See Chapter 9.
- Did you bite your tongue? Did you lose bladder control?

    This suggests seizures, especially if there was a prodrome, e.g. abnormal smell in temporal lobe epilepsy. Longer duration of LOC with tonic-clonic movements and cyanosis and slow recovery with confusion also suggest fits. See Chapter 8.

- Do you have any numbness in your feet or fingers?

    This suggests peripheral neuropathy. Common causes are diabetes, B_{12} deficiency and alcoholism.
- Have you noticed changes in your eyesight?

    Visual impairment (cataracts, glaucoma and inappropriate or dirty glasses) makes detection of hazards difficult. Slowed dark adaptation increases risk of falls at night.
- Do you have difficulty getting going, turning over in bed or freezing in doorways?

    These are symptoms of Parkinson's disease. See Chapter 8.
- Ask about all the drugs the patient is taking; remember over-the-counter medications. See Table 5.1.
- Take a full alcohol history.

Previous falls?

- A history of falls is highly predictive of future falls. Fifty percent of falls are recurrent.
- If this was the first fall, it may have been caused by hypotension secondary to an acute serious event such as an MI, GI bleed, sepsis associated with pneumonia or delirium.
- Recurrent falls are more likely to be caused by frailty, chronic diseases and dementia.

Location

- Patients who fall outside are fitter than their house-bound peers and have a better prognosis.
- Falls in the bathroom may be related to a slippery floor or use of emollients.

Activity

- What were you doing when you fell?
- Postural dizziness getting out of bed or standing up after sitting for some time suggests orthostatic hypotension.
- Situational syncope, e.g. blacking out after eating (post-prandial syncope), when passing urine (micturition syncope). See Chapter 9.
- Falling over is associated with urinary incontinence; both are markers of frailty.
- Falling after turning the head to one side might suggest carotid sinus hypersensitivity.
- Hanging clothes on washing line and going to the hairdresser are risky activities!

Table 5.1 Drugs associated with a high risk of falling

Drug	Examples	Mechanism	Management strategy
Antihypertensives	Diuretics, calcium channel blockers Beta-blockers	Postural hypotension May also exacerbate bradycardia secondary to conduction disorders	Regularly check blood pressure lying and standing Consider ambulatory blood pressure to exclude white coat hypertension or overtreatment of hypertension
Opiate analgesics	Codeine, morphine	Cross the blood–brain barrier, slow central processing and cause drowsiness	Start low, go slow
Long-acting hypoglycaemic agents	Chlorpropamide, glibenclamide	Hypoglycaemia	Choose short-acting agents, e.g. gliclazide
Antipsychotics	Haloperidol, chlorpromazine, risperidone	Extrapyramidal side-effects	Use non-pharmacological methods of reducing delirium/agitation Start low, go slow; reassess need frequently and aim to stop
Hypnotics	Long-acting benzodiazepines	Slow central processing; drowsiness persisting following morning	Avoid; if not possible, restrict to short-term use Abrupt discontinuation may lead to withdrawal syndrome, so switch to diazepam and wean slowly as per BNF guidelines
Antidepressants	Tricyclic antidepressants: more strongly associated with falls than SSRIs and SNRIs	Slow central processing Risk factor for hyponatraemia, which causes delirium associated with high risk of falls Long QT syndrome: amitriptyline, citalopram	Prescribe for the individual, if there is a past history of hyponatraemia, avoid citalopram, consider mirtazepine Check ECG
Anti-epileptics	Phenytoin, carbamazepine	Associated with dizziness Narrow therapeutic window Effect on vitamin D metabolism	Check drug levels as dizziness might be a sign of toxicity Ensure the patient is treated with calcium and vitamin D plus antiresporptive where appropriate
Group 1A anti-arrhythmic drugs	Digoxin	May promote arrhythmias	Avoid where possible
Alcohol	Greater than 1 unit per day	Acute intoxication Chronic subdural haematoma, cerebellar disease Wernicke–Korsakoff syndrome Withdrawal	Get accurate alcohol history Ensure thiamine and magnesium levels are replete Prescribe chlordiazepoxide
OTC	Dextromethorphan, e.g. 'Night Nurse'	Drowsiness	Educate patients and carers that just because a drug does not need to be prescribed does not mean it is safe

OTC, over-the-counter drugs; SNRIs, serotonin and noradrenergic reuptake inhibitors; SSRIs, serotonin reuptake inhibitors; TCA, tricyclic antidepressants.

> Remember:
>
> **60%** of over 60-year-olds taking four or more medications will fall in a year.

Time

- Falling in the morning when getting up or following getting up after sitting for some time is suggestive of postural hypotension usually related to medications, but also secondary to Lewy body disease, Parkinson's disease and diabetic autonomic neuropathy. See Chapter 9.
- Falling during the night may be secondary to nocturia due to BPH (see Chapter 13) in combination with postural hypotension, poor lighting in hallways plus drowsiness secondary to hypnotics.

Trauma sustained

- Minor soft tissue injury in 40–60% of falls: haematoma, skin tear, laceration.
- More serious soft tissue injury in 5% of falls: but would include subdural haematoma (see Figure 5.1), large haematoma requiring blood transfusion.
- Humeral fracture in 5% of falls.
- Wrist fracture.
- Vertebral fracture.

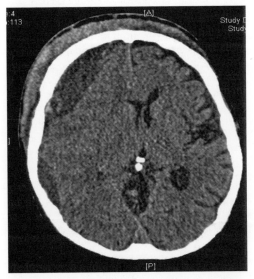

Figure 5.1 CT of the head demonstrating subdural haematoma. Note subcutaneous haematoma over right side of forehead, old darker subdural blood and newer brighter blood from new subdural haematoma.

- Pelvic fracture.
- Fractured neck of femur in 2% of falls.

Determining the causes of falls

This requires a corroborative history. It is essential to get a witness report of the events surrounding the fall because:

- The patient may play down the number and severity of the falls because of fear of consequences, for example being persuaded to move to institutional care.
- The patient may not remember blacking out, especially if the event was transitory.
- The witness can give information about the length of unconsciousness, whether there were tonic-clonic movements and post-ictal drowsiness, helping to differentiate syncope from epilepsy.
- The patient may have cognitive impairment. This may both contribute to the falls and prevent the patient from remembering the details.
- Research shows that even cognitively intact older people living in the community do not remember falls after 3 months.

Examination

Examination must be thorough but pay particular attention to the following:

- Does the patient look ill? If so, consider acute problems such as GI bleed, MI or PE.
- Check pulse rate and rhythm.
- Perform carotid sinus massage with pulse, BP and ECG monitoring if history suggests CSH. See Chapter 9 for method and contraindications.
- Check for postural hypotension: measure the BP – lying and after standing for 3 min. The drop is significant if it is > 10 mmHg diastolic or 20 mmHg systolic and accompanied by symptoms. Note whether there is a compensatory tachycardia. See Chapter 9.
- Listen for murmurs, especially aortic stenosis, carotid bruits.
- Assess the CNS and look for lateralizing signs.
- Look for signs of PD: mask facies, tremor, rigidity and bradykinesia. Examine the gait: shuffling, retropulsion and festination.
- Does the patient have myxoedema?
- Check for peripheral neuropathy.
- Check vision with a Snellen chart. Ask the patient whether they have had their eyes checked recently. Cataracts are easily treated.
- Bifocal and varifocal lenses are associated with falls; the view ahead in the lower portion of the

lens may be blurred and impair depth perception and contrast sensitivity. This makes it difficult to negotiate steps and uneven pavements safely.
- Is there evidence of hearing impairment? Are the hearing aids correctly positioned? This does not have a direct bearing on falls risk, but it is helpful to hear shouted warnings! See Chapter 15.
- Examine the neck movements. Does this cause dizziness? If the patient describes true vertigo, do the Hallpike manoeuvre. Sit the patient on the bed and turn their head 45° towards the side producing the most symptoms. Then help them to lie down quickly until their neck is extended by 20°. The test is positive if there is rotational nystagmus towards the floor. Treat using the Epley manoeuvre to reposition the otoliths in the utricle. The patient sits on the bed with their head turned to 45° on the positive side. They then lie flat, keeping the head turned for 30 s. Next they turn their head 90° again, holding the position for 30 s. They roll onto the side they are facing for 30 s more and then sit up, still with the head turned for 30 s more. This process should be repeated three times. Warn the patient that it might provoke nausea and vertigo.
- Check for dementia/delirium. See Chapter 4.

Abnormal gait
- **Frontal-related gait pattern**: common in cerebrovascular disease, vascular dementia and Alzheimer's disease. The gait is wide-based and apraxic and the patient may freeze; there is increased risk of falling when the patient turns. These patients fall when distracted as they cannot dual-task.
- **Normal pressure hydrocephalus**: a wide-based ataxic gait, associated with urinary incontinence and cognitive impairment. Head CT head shows dilated ventricles.
- **Hemiplegic gait**: steps are slower and shorter and the gait is less smooth because the affected leg is circumducted, i.e. the foot scrapes the floor in an arc.
- **Spastic paraparesis**: e.g. secondary to cervical myelopathy, bilateral scissoring of stiff legs.
- **Cerebellar disease**: an irregular, wide-based, unsteady gait.
- **Sensory ataxia**: e.g. peripheral neuropathy secondary to diabetes, the patient watches the ground and their feet rather than looking ahead. Romberg's test is positive. The patient may stamp their feet.
- **Vestibular ataxia**: think of this if the patient complains of nausea, vomiting and vertigo.

- **Parkinsonian gait**: hypokinetic, festinant, shuffling gait with reduced arm-swing.
- **Antalgic gait**: e.g. secondary to osteoarthritis, asymmetrical because the patient puts their weight on the side with the painful joint as briefly as possible.
- **Waddling gait**: weakness of the hip girdle muscles and difficulty getting out of a chair caused by proximal myopathy, e.g. secondary to steroids and osteomalacia.
- **Trendelenberg gait**: weakness of one side of hip girdle due to gluteal medius weakness causes dipping of the affected side which is compensated for by the trunk leaning over the affected side.
- **Foot drop**: high-stepping, foot-slapping gait, e.g. secondary to common peroneal nerve palsy caused by compression from a tight lower leg plaster.

Baseline tests
- Full blood count.
- Thyroid stimulating hormone.
- B_{12}.
- ECG.

Further investigations
Most falls are caused by problems with gait and balance. Further investigations depend on findings from the history and examination. If falls continue or remain unexplained, investigate more aggressively:

- Holter monitor: may show arrhythmias if the symptoms are frequent. If not, but the history is highly suggestive of an arrhythmia, consider an implantable loop recorder.
- If there are features of structural or valvular heart disease on examination or an abnormal ECG, echocardiography will be useful.
- Tilt table: measuring beat-to-beat variation in pulse and BP with the patient tilted (head up) to 70°. See Chapter 9.
- CT scan if multi-infarct disease suspected.
- If seizures are suspected, consider EEG and CT.

Extrinsic risk factors
- Older people tend to live in older housing, which may need repairs.
- Poor lighting, especially near stairs.
- A lifetime's clutter, especially if the patient has Diogenes' syndrome.
- Inappropriate footwear; slippers are well-named and shoes with high heels impair balance. Shoes

should fit correctly, have a small heel and a firm sole not so thick that it reduces proprioception.
- Incorrect use of walking aids.
- Pets underfoot.
- Trailing electrical cables.
- Slippery floor with loose rugs.
- Bathroom with low toilet, lack of grab rails by bath or shower.
- Unfamiliar environment, e.g. hospital or a care home.
- Wet, icy or uneven pavements.

Sequelae of falls

Sequelae occur in about half of reported falls. In addition to the traumatic complications above, falls may cause:

- Friction burns from carpet.
- Burns needing grafting (fall onto a fire or radiator).
- Quadriplegia due to a central cord lesion in a patient with spinal cord compromised by spondylosis (fortunately rare).
- Fear of further falls is common (up to 30% of fallers) and disabling, leading to loss of confidence, immobility (see Table 5.4) and even institutionalization.
- Anxiety/depression about the future.
- Anxiety in carers (formal and informal) may become intolerable, leading to the potential for elder-abuse.
- The need to move to safer surroundings may separate the faller from their support network. Well-meaning families may move their parents away from where they have been based for many years.

Sequelae of a long lie

That is, remaining on the floor for 1 h or more after falling:

- Pressure sores (see Chapter 15).
- Rhabdomyolysis.
- Hypothermia may result if the fall occurs in the cold, e.g. outside or in an unheated room (see Chapter 12).
- Hypostatic pneumonia.
- Fifty percent of those who lie on the floor for >1 h are dead within 6 months, even if no injury was sustained from the fall.

People with dementia are eight times more likely to fall than their cognitively intact peers due to:

- Inappropriate risk taking.
- Abnormal gait/balance due to impaired central processing.
- Extrapyramidal side-effects of antipsychotic drugs.
- Sedation secondary to benzodiazepines.
- Orthostatic hypotension in PD or Lewy body dementia.
- Visuo-spatial abnormalities in vascular dementia.
- Carotid sinus hypersensitivity may be secondary to atherosclerosis and might be an early indicator of vascular dementia.
- A treatable cause may be overlooked because of the limited history.
- Vitamin D deficiency.

- Up to 25% of frequent fallers are dead within 1 year of presentation, not directly due to injuries but because of the underlying cause of falls.

Management

This needs to be multidisciplinary and multi-agency. The local council should ensure good maintenance of paving and lighting outside warden-controlled flats and arrange early gritting of the pavements in icy weather. Many hospitals now offer Falls Prevention Clinics.

- Identify and treat *all* contributing causes and risk factors.
- Refer patients with significant bradycardia, heart block and cardioinhibitory disease for pacing.
- Refer patients with significant aortic stenosis for cardiological evaluation.
- Refer people with PD to your local specialist service.
- Stop unnecessary drugs; the strongest evidence is the risk reduction achieved by stopping antipsychotics.
- Remember osteoporosis prevention and treatment; see Chapter 6.
- Refer for physiotherapy. The aims are:
  o Correct prescription and use of walking aids. For example, people with PD do better with wheeled frames than Zimmer frames which disrupt the flow of walking. See Table 5.5.

○ Improve gait pattern, e.g. encourage people with PD to take longer steps and to stand straighter.

○ Teach the patient how to get up from the floor.

○ Current evidence shows that individually tailored exercise plans which incorporate strength, balance, flexibility and endurance do prevent future falls, for example, the Otago exercise plan and Tai Chi.

• Refer for occupational therapy assessment to identify and remove environmental hazards and provide equipment to facilitate mobility at home. Consider getting a stair-lift or moving downstairs. Home hazard reduction is not evidence-based but is pragmatic.

• Give advice on appropriate footwear.

If falls cannot be prevented, reduce their consequences:

• Prescribe calcium and vitamin D and bisphosphonates if osteoporosis is present.

• Recommend maintaining an adequate environmental temperature.

• Soften floor coverings, i.e. carpet rooms.

• Remove obstacles and dangers, e.g. guard fire.

• Place emergency bedding where it can be reached from the floor.

• Arrange for a personally worn alarm system or for frequent visitors.

• Educate the patient and their relatives about safety in the home and the risk of falls: the Royal Society for the Prevention of Accidents (RoSPA) and Age UK produce very helpful leaflets.

Hip protectors

• Pads made from the same material as motorcycle helmets diffuse the impact of a fall away from the femoral neck.

• Worn over the greater trochanter in tight-fitting underpants.

• Good standing balance is needed to get the pants on and off unaided.

• May result in incontinence as they are difficult to get off quickly.

• Current evidence does not show that they decrease the incidence of hip fractures.

• May have a role in motivated community dwelling by older people who understand their use, or in care homes where the staff supervise dressing and toileting.

Falls in hospital

• Very common: 2–7 per 1,000 patient days.

• Eleven percent of falls occur within 24 h of admission, and 50% occur within the first 2 weeks.

• The majority of these are recurrent falls.

• This suggests a first peak due to the acute illness and the unfamiliar environment, with a second peak owing to dementia and chronic instability.

• Falls in hospital are strongly associated with cognitive impairment/acute delirium.

• Hospitals are unfamiliar surroundings with different routines, noise and light at night, all of which leads to disturbed sleep and drowsiness the following morning when the physiotherapist arrives.

• In hospital, patients are encouraged to take all their medications. They may have wisely been omitting their diuretics and antihypertensives, so become profoundly hypotensive when given them all together!

• Remember, older people are often admitted with vomiting, diarrhoea and sepsis and may already be dehydrated, so omit their antihypertensives and watch the BP.

• Falls in hospital result in soft-tissue injuries and fractures, the majority of which are minor, but patients do sustain fractured hips and subdural haematomas which can be fatal.

• Patients who fall have a longer length of stay, are at increased risk of nosocomial infection and are less likely to return to their own homes.

• Understandably, relatives are upset when a patient falls in hospital, as it is supposed to be a place of safety. This leads to complaints and sometimes litigation. Therefore it is in everybody's interest to reduce the risk of falls.

• Various risk assessment tools have been developed to identity those at high risk, e.g. STRATIFY, but current experience is that all older people should be considered high-risk and managed as such.

• Ensure that there are no ongoing reversible medical problems.

• There will always be a balance between the risk of falls and the benefits of encouraging rehabilitation.

Dizziness

This can be a heart sink symptom because there are many and varied causes, but use it as an opportunity to employ your detective skills! Think of dizziness as a syndrome, i.e. having multiple causes. One approach is to consider which factors might affect each system, as in Table 5.2.

Table 5.2 Causes of dizziness

Type	Disease	Symptoms	Diagnosis	Treatment
Labyrinth	Benign Positional Paroxysmal vertigo (BPPV)	Subjective sensation of rotation, lasts less than 5 min, provoked by change in position	Hallpike–Dix manoeuvre	Epley/Brandt–Daroff manoeuvre
VIII nerve lesion	Acoustic neuroma	Unilateral tinnitus	MRI internal auditory meatus	Surgical excision where appropriate
Cochlea and labyrinth	Ménière's disease	Triad of vertigo, hearing impairment and tinnitus, often unilateral		Prochlorperazine for short-term only, betahistine
Labyrinth, vestibule	Acute vestibular failure	Single episode of rotatory vertigo lasting 1 day	E.g. viral, labyrinthitis, vestibular neuronitis	
	Drugs		Streptomycin	
CNS	Vertebro-basilar syndrome	History of acute or chronic vertigo associated with headaches, aura, sensory and motor features		
	Cerebellar diseases: stroke, tumour	May be other features including ataxia, past-pointing	CT/MRI head	Surgery, radiotherapy, good symptom control
Peripheral	Neuropathy, e.g. diabetic, B_{12} deficiency	Loss of sensation in feet, may be cognitive decline	HbA1c, B_{12}, folate, TSH	Improve diabetic control, check feet, replace haematinics and levothyroxine
	Migraine	May be accompanied by headache, visual fortification spectra	Usually from history, CT head will be normal for age	
Cardiovascular causes	Orthostatic hypotension: drugs, autonomic neuropathy, Shy–Drager syndrome	Dizziness, muzziness triggered by getting out of bed, standing up after sitting for a long time	Lying and standing BP	See Chapter 9
	Medications Alcohol Antihypertensives Diuretics Older antidepressants PPIs	Light headed, muzzy headed	History	Stop medications where possible

Tachyarrhythmia/bradyarrhythmia	Palpitations, falls	ECG, Holter monitor, Reveal device	'Pace and block'
Syncope/presyncope	Light-headedness, nausea, sweatiness, TLOC	Tilt table, Holter monitor, Carotid sinus massage	Treat underlying cause, see Chapter 9
Aortic stenosis	Muzzy, especially on exertion	Echo	Aortic valve replacement, TAVI
Metabolic — Hypoglycaemia	Dizziness after not eating	Low BM	Sugary drink, Hypostop, review diabetic medications
Hypothyroid	Cold intolerance, weight gain	High TSH, low T4	Oral levothyroxine replacement
Addison's disease: primary adrenal failure, usually autoimmune in origin	Light-headedness, weight loss, fatigue	Synacthen® test, hyponatraemia and hyperkalaemia	Replace glucocorticoid, usually hydrocortisone 20mg a.m., 10mg noon and mineralocorticoid, usually fludrocortisone 100mcg
Psychiatric — Anxiety/depression	Constant, unrelieved dizziness. Additional symptoms of low mood, poor sleep, anxiety	Exclude organic causes, determine whether depression or anxiety is most prominent disease	Treat as in Chapter 4
Other — Anaemia	Insidious blood loss, e.g. secondary to colonic tumour, may present with dizziness	FBC, haematinics, gastroscopy, CT abdomen, colonoscopy, as indicated	Treat cause
Carbon monoxide toxicity	Headache and dizziness	COHb level	High flow oxygen, via a face mask. See Chapter 10
Wax in ears		Direct visualization with otoscope	Soften with eardrops such as sodium bicarbonate and microsuction if necessary

BPPV, benign paroxysmal positional vertigo; MRI, magnetic resonance image; HbA1c, glycosylated haemoglobin; PPI, proton pump inhibitor; TAVI, transcatheter aortic valve implantation; COHb, carboxyhaemoglobin level.

Patients sometimes describe dizziness as muzziness, light-headedness or 'funny head'. The illusion of rotation is more suggestive of vertigo. Associated nausea points to a peripheral cause whereas absence of nausea points to a central cause.

Immobility

- Reduced mobility ranges from not being able to drive, to being housebound or wheelchair-dependent.
- Immobility increases with increasing age:
- More than 50% of over 75s have difficulty getting around their own homes.
- Among ambulant over 80-year-olds, at least 25% need a walking aid such as a stick or frame.
- Twenty percent are totally housebound.
- Many older people find it difficult to climb on to a bus, and if they do manage it, there are other pitfalls: getting up from the seat, walking down the crowded aisle possibly whilst the bus is still in motion and getting off at the correct stop.
- This coincides with the time that people are no longer able to drive because of failing vision, cognitive impairment, recurrent syncope, etc. (see Chapter 16).

Reasons for immobility

- Pain and stiffness in bones, joints and muscles (Table 5.3). This is the most common reason.
- Weakness, e.g. neurological or endocrine (see Table 5.4), but also generalized systemic disease.
- Visual impairment.
- Breathlessness secondary to pulmonary and cardiac disease.
- Psychological problems: fear/anxiety/depression/dementia (see box below).
- Frequent falls and fear of falling.

Table 5.3 Immobility caused by pain/stiffness

In joints	In muscles	In bones
Osteoarthritis	Myositis	Osteoporosis
Rheumatoid arthritis	Polymyalgia rheumatica	Osteomalacia
Gout	Myxoedema	Paget's disease
Pseudogout	PD	Malignant disease
Infection	Spasticity	Metastases

Table 5.4 Immobility caused by weakness

Neuronal damage	Muscle damage	Reduced effort tolerance
Hemiplegia	Disuse atrophy	Loss of fitness
Peripheral neuropathy	Myopathy	Dyspnoea
Motor-neuron disease	Amyotrophy	Anaemia
Paraplegia	Hypokalaemia	Reduced cardiac output

- Iatrogenic, e.g. sedation, surgery (amputations and unsuccessful orthopaedic procedures).
- Foot-care disorders, e.g. bunions and nail neglect; also severe ischaemia and infection.

Complications of immobility

Physical
- Muscle wasting (see Chapter 6).
- Muscle contractures.
- Osteoporosis (see Chapter 6).
- Pressure sores (see Chapter 15).
- Hypothermia (see Chapter 12).
- Hypostatic pneumonia.
- Constipation.
- Incontinence.
- Deep-venous thrombosis (see Chapter 9).

Psychological
- Depression.
- Loss of confidence.

Social
- Isolation.
- Risk of institutionalization.

Management of immobility

- Treat reversible medical problems.
- Refer fit patients with severe OA of the hips or knees for joint replacement.
- Optimize analgesia for painful joints/backs.
- Look for and treat dementia, delirium and depression.
- Review medication to ensure patient is not over-sedated or has become parkinsonian secondary to psychotropic medication or prochlorperazine.
- Refer to physiotherapy for review of posture, gait practice and use of correct walking aids. See Table 5.5.

Table 5.5 A comparison of types of walking aids

Walking aid	Description	Use	Disadvantages
Stick	Wood or aluminium. Correct length essential for functional gait pattern. Can be used singly or in pairs. Fisher grip: moulded hand grip may improve function.	Widens base of support and supports up to 25% of body weight. Use on same side for generally improving balance. Use on opposite side for weakness or painful/unstable joint.	Has to be propped up/laid flat when not being used and becomes a trip hazard! Check ferrules for wear.
Tripod/quadrupod	Aluminium with three or four feet.	Gives more support than a stick and stands up on its own. The wider the base of the device, the wider the base of support. Used on opposite side of hemiplegia.	Can be large and ungainly.
Elbow crutches	Aluminium crutches with forearm support. Used in pairs.	Can support 80% of body weight. Useful for non-weight-bearing on a lower limb, e.g. because of amputation, or fracture.	Risk of tripping as above. Patient needs to have enough cognitive function to use them safely.

(*Continued*)

Table 5.5 (*Continued*)

Walking aid	Description	Use	Disadvantages
Axillary crutches	Crutches which bear the weight under the arms.	More often used for younger patients. Can achieve speed greater than normal walking!	Brachial nerve palsy if used too much.
Zimmer frame	Aluminium tubing with four rubber feet.	Offers maximum support to patient. Bag may be attached.	Patient has to be able to learn new gait pattern: the frame is lifted up and forward, and the patient then steps into the frame. This can be especially difficult on carpet. Encourages poor posture, especially forward flexion.
Rollator	As above, but there are wheels on the two front legs.	Patient can push the frame continuously; especially useful for patients with PD.	Poor posture, slow gait, problems walking outdoors.

Gutter frame

Has support for the forearms.

Useful for patients with rheumatoid affecting their wrists, and wrist injuries.

As above.

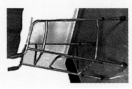

Delta frame

Usually a three-wheeled foldaway frame, often with a seat/space for shopping.

More robust so can be used outside. Feet should be in line with the back wheels when walking.

Heavy. Must be fully opened out and locked for safety. Patients pay for their own.

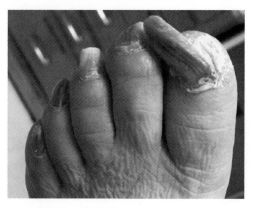

Figure 5.2 Onychogryphosis.

- Check seating is appropriate – correct seat height and arms.
- Ask podiatrist to help with painful ingrowing toe nails, onychogryphosis (Figure 5.2), bunions, and corns, etc.
- If the patient is likely to remain immobile, ensure that they are assessed for pressure-relieving equipment on the bed and chair. Monitor skin condition and nutrition. See Chapter 15.

Wheelchairs

- These improve the patient's independence and quality of life.
- Patients are assessed for the most appropriate wheelchair by the physiotherapy team.
- Usually, non-specialist equipment is provided by the hospital, but specialist equipment is ordered from NHS wheelchair services.
- If the patient has sufficient upper limb strength and stamina, provide with a self-propelling wheelchair.
- If not, an attendant-propelled wheelchair may be appropriate. Short term, such wheelchairs can be borrowed from the British Red Cross for a deposit (donations appreciated).
- Electric wheelchairs are ideal for cognitively intact but physically impaired patients with conditions such as multiple sclerosis and MND.
- Specialist wheelchairs are needed for patients with no sitting balance, for example after a stroke.

- The wheelchair assessment should include appropriate pressure-relieving cushioning.
- Outdoor buggies can improve the independence of cognitively intact, community dwelling patients. Obtain from Motability (www.motablitiy.co.uk).
- Consider how the patient will transfer in and out of the chair.
- If the patient is being discharged home, it may be necessary to install a ramp up to the front door; the front and internal doors and passages will need to be wide enough to accommodate the wheelchair.

 REFERENCES

NICE (2004) *Clinical Guideline 21. Falls.* www.nice.org.uk/CG21

Royal College of Physicians (2011) *Falls and Bone Health.* www.rcplondon.ac.uk/resources/national-audit-falls-and-bone-health-older-people

 FURTHER INFORMATION

Age UK: www.ageuk.org.uk.

American Geriatrics Society, British Geriatrics Society, American Academy of Orthopedic Surgeons Panel on Falls Prevention (AGS, BGS, AAOS) (2001) Guidelines for the prevention of falls in older persons. *Journal of American Geriatrics Society*, 49 (5): 664–672.

Lord SR, Sherrington C, Menz HB, Close JC (2007) *Falls in Older People: Risk Factors and Strategies for Prevention.* Cambridge University Press, Cambridge.

National Hip Fracture Database: http://www.nhfd.co.uk/.

National Patient Safety Agency (2007) *Age Slips, Trips + Falls in Hospital.* www.nrls.npsa.nhs.uk/resources/?entry45=59821

Prevention of Falls Network Europe (PROFANE): www.profane.eu.org.

Royal Society for the Prevention of Accidents: www.rospa.co.uk.

SIGN (2009) *Guideline 111 Management of Hip Fracture in Older People.* http://www.sign.ac.uk/guidelines/fulltext/111/index.html

University of York (2000) *The Economic Cost of Hip Fractures in the UK.* http://www.viewcare.co.uk/Publications/hipfracture.pdf.

6

Bones, joints and muscles

Bones

Age changes

Bone structure changes throughout life owing to ongoing bone resorption by osteoclasts and bone growth by osteoblasts. With increasing age, the balance is lost, leading to a net increase in bone resorption. This in turn leads to gradual and progressive loss of bone from the age of 35 onwards. This process affects trabecular bone more than cortical bone. In osteoporosis, the molecular composition is similar to normal bone, but the microarchitecture is disorganized so that the bone is fragile and at increased risk of fractures.

Bone loss per year is 0.2% of the total from the age of 35. This rate of loss increases to 1% after the menopause in women. Therefore, on average, by the age of 80 a woman will have lost 30% of her bone mass, whilst a man of the same age will have lost 10%.

The shape of long bones changes with increasing age; the internal cavity increases in diameter, the outer cortical layer becomes thinner and the total bone diameter becomes expanded. These changes result in weaker bones.

Osteoporosis

Risk factors

- Age > 65.
- Female sex.
- Family history, especially maternal hip fracture.
- Failure to maximize by early adulthood because of poor nutrition or oestrogen deficits, e.g. secondary to anorexia nervosa.
- Hormonal changes at the menopause: the fall in oestrogen causes a marked acceleration of bone loss. Fractures secondary to osteoporosis affect one in two post-menopausal women.
- Previous fragility fractures.
- Low body weight (BMI $< 19 \, kg/m^2$).
- Physical inactivity, e.g. following a stroke.
- Use of corticosteroids for 3 or more months.
- Other drugs especially antiepileptics, aromatase inhibitors for breast carcinoma, anti-androgen treatment and caffeine.
- Alcohol intake > 3 units/day.
- Smoking.
- Endocrine disorders, e.g. thyrotoxicosis, Cushing's disease, hyperparathyroidism and hypopituitarism.
- Chronic disease: CKD, liver disease and COPD.
- Malabsorption.
- Falls are not a cause of osteoporosis but are strongly predictive of osteoporotic fractures.
- Older people often have vitamin D deficiency and secondary hyperparathyroidism, and these are likely to contribute.

Osteoporosis in men

- Affects 20% of men over 70.
- One in five men over the age of 50 will sustain a fracture.
- Fifty percent of men affected have idiopathic osteoporosis.
- Of the remaining 50% with secondary osteoporosis, the most common causes are:
  - hypogonadotrophic hypogonadism;
  - steroids;
  - alcohol;
  - hyperparathyroidism;
  - malabsorption, e.g. secondary to Crohn's disease, gastric surgery and coeliac disease.

Lecture Notes Elderly Care Medicine, Eighth Edition. Claire G. Nicholl and K. Jane Wilson.
© 2012 John Wiley & Sons, Ltd. Published 2012 by John Wiley & Sons, Ltd.

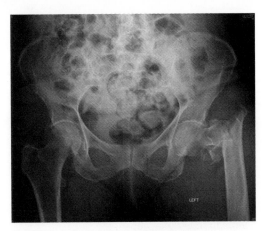

Figure 6.1 Radiograph of a comminuted intertrochanteric fracture of the left hip.

- The reduction of insulin-like growth factor production is also being investigated as a risk factor.

Clinical features

Osteoporosis is usually asymptomatic until there has been a fracture:

- Often the first presentation is a Colles' wrist fracture in women aged 50–65.
- Vertebral fractures may present as severe mid-thoracic or low back pain often with no history of trauma.
- Loss of height and dorsal kyphosis secondary to multiple vertebral fractures. A loss of > 4 cm suggests at least one vertebral fracture.
- Contact between ribs and iliac crests.
- Hip fractures: rising incidence with increasing age. See Figure 6.1 showing a comminuted fracture of the left hip. The incidence is rising faster than expected from demographic changes. There are now 57,000 cases per annum in the UK – 75% of which are aged over 75.
- Other fractures associated with osteoporosis include neck of humerus, pelvis and distal tibia/fibula.

Investigations

The WHO Fracture Risk Assessment Tool (FRAX) collates clinical information and risk factors to stratify the patient's risk and determine whether a dual-energy X-ray absorptiometry (DXA) scan would give extra information.

Bone mineral density

The DXA scanner measures bone density usually at the proximal femur and lumbar vertebrae (because

Fractured neck of femur

- Increasingly common in the ageing population.
- The number predicted worldwide in 2050 is 6.26 million.
- Presents as pain in the hip with inability to weight bear; however, if the fracture is impacted, the patient may still be able to walk.
- The affected leg is shortened because the hip is flexed and externally rotated.
- The fracture is surgically fixed according to its site.
- Evidence suggests that patients should have their surgery within 48 h of admission, during the normal working day. Pre-operative delay leads to a longer length of stay which in turn leads to a higher risk of nosocomial adverse events.
- The patient does best if mobilized early.
- The reasons for the fall should be sought and treated.
- Women over 75 who sustain a fracture should be treated for osteoporosis (NICE).
- The mortality rate at 1 month post fracture is 10%.
- At 1 year, the mortality rate is 25%.
- Twenty percent of people with hip fractures require institutional care.
- Forty percent never regain their full premorbid function.

Fractured pelvis

- Usually the pubic rami. As the pelvis is a ring it is likely to fracture in two places. See Figure 6.2.
- Often caused by trivial trauma.
- Produces pain in the groin that is worse on getting up from sitting and walking.
- Treatment is conservative with analgesia and early mobilization.
- Most heal within 6–8 weeks.
- The mortality rate at 1 year is 15–20%.
- Sadly, patients who have sustained a pelvic fracture are less likely to be considered for treatment of osteoporosis than those with hip fractures.

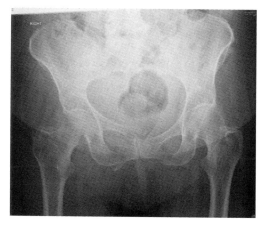

Figure 6.2 X-ray of fractured pelvis.

these are clinically important fragility fractures). Osteoporosis is defined as a bone mineral density (BMD) of greater than 2.5 standard deviations below that of a normal pre-menopausal woman and is expressed as a T score (i.e. T –2.5 SD).

Ultrasound of the calcaneum
This has the advantage of being inexpensive and portable so that it can be used in the primary-care setting, but it has not been fully validated. It is probably most useful for risk stratification; if the result suggests low bone density, the patient should have DXA scan.

Excluding causes of secondary osteoporosis

If serum calcium is raised, check PTH level to exclude primary hyperparathyroidism (see later).

- Thyroid function tests to exclude thyrotoxicosis (see Chapter 12).
- Liver and renal function tests.
- Bone function tests.
- Testosterone: in men with suspected hypogonadotrophic hypogonadism.
- ESR, serum immunoglobulins and urinary Bence–Jones protein to exclude myeloma.
- Dexamethasone suppression test to exclude Cushing's disease.

Complications

- Fractures, as above.
- Pain and reduced mobility.
- Deformity: kyphosis, loss of height, abdominal protrusion. Cord compression is very uncommon in this context.

- Loss of independence and increased risk of being admitted to a care home.
- Use of resources: 25% of UK orthopaedic beds are occupied by patients with fractured hips. The average cost is £25,000 per patient. Fractures in osteoporotic bones now account for over 1 million bed-days annually in the NHS. The cost of treatment of these patients is now more than £5 million per week.

Prevention

- Adequate nutrition.
- Calcium and vitamin D.
- Hormone replacement therapy is most useful in women in early menopause.
- Exercise: should be regular and weight-bearing, e.g. brisk walking, Tai Chi.
- Stop smoking and moderate alcohol intake.
- Prophylactic use of bisphosphonates: if treating with steroids at > 7.5 mg prednisolone for three or more months.

Treatments

Calcium and vitamin D
The debate regarding the role of calcium and vitamin D in the treatment of osteoporosis rages on. Questions surround the efficacy of both elements and the optimum dose. It has been shown that treatment with calcium and vitamin D prevented hip fractures in older people living in care homes. There is controversy about the role in other populations; research is ongoing. A large meta-analysis of women given calcium and vitamin D demonstrated a modest increase in cardiovascular events. The Scientific Advisory Committee on Nutrition is undertaking a new review of this controversial area.

What is certain is that all the trials demonstrating the efficacy of bisphosphonates, strontium and teriparatide have co-prescribed calcium and vitamin D preparations.

Bisphosphonates
Bisphosphonates, e.g. risedronate and alendronate, work by binding to hydroxyapatite in the bone, which inhibits recruitment of osteoclasts and apoptosis, thus inhibiting bone resorption. Effects are seen in the first 12–18 months of use. Both are shown to increase bone mass of the spine and the hip and to reduce fractures and are indicated in women and men. Weekly preparations are available. This is an advantage because bisphosphonates have to be taken on an empty stomach to ensure absorption. Thus, patients only miss

their early morning cup of tea once a week! The patient also has to remain upright for 30 min to reduce the risk of oesophageal ulceration. Ibandronate has the added advantage of being a monthly oral preparation or a 3-monthly injection.

Intravenous zoledronate is given annually. The infusion is usually given in hospital because a few patients developed atrial fibrillation in the drug trials. More common side-effects include flu-like symptoms, fever, headache, diarrhoea and vomiting. Zoledronate is more potent than the other bisphosphonates.

Osteonecrosis of the jaw is a rare complication that seems more likely in patients on high-dose bisphosphonates for carcinoma; however, it is sensible to warn patients to inform their dentists if they are planning any invasive dental treatment.

There is also concern that bisphosphonates may be the cause of atypical subtrochanteric fractures below the neck of femur which produce a characteristic 'beak' appearance on the radiograph of the fracture site. Current advice is to reassess the patient's risk-benefit after 5 years of treatment and consider stopping the bisphosphonate. Bisphosphonates are not recommended if the creatinine clearance is less than 35 ml/h.

Strontium ranelate

This is thought to increase bone growth and reduce bone loss, although the precise mode of action is unknown. It comes in a sachet to be mixed with water and usually is taken at bedtime. It is an alternative for women over 75 years old who do not tolerate bisphosphonates. Side-effects include diarrhoea, nausea and increased thromboembolic risk.

Teriparatide, recombinant 1-34 PTH

This is given daily by subcutaneous injection for 18 months. Given intermittently, PTH is anabolic and stimulates osteoblast activity (contrary to the effect of endogenous PTH which is catabolic). Use of teriparatide is restricted to patients with severe disease who have not tolerated or responded to other treatments because it is extremely expensive. Side-effects include gastrointestinal upset. It is contraindicated in renal impairment.

Selective oestrogen modulators (SERMs)

SERMS, e.g. raloxifene, act as oestrogen agonists in the bone and liver, but as oestrogen antagonists in the breast and uterus, and therefore increase bone density without increasing the risk of breast or uterine cancer. It reduces the risk of vertebral fractures only. HRT is now only used second line because of the high risk of cancer and heart disease in older women.

Synthetic analogues of calcitonin

Given as intramuscular injections, synthetic analogues of calcitonin also inhibit bone resorption. They are not as effective as other agents, so are used as second line. However, they may be a useful adjunct in pain control following an acute vertebral wedge fracture.

Denosumab

A monoclonal antibody to RANK ligand (receptor activator of nuclear factor kappa-B), denosumab is given by subcutaneous injections 6 monthly to post-menopausal women. The mechanism of action is shown in Figure 6.3.

Side-effects include cellulitis, eczema and a few reports of osteonecrosis of the jaw. Denosumab

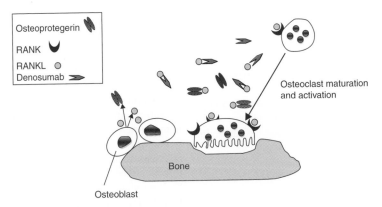

Figure 6.3 The mechanism of action of denusomab. Osteoblasts build bone and have a role in bone resorption by producing RANK ligand (RANKL) and osteoprotegerin. RANKL binds to its receptor RANK and mediates osteoclast differentiation, activation and survival. The protein osteoprotegerin binds to RANKL and functions as an endogenous inhibitor of this pathway. Denosumab is a monoclonal antibody to RANKL and functions like osteoprotegerin, mopping up RANKL and reducing osteoclast activity and decreasing bone resorption.

must not be given without correcting calcium and vitamin D levels. If denosumab is discontinued, the patient must be treated with another preparation, e.g. IV zoledronate, or there is profound rebound bone-remodelling.

Analgesia
This is essential for all osteoporotic fractures.

Secondary osteoporosis
Treat causes of secondary osteoporosis.

Internal fixation of hip fractures
The most appropriate type of fixation depends on the fracture site.

Balloon kyphoplasty
This is a treatment for vertebral collapse; it restores the vertebral body height, reduces pain rapidly and thus enables the patient to mobilize early.

Concordance

Concordance with calcium and vitamin D preparations and bisphosphonates is extremely poor even 3 months after they are first prescribed. Explaining the rationale to patients may improve this. Different preparations of vitamin D and calcium are available including soluble and capsule forms as well as the familiar chalky tablets, so it is worth trying to find the most palatable for an individual. It may be worth considering monthly or yearly bisphosphonates or denosumab injections; as expensive as these treatments are, they are cheaper than hospital admissions following fractures.

Patient education

Encourage patients to stop smoking, reduce their alcohol intake and increase their weight-bearing activity.

Prevention of further fractures

- Treatment of osteoporosis.
- Exercise programmes.
- Falls prevention strategies (see Chapter 5).
- The benefit of hip protector pads is controversial (see Chapter 5).

Osteomalacia

This is reduced calcification of the osteoid matrix due to vitamin D deficiency. The amount of bone is normal, but it is soft and weak compared with normal bone.

Incidence

Incidence is uncertain and depends on the population studied:

- Admissions to Scottish departments of geriatric medicine, 4%.
- Post-mortem study of elderly patients, 12%.
- Biopsies on fractured neck of femur patients, 25%.

Causes

Reduced vitamin D availability
- Deficient diet.
- Reduced sun exposure: most common in Muslim and Hindu cultures (where women cover their heads) and in institutionalized elderly people. Ultraviolet light converts 7-dehydrocholesterol to previtamin D_3 and then to vitamin D_3 (cholecalciferol).
- Ten to fifteen minutes' exposure to sunlight is sufficient to replenish the body's stores.
- Vitamin D binding protein carries D_2 and D_3 to the liver which converts it to 25-hydroxyvitamin D. Then 1-alpha-hydroxylase in the proximal tubule of the kidney converts it to 1, 25-dihydroxycholecalciferol.
- Malabsorption of vitamin D in food and medications occurs in coeliac disease, diverticular disease of the small bowel and post-gastrectomy.

Impaired vitamin D metabolism
- Chronic kidney disease (reduced activity of 1-hydroxylation).
- Drugs that induce liver enzymes, e.g. phenytoin and carbamazepine.

Clinical features

- Pain in the axial skeleton (spine, shoulders, ribs and pelvis).
- Muscle weakness.
- Waddling gait and difficulty standing from sitting secondary to osteomalacic myopathy.
- Fragility fractures.

Investigations

- X-rays may show insufficiency fractures, Looser's zones.
- Bone scintigram may show 'hungry bones', so-called because the bones take up the isotope so readily that they are very bright and the kidneys may not be visible.

- Blood tests: raised alkaline phosphatase, low corrected calcium and low phosphate.
- Serum 25-hydroxyvitamin D_3 will also be low.
- Bone biopsy will clinch the diagnosis where there is doubt.

Treatment

- Oral vitamin supplements, e.g. Calcichew D3 Forte.
- In the case of abnormal metabolism, e.g. renal disease, give a hydroxylated preparation, i.e. alfacalcidol or calcitriol.
- Watch for hypercalcaemia.

Paget's disease of the bone

This is a localized abnormality of bone that arises because of increased activity of the osteoclasts and osteoblasts. The net result is an increase in bone turnover, which produces bone that is expanded, but is paradoxically weaker than normal bone. Paget's disease of the bone most frequently affects the pelvis, spine, skull and the femur, although any bone can be affected. A single bone is affected in 10% of cases. The adjacent bone may also be affected.

Incidence

The incidence increases with age. The prevalence is 5% of over 40 year olds, rising to 10% of over 80 year olds. There is a slight male preponderance. It is more common in northern Europe, Australia and New Zealand and much less common in Asian countries.

Aetiology

This is still unknown, but there is likely to be a link between environmental and genetic factors. There have been studies linking it to various viruses including measles and the respiratory syncytial virus. Some families possess a candidate gene on chromosome 18q2. There may be a link with HLA DQW 1 antigen. RANK ligand has also been implicated and upregulation may account for the localization of the abnormal bone.

Clinical features

- Usually asymptomatic and is diagnosed incidentally on X-rays, or because of a raised alkaline phosphatase.
- Pain, which might be localized to the affected bone or secondary to nerve entrapment.

- Deformity, e.g. enlargement of the skull, anterior bowing of the tibia or lateral bowing of the femur.

Investigations

- Raised serum alkaline phosphatase.
- Raised urinary hydroxyproline suggests active disease.
- Serum calcium is raised in patients who are immobile.
- X-rays show affected bones to be enlarged, abnormally dense and distorted, e.g. cottonwool appearance of the skull, picture frame appearance of vertebrae.
- Bone scintigraphy.

Complications

- Fractures of abnormal bone, usually the femur or tibia.
- Secondary osteoarthritis of adjacent joints.
- Neurological: compression of the cranial nerves as they exit the skull, most commonly affects the eighth nerve, but can also affect the second and the fifth; or paraplegia if the spinal cord is compressed.
- Hydrocephalus.
- High-output heart failure caused by Paget's disease of the bone is very rare.
- The development of malignant tumours is also rare, but examples include osteosarcoma (incidence is < 1%) and chondrosarcoma.

Treatment

- Aimed at treating pain and preventing deformities and fractures.
- Acute disease is treated with a bisphosphonate, usually risedronate, which reduces disease activity (mirrored by a fall in serum alkaline phosphatase and urinary hydroxyproline) and pain within days of starting treatment.
- Risedronate is usually given for 2–6 months.
- Treatment can be repeated if necessary.
- Intravenous pamidronate can be given if an oral preparation is not tolerated or if the disease is rapidly progressing.

Primary hyperparathyroidism

Incidence

- Common, affecting 1 in 500 women and 1 in 2,000 men per year.

- Occurs worldwide.
- Fifty-five percent are women over 70 years of age.
- Should be considered in any patients with hypercalcaemia in the context of normal renal function and no history of malignancy.

Clinical features

- The majority of elderly patients (up to 80%) will be asymptomatic and the problem will have been discovered on biochemical testing done for other reasons.
- Asymptomatic patients should simply be observed and their biochemistry monitored.
- However, 12% of cases with a raised calcium level will have had documented episodes of confusion and dehydration and will merit treatment unless there are other major co-morbidities.
- Check PTH level.
- Serum phosphate may be low.
- Primary hyperparathyroidism is usually due to an adenoma in a single parathyroid.
- Sestamibi scan: technetium[99] is preferentially taken up by the overactive parathyroid gland; used to demonstrate anatomy prior to surgery.
- Minimally invasive parathyroidectomy is now available, with good results and short hospital stays.

Hypercalcaemia

There are many causes of hypercalcaemia. In practice, the following are the main groups affecting older people:

- Primary hyperparathyroidism, as above.
- Hypercalcaemia of malignancy may be due to bone metastases but also non-metastatic manifestation of malignant disease. PTH is suppressed in this context.
- Myeloma (see Chapter 14).
- Drug induced: thiazide diuretics, lithium and vitamin D.
- Chronic kidney disease (see Chapter 13).
- Sarcoidosis, hyperthyroidism and Addison's disease are all rare causes in this age group.

Emergency treatment involves rehydration with intravenous normal saline. If the patient is fluid overloaded, loop diuretics are useful to facilitate urinary excretion of calcium. Intravenous pamidronate is an effective treatment especially in malignancy.

Joints

Many people accept joint problems as a part of growing older, but arthritis is not universal, and in old age it must be diagnosed accurately for appropriate management (Table 6.1).

Osteoarthritis

- Osteoarthritis (OA) is the most common joint disorder and the incidence increases with increasing age.
- Eighty percent of 80 year olds will have some X-ray evidence of OA, but not necessarily symptoms.
- Small changes in management may produce big improvements in quality of life and symptom control.
- Long-standing, complicated and burnt-out rheumatoid arthritis may be difficult to differentiate from generalized OA in old age.
- Aetiology usually unknown, i.e. primary osteoarthritis.
- May be secondary to:
  o Genetic predisposition.
  o Repetitive heavy loading of the joints.
  o Obesity.
  o Trauma leading to articular deformity.
  o Inflammatory disease, including gout and rheumatoid arthritis.
  o Aseptic necrosis.
  o Endocrine disease, e.g. myxoedema and acromegaly.
  o Neuropathy, e.g. diabetic, and therefore painless.
  o Hereditary disease, e.g. haemophilia, hypermobility syndromes.
  o Metabolic disease, e.g. Wilson's disease, haemochromatosis, homocysteinuria.

Table 6.1 Patient consulting rate per 1,000 persons (by age in years) for patients with joint diseases

	Joint diseases: consulting rate				
All ages	0–14	15–44	45–64	65–74	75
34	2	14	62	105	114

Pathophysiology

Current understanding is that wear and tear combines with the loss of normal homeostasis of cartilage which sets off an inflammatory response (secondary to the release of metalloproteases, IL6 and TNFα) which leads to degradation of the matrix of the cartilage. Water makes up 80% of normal cartilage matrix. This is reduced to 60% in damaged cartilage. Early in the disease, the cartilage is expanded, but as time goes by it softens and loses elasticity. Eventually the edges of the cartilage are weakened and become fibrillated. This exposes the subchondral bone which then articulates with bone on the other side of the joint. The subchondral bone becomes more cellular and may develop cysts. Abnormal new bone formation produces osteophytes.

Symptoms

- Pain: gradual in onset, intermittent, worse on movement and relieved by rest.
- Sleep may be disturbed in severe cases.
- Joints most often affected are DIPs, PIPs, base of thumb (painless but unsightly), hips, knees and cervical and lumbar spine.
- Hip pain is worse in the anterior groin and may radiate into the buttock or thigh.
- Knee pain is worse in the anterior knee and patellofemoral joint, but may be referred to the hip.
- Early morning stiffness should last no longer than 15 min.
- Functional problems include difficulty bending down to put on shoes, getting out of a chair and walking long distances, which eventually leads to immobility.

Signs

- Tenderness and bony swelling secondary to osteophytes and swelling due to effusion.
- Painful, reduced range of movement.
- In OA of the hip, the leg may be shortened because the hip is flexed and externally rotated and there may be marked quadriceps wasting.
- Crepitus.
- Eventually the joint may become deformed, e.g. genu valgus (knock knees) and varus (bow knees), and hallux valgus (bunion).
- Gait may be antalgic, i.e. less time is spent with weight on the affected side.

Radiological features

- Loss of joint space secondary to loss of cartilage (see Figure 6.4).

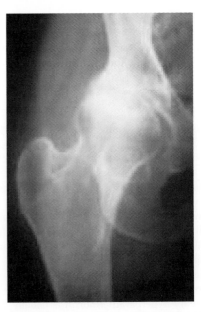

Figure 6.4 Radiograph of the right hip showing severe loss of joint space.

- Osteophytes.
- Subchondral erosions and cysts.

Treatment

Pharmacological
- Simple analgesia, such as paracetamol taken regularly, can be enough to control pain.
- NSAIDs should be reserved for flare-ups because of multiple side-effects. COX-2 inhibitors, e.g. celecoxib, are designed to preferentially treat inflammation without causing GI symptoms. However, they have been associated with increased risk of thrombotic heart disease, leading to rofecoxib being withdrawn.
- Topical NSAIDs may be very effective, as the patient perceives improvement by applying it directly to the affected joint, and there are fewer side-effects than oral NSAIDs.
- Capsaicin, derived from chilli peppers and applied topically, can give good pain relief.
- Intra-articular steroid injection can produce pain relief for a period of 2-4 weeks, sufficient to allow a patient to enjoy a special occasion, but is not indicated for long-term treatment.

Non-pharmacological
- Weight loss relieves the strain on the joints.
- Physiotherapy is aimed at improving the range of movement and strengthening muscles

surrounding the joint, thus stabilizing it, for example to reverse quadriceps wasting to protect the knee.

- Encourage older people to exercise regularly; swimming is good because it unloads the joints.
- Using a stick in the opposite hand or a frame can reduce the load on an affected hip or knee by 50%.
- Hot and cold packs for temporary relief of pain.
- Some patients swear by glucosamine and chondroitin supplements.
- There is evidence from two small trials to support knee-taping in OA to improve proprioception and reduce knee pain.
- Joint replacement.

Complications of joint replacement

- Infection: affects about 1% of hip replacements. Usually prophylactic antibiotics are given. The most common infection is a simple wound infection. A deeper infection may be more difficult to diagnose; a gallium scan can be helpful.
- DVT: subcutaneous enoxaparin is usually given as prophylaxis.
- Loosening of prosthesis: X-ray or bone scan may demonstrate this.
- Fracture of adjacent bone: visible on X-ray.
- Patient outlives prosthesis and a second operation is needed.
- Increased mobility reveals an additional pathology, e.g. angina results from the increased activity.

The ideal patient for joint replacement

- Refractory pain in single joint or only one severely affected joint.
- Physically fit.
- Well motivated.
- Mentally alert and orientated.
- Well nourished, but not obese.
- Unlikely to place unreasonable demands on new hip, i.e. normal mobility anticipated post-operatively and not excessive activity.
- Of sufficient age so that patient is unlikely to outlive the new joint. About one-quarter of replacement hips need revision after 10 years.

Rheumatoid arthritis (RA)

- The incidence is about 1% worldwide in older people.
- RA is a systemic auto-immune inflammatory disorder, which may be present in older people in one of the following patterns of disease:
  - *Inactive disease:* an episode in earlier life which has burnt itself out but left many deformities and disabilities, sometimes progressing to a mixture of old RA and more recent OA. The treatment is the same as for OA.
  - *New disease* arising in old age for the first time can be difficult to differentiate from polymyalgia rheumatica (PMR). Both present with severe early-morning stiffness and shoulder and hip involvement and produce a raised ESR. Both may respond briskly to steroids. It is important not to miss RA, so that patients are offered disease-modifying anti-rheumatic drugs (DMARDs) where appropriate. See Figure 6.5.
  - Exacerbation of chronic disease.

Potential problems in the treatment of rheumatoid arthritis in elderly patients

Splinting of joints

If bulky and heavy, this may significantly interfere with a frail person's ability to maintain personal independence. Night splints are more acceptable to some patients.

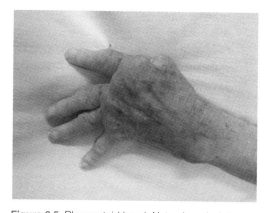

Figure 6.5 Rheumatoid hand. Note ulnar deviation of the fingers, swelling of the metacarpophalangeal joints and over the ulna styloid process, and subluxation of the proximal phalanges on the MCP joints. Source: http://uk.wikimedia.org/wiki/File: Rheumatoid_Arthritis.JPG.

Active rheumatoid disease

- May have very sudden and severe onset in old age.
- May be self-limiting.
- Rheumatoid factor is more often positive in older age so is less specific.
- Older onset RA may affect proximal large joints more than smaller joints.
- Older onset RA may cause pitting oedema of the hands.
- Positive autoantibodies such as anticitrullinated peptide antibody (anti-CCP) may be useful in distinguishing RA from PMR.
- Equal sex incidence (females no longer predominate).
- Fewer systemic complications.
- Treatment may be more hazardous in old age.

Rehabilitation

The presence of severe upper-limb problems and other disorders will significantly hinder a patient's ability to cooperate fully in an intensive physiotherapy programme.

Drugs

Drugs are often toxic in old age but can be helpful in controlling disease and therefore preventing pain and deformity:

- Quick symptom relief may be the best way to preserve mobility and independence; therefore steroids (in spite of disadvantages) may be used earlier than in younger patients. Remember the usual precautions of proton pump inhibitors (PPIs) and bisphosphonates.
- DMARDs may act too slowly to benefit very elderly people. Also, there is increased risk of side-effects because of age and pathological changes in other systems, e.g. renal impairment worsened by penicillamine and gold, and visual impairment potentiated by chloroquine. Methotrexate is used as once-weekly monotherapy. Folic acid is prescribed also to protect the liver. Careful monitoring of blood counts, creatinine, aminotransferase and chest symptoms is essential to detect toxic side-effects early. The patient must be educated to take it once *weekly* only. Consider giving *m*ethotrexate on *M*ondays and *f*olate on *F*ridays! The role of antitumour necrosis factor agents, such as infliximab and etanercept, is being assessed in the older population, and early signs are that they are likely to be no more toxic than in younger patients.

- The mainstay of treatment in active disease is with NSAIDs, but all complications of treatment are more pronounced in the elderly, including renal impairment, fluid overload and risk of GI bleeds.
- It was hoped that COX-2 inhibitors would inhibit synovial prostaglandins without inhibiting intestinal prostaglandins, thus relatively sparing the GI tract. Unfortunately, their use has been associated with an increased risk of thrombotic cardiovascular events.

Crystal arthropathy

Recurrent episodes of sudden severe pain causing immobility are often due to an acute inflammatory response to either urate (gout) or calcium crystal (pseudogout) deposition in a joint. All causes are more common in older age, and both sexes are affected equally. See Table 6.2 for a comparison between the two types.

Note that both gout and pseudogout may be confused with acute joint sepsis. Aspiration for pus and crystals is the best technique for differentiation.

Infective arthropathy

- Should be considered when a single joint is painful.
- May be difficult to diagnose in the presence of old joint deformities.
- May be confused with gout or pseudogout.
- Systemic toxic effects may be minimal in the elderly.
- Concurrent treatment may mask the problem, e.g. steroids, analgesics and antibiotics.
- Aspirate if in doubt.

Muscle pain
Polymyalgia rheumatica (PMR)

PMR presents with generalized muscle pain and tenderness, usually affecting the shoulder girdle, then the pelvic girdle with marked stiffness. It does not cause muscle weakness. It is probably due to an arteritis and is likely to be part of a spectrum of giant-cell arteritis. It is usually idiopathic, but may be triggered by a viral infection or may indicate the

Table 6.2 Clinical features, precipitating factors and treatment of crystal arthropathies

	Gout	Pseudogout
Type of crystal	Urate	Pyrophosphate
Appearance under polarized light	Negatively birefringent	Positively birefringent
Joints most commonly affected	MTP joint of great toe, ankle, PIP joints of fingers	Large joints, most commonly knee
Precipitating factors	Diuretics, overindulgence, fasting, uric acid containing foods such as strawberries, acute illness or surgery, blood malignancies	No acute precipitant may be identified, but acute illness or surgery often responsible, due to dehydration
Extra-articular features	Tophi may be present around the affected joint or on the pinna	None
Serum uric acid	May be raised or normal in an acute attack	Normal
X-ray appearance	Erosions	Linear opacification of articular cartilage
Treatment of acute episode	NSAIDs, colchicine, steroids, rest, ice-pack	NSAIDs, rest
Prevention	Allopurinol (febuxostat in CKD)	None
Associated conditions	Obesity, hypertension, CAD	Diabetes, myxoedema, hyperparathyroidism
Family history	Common	Less common

CAD, coronary artery disease; CKD, chronic kidney disease,

presence of an underlying malignancy. PMR may be associated with a low-grade fever, and fatigue.

Epidemiology

- Most common in people aged 60–70.
- Female to male ratio is 2:1.
- Incidence is 20/100,000 per annum.
- It is the most common reason for commencing older people on steroids.

Diagnostic criteria

- Bilateral shoulder pain and/or neck stiffness.
- Onset of illness of less than 2 weeks.
- Initial ESR greater than 40.
- Duration of morning stiffness of more than 1 h.
- Age greater than 65 years.
- Depression and/or weight loss.
- Bilateral tenderness in upper arms.

Three positives are suggestive of PMR. Those features higher in the list are most strongly predictive. A successful therapeutic trial with steroids will confirm diagnosis: the response is often dramatic and within 3 days.

NB: Creatine kinase, muscle biopsy and EMG are all usually normal.

Complications of untreated PMR

- Chronic disability.
- Normochromic anaemia.
- Hepatitis with raised alkaline phosphatase.
- The patient may become immobile.
- Progression to giant-cell arteritis with major-vessel occlusion, leading to blindness, stroke or myocardial infarction.

Treatment

- Steroids: 20 mg prednisolone daily is sufficient for PMR. Higher doses are necessary if giant-cell arteritis is suspected (see Chapter 9). Rapid improvement in symptoms helps to confirm the diagnosis. If the patient is not sure that they are better, then the diagnosis is not PMR.
- Dosage should be monitored according to symptoms and level of ESR. Once symptoms are controlled and ESR has fallen to normal, reduce the dose slowly.
- Bone protection should be given.
- Treatment may be necessary for 2 years or more and disease may recur and require a further course of steroids.

- NSAIDs may help to resolve symptoms of PMR, but will not protect the patient from vascular occlusion.

Muscle weakness

Ageing changes

Muscle bulk and efficiency decline with increasing age. Muscles become atrophic and paler in colour due to a decrease in the number of muscle fibres, an increase in fat and fibrous tissue and increased deposition of lipochrome pigment. These changes are not exclusively due to ageing, but merely reflect the more sedentary life in old age in developed countries. Muscle bulk can still be increased in old age by regular exercise. Neuronal impairment may be another explanation for the 'ageing changes'. The loss of muscle mass and strength associated with age is thought to play a major role in the pathogenesis of frailty and loss of function.

Muscle pathology in old age

Sarcopenia

- Sarcopenia is loss of skeletal muscle mass and strength associated with age.

- The prevalence is likely to be rising as the population ages. It is estimated that 50% of over 80 year olds have sarcopenia.
- Sarcopenia is different from cytokine-mediated cachexia due to cancer or muscle loss associated with starvation.
- It can develop alongside atrophy due to disuse, disease and poor nutrition.
- Sarcopenia leads to loss of function such as getting out of a chair and walking upstairs and is associated with increased risk of falling over.
- Mechanisms include age-related loss of muscle mass, atrophy of muscle fibres especially the fast twitch type IIa and IIb fibres, reduced mitochondrial function and reduced synthesis of muscle protein. See Figure 6.6.
- There is no universally agreed diagnostic tool, but using DXA to measure lean muscle mass has the advantages of being widely available, no radiation exposure and being cheaper than MRI or CT scanning.
- The mainstay of treatment is resistance exercise, which has the added advantage of improving bone strength, reducing falls and social contact for the patient.
- There is no evidence that oestrogen works. Testosterone does increase muscle mass but has many side-effects.

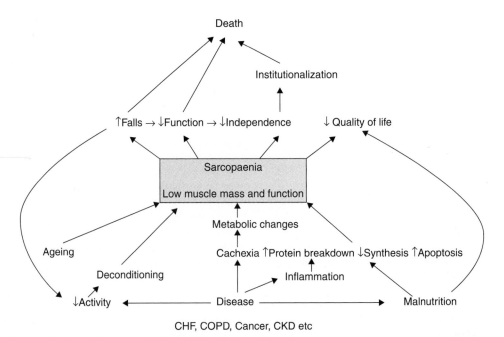

Figure 6.6 Pathogenesis and consequences of sarcopenia.

- Currently, there is much research into the role of ACE inhibitors thought to prevent mitochondrial decline and improve endothelial function.

Myopathies

- Usually cause symmetrical proximal muscle weakness without tenderness.
- Endocrine causes: Cushing's disease, thyrotoxicosis, hypothyroidism and Addison's disease.
- Drug-induced: e.g. statins, steroids, ciprofloxacin, colchicine and alcohol.
- Metabolic: usually due to hypokalaemia (endocrine or drug induced).
- Vitamin D deficiency (part of osteomalacia).
- Symptoms more profound if several causes co-exist.

Myositis

- Proximal muscles are tender and weak.
- Serum creatine kinase usually elevated.
- EMG demonstrates spiky polyphasic muscle action potentials and occasional spontaneous fibrillation.
- Muscle biopsies show inflammation.
- Rarely infective in old age, but transient post-viral symptoms are common.
- Polymyositis is often associated with underlying malignancy.
- Dermatomyositis: dermatological signs occurring with the muscle features include Gottron's papules (pink papules on the knuckles) and a heliotrope rash (patchy red/purple rash and oedema of the eyelids). Jo-1 antibodies often positive.
- Symptoms may respond to steroids, azathioprine or cyclophosphamide.

Myasthenia gravis

- This is an acquired autoimmune disease.
- Antibodies are formed to acetylcholine receptors (AChR) at the neuromuscular junction of skeletal muscle.
- It is uncommon; annual incidence 2 per 100,000.
- Ten percent of all cases occur in older age.
- The majority in this age group are idiopathic.
- Symptoms include exaggerated fatigue, e.g. of the eye muscles, causing ptosis or diplopia, bulbar weakness leading to dysphagia.
- An intercurrent infection may precipitate a crisis.
- Diagnosis is by correction of the symptom with use of the short-acting anticholinesterase edrophonium chloride (Tensilon® test).

- Anti-AChR auto-antibodies are present in 74% of cases.
- May be drug induced (penicillamine and aminoglycosides).
- Eaton–Lambert (myasthenic) syndrome may present in a similar way, and often causes proximal leg muscle weakness so the patient finds it difficult to get up out a chair. However, there is an underlying carcinoma in up to 70% of cases, frequently small cell lung carcinoma. Autoantibodies develop to the voltage-gated calcium channels (VGCC) in the muscle. The response to Tensilon® is poor.

Investigation of muscle disease

- Raised creatine kinase indicates muscle damage.
- An EMG helps differentiate neurogenic from primary muscle disorders.
- Muscle biopsies are difficult and require skilled and experienced interpretation; therefore best results are from specialized centres.
- Tensilon® test and anti-AChR antibodies in suspected myasthenia, anti-VGCC antibodies in Eaton–Lambert syndrome.
- Specific tests to confirm underlying cause, e.g. thyroid-function tests.

Treatment

- Correct precipitating cause, if possible.
- Anticholinesterases in myasthenia, e.g. pyridostigmine.
- Steroids are worth trying in malignant myopathy, especially polymyositis/dermatomyositis, but beware of causing steroid myopathy.

→ FURTHER INFORMATION

American College of Rheumatology (2000) *Recommendations for the Medical Management of OA of the Hip and Knee.* http://www.rheumatology.org/practice/clinical/guidelines/oa-mgmt.asp.

British Orthopaedic Association (2007) *The Care of Patients with Fragility Fracture.* http://www.fractures.com/pdf/BOA-BGS-Blue-Book.pdf.

DTi (2000) *The Economic Cost of Hip Fracture in the UK.* www.dti.gov.uk/files/file21463.pdf.

Kavanaugh AF (2005) *Rheumatic Diseases in the Elderly. Clinics in Geriatric Medicine (The Clinics: Internal Medicine).* Elsevier, Amsterdam.

National Osteoporosis Society and Royal College of Physicians (2002) *Guidelines of the Working Group for the Bone and Tooth Society. Glucocorticoid Induced Osteoporosis: Guidelines for Prevention and Treatment.* http://bookshop.rcplondon.ac.uk/contents/pub89-64206b70-b147-4976-9ee1-bf4948458468.pdf.

National Hip Fracture Database: http://www.rcseng.ac.uk/news/docs/NHFD%20(final).pdf.

NICE (2010) *Alendronate, Etidronate, Risedronate, Raloxifene and Strontium Ranelate for the Primary Prevention of Osteoporotic Fragility Fractures in Postmenopausal Women (amended). Technology Appraisal Guidance 160.* www.nice.org.uk.

National Osteoporosis Guideline Group (NOGG): www.shef.ac.uk/NOGG/.

NICE (2011) *Osteoporosis – Primary Prevention.* http://guidance.nice.org.uk/TA160.

NICE guidance regarding DXA scanning – CKS online tool: http://www.cks.nhs.uk/osteoporosis_prevention_of_fragility_fractures/management/scenario_diagnosis/opportunistically_suspecting_osteoporosis#-- − 473484.

Poole KES, Compston JE (2007) Osteoporosis and its management. *BMJ* 333: 1251–1256.

Scientific Advisory Committee on Nutrition (2007) *Update on Vitamin D. Position Statement by the Scientific Advisory Committee on Nutrition.* www.sacn.gov.uk.

SIGN (2003) *Management of Osteoporosis: A National Clinical Guideline.* http://www.sign.ac.uk/pdf/sign71.pdf.

7

Stroke made simple

Importance

Anyone can have a stroke, including babies and children, but the vast majority (90%) of strokes affect people aged over 55. Each year over 150,000 people in the UK have a stroke. Stroke is the third most common cause of death, after heart disease and cancer (11% of all deaths). Stroke is the largest single cause of severe adult disability in developed countries and is very expensive as patients need prolonged rehabilitation and, sometimes, care for life. Half a million people in the UK are living with long-term disability as a result of stroke. Managing stroke in a stroke unit (multidisciplinary, coordinated care) produces marked benefit.

Definitions

A stroke is defined as 'rapidly developing clinical signs of focal disturbance of cerebral function, with symptoms lasting 24 h or longer or leading to death, with no apparent cause other than of vascular origin'. This includes subarachnoid haemorrhage (SAH) but excludes subdural haematoma and haemorrhage into a tumour. By definition, a transient ischaemic attack (TIA) lasts less than 24 h, so TIAs are classified separately, but the causes of TIA and stroke are very similar. TIAs are a risk factor for stroke. The term 'stroke' is now used in preference to cerebrovascular accident (CVA).

Outcome of stroke

The outcome of a stroke (Table 7.1) depends on the aetiology, volume and part of the brain that is affected, the age and fitness of the patient and co-morbidities. You will see a range of figures for outcome, depending on the population in the study. The case fatality rate has fallen steadily since the 1980s but it remains higher in women and for haemorrhagic stroke.

Aetiology and pathology

A stroke results from interruption to the brain's blood supply due to an infarct or a haemorrhage. An infarct is an area of ischaemia, usually due to thrombosis *in situ* or an embolus from the carotids or heart but occasionally due to low BP from any cause or damage to the blood vessel wall with dissection. A primary haemorrhage may be due to an arterial abnormality, such as an aneurysm, but most infarcts and bleeds occur in vessels damaged by hypertension and atheroma. Cerebral amyloid angiopathy (see Chapter 4) is increasingly recognized as a cause of lobar intracerebral haemorrhage (ICH) in elderly patients. $T_2{}^*$-weighted MRI demonstrating chronic cerebral microbleeding at the white/grey matter junction supports this diagnosis. Secondary bleeding may occur in an area of brain damaged by an infarct. The proportions of the types of stroke vary in different countries: in the UK atherothrombotic strokes comprise 85% of

Lecture Notes Elderly Care Medicine, Eighth Edition. Claire G. Nicholl and K. Jane Wilson.
© 2012 John Wiley & Sons, Ltd. Published 2012 by John Wiley & Sons, Ltd.

Table 7.1 Outcome of stroke

Outcome	Percentage
1-month mortality (UK)	15–20
• ischaemic	10
• haemorrhagic	50
1-year mortality of survivors	25
Around 3 months:	
Dead	15
Full or almost full recovery	10
Minor impairment	25
Moderate to severe impairment (need significant help)	40
Long-term high-dependency care	10
Further stroke in the first year	15
Return to work if previously working	35
Unable to walk unaided	20
Unable to walk outdoors	40

cases whereas in Japan haemorrhagic strokes are much more common. The biggest risk factor for stroke is increasing age. AfroCaribbean and SE Asian ethnicity and apolipoprotein E ε2 or ε4 carriage (for ICH) also increase risk, but it is more useful to consider risk factors that can be modified.

Risk factors for stroke are similar to those for other vascular diseases such as coronary artery disease (CAD) and peripheral vascular disease (Table 7.2). However, there are differences in relative risk that are not understood, e.g. smoking is a bigger risk for CAD and hypertension is a bigger risk for stroke. In future, there may be increased understanding of the role of inflammation: a high CRP on a sensitive assay is emerging as a risk factor for vascular disease. Primary and secondary risk factors are similar. Risk factors tend to be multiplicative. As there is more chance of another vascular event once one has occurred, the risk–benefit ratio for treatments changes. (This is why healthy 40 year olds are advised not to take aspirin as their chance of a bleed outweighs the likely benefits.)

The CHADS$_2$ score (see Table 7.3) is a clinical prediction rule for estimating the risk of stroke in patients with non-rheumatic atrial fibrillation, based on age and major clinical risk factors.

The inclusion of additional 'stroke risk modifiers' has been proposed, giving the following CHA$_2$DS$_2$-Vasc score:

- Age: 65–74 scores 1, 75+ scores 2
- Sex: female gender scores 1
- Vascular disease present scores 1

A total score of 0/9 is so low risk that even aspirin is not indicated, a score of 1 indicates aspirin would be beneficial, and a score of 2 and above indicates oral anticoagulation should be used.

Older people should be considered for warfarin, though contraindications include recurrent falls and dementia. In the BAFTA (Birmingham Atrial Fibrillation Treatment of the Aged) study (mean age 81.5 years) warfarin was much more effective than aspirin and actually had a trend towards causing fewer haemorrhages. A risk score for bleeding had been devised (HAS-BLED). See atrial fibrillation (AF) in Chapter 9.

Because of the complexity of dosing with warfarin (vitamin K antagonist) and the need for regular blood tests (INRs) huge effort has been put into developing easier to use anticoagulants. Dabigatran [a direct thrombin (IIa) inhibitor] is the newly licensed front runner and factor Xa inhibitors (e.g. rivaroxaban and apixaban) are near to market and may offer more consistent anticoagulation and decreased risk of ICH, albeit at a high cost.

Presentation

Typically, the onset is abrupt. Occasionally a hemiparesis develops over 12 or more hours. If symptoms progress over days/weeks, suspect an alternative diagnosis such as tumour or subdural haematoma. Other common stroke mimics include hypoglycaemia, partial seizures, Todd's paresis after a partial seizure, hemiplegic migraine and metabolic disturbances.

Reduced conscious level at presentation usually indicates non-stroke pathology but a stroke may present with coma, in which case neurological examination requiring cooperation is impossible. Stroke **presents** with coma in three situations:

1 Brain stem infarct.
2 Large cortical infarct with brain stem compression.
3 Seizure after stroke.

In a brain stem stroke, signs are often bilateral and the pupils may be small. In a major cortical stroke, the cheek on the paralysed side may flap in and out with respiration and the limbs on that side are likely to have completely lost all tone. Reflexes may be unhelpful at this stage. An almost

Table 7.2 Management and goals for risk factors for stroke and primary and secondary prevention

Risk factor	Management	Goal
BP high	Promote healthy lifestyle; diet (see below), reduce alcohol intake and increase exercise. Treat BP if still high with drugs individualized to patient (but ACE inhibitor/diuretic combinations may have a particular role)	< 130/90 mm/Hg; < 130/85 mm/Hg if renal insufficiency or heart failure; < 130/80 mm/Hg if diabetic
Heart disease	As appropriate for the condition, also aiming to reduce platelet stickiness, minimize LVH and maintain sinus rhythm	Reduce chances of embolization
Atrial fibrillation	Verify AF on ECG or paroxysmal AF (PAF) on 24-h tape. For patients in chronic or intermittent AF, use warfarin aiming for INR 2.0–3.0. Aspirin is used if there are contraindications to oral anticoagulation or the patient is low-risk (CHADS$_2$ score)	Antiplatelet drugs if 'low risk' but anticoagulation for AF or PAF
Sticky platelets	Secondary prevention. Aspirin (75–300 mg) except in intolerance and brain haemorrhage, caution with asthma and history of GI haemorrhage, with modified release dipyridamole for 2 years after vascular event. Clopidogrel if aspirin intolerant. However, a recent review suggests clopidogrel should be used first-line in stroke or multivascular disease (NHS HTA 2011)	Concordance with long-term antiplatelet therapy
Carotid stenosis	Antiplatelet therapy, document degree of stenosis and offer endarterectomy if CT confirms stroke in ipsilateral hemisphere, function worth preserving and stenosis > 70% or > 50% in men with cortical symptoms	Ensure eligible patients with anterior circulation strokes are screened: the fit elderly have most to gain
Smoking	Advise quitting and refer for support, e.g. clinic/pharmacological help (nicotine or buproprion, varenicline)	Quit and avoid passive smoking
Unhealthy diet	Advocate low-fat, low-salt, high fruit and vegetable diet with weight loss if needed. Discourage excess consumption of any food, however 'healthy', to avoid health scares, e.g. heavy metals in oily fish	Varied healthy diet, evidence for 'Mediterranean diet'
Obesity	Calorie restriction and increased caloric expenditure	Achieve and maintain desirable weight (BMI 20–25 kg/m^2). Higher BMI is less of a risk if central obesity is not present
Excess alcohol	Low/moderate alcohol intake protects from atherothrombotic stroke (amount probably depends on individual as increase in BP and obesity may be adverse) but high or binge intake is a risk for haemorrhage	Avoid binge or excessive drinking
Adverse lipid profile	Advice about diet, weight and exercise. For 2° prevention start simvastatin 40 mg regardless of cholesterol. Refer to specialist if triglycerides/total cholesterol remain high	It is likely that the lower the total cholesterol, the better
Diabetes and impaired glucose tolerance	After diet and exercise, use oral hypoglycaemic drugs, particularly metformin, unless contraindicated; insulin if adequate control not achieved	Normal fasting plasma glucose (< 7 mmol/L) and near normal HbA1c (< 7%)
Lack of exercise	Medical check before initiating vigorous exercise programme: start slowly if older or unfit. Moderate-intensity activities (40–60% of maximum capacity) are equivalent to a brisk walk. Additional benefit from vigorous (> 60% of maximum capacity) exercise for 20–40 min on 3–5 days/week	At least 30 min of moderate-intensity physical activity on most days of the week
Previous TIA	Treat all risk factors	

Table 7.3 CHADS$_2$ score for predicting risk of stroke in 1 year in non-valvular atrial fibrillation

CHADS attribute	Point allocation	CHADS$_2$ Score	Stroke risk (%)	95% CI	Risk category	Treatment
Congestive heart failure	1	0	1.9	1.2–3.0	Low	Aspirin
Hypertension	1	1	2.8	2.0–3.8	Moderate	Aspirin or warfarin (choice)
Age > 75 years	1	2	4.0	3.1–5.1	High	Warfarin (unless contraindicated)
Diabetes mellitus	1	3	5.9	4.6–7.3		
Prior **S**troke/TIA (given 2 points, hence the **2** in the score)	2	4	8.5	6.3–11.1		
	Max = 6	5	12.5	8.2–17.5		
		6	18.2	10.5–27.4		

pathognomonic sign is conjugate deviation of gaze towards the side of the lesion, due to the unopposed effect of the contralateral frontal eye field (remember, the patient 'looks away' from a tumour but 'towards' a stroke). Loss of consciousness points towards a severe stroke, but there are no reliable clinical predictors to distinguish haemorrhage from infarct.

The conscious or slightly drowsy patient usually presents little diagnostic difficulty. The peak time of onset for stroke is in the early hours of the morning and the patient will describe waking up and trying to get out of bed, only to find themselves unable to walk. An eyewitness may relate that the patient dropped their cup and developed facial asymmetry and difficulty with speech and then became unable to stand or perhaps even sit properly. Examination will then usually reveal characteristic deficits: in the early stages, the paralysed limbs are more often flaccid than spastic and in some cases they stay that way. Establish the exact time of onset (unfortunately impossible if the patient woke from sleep, around 25% cases). If it is less than 4.5 h, act fast as thrombolysis may be possible (see subsequent text).

Educational programmes are encouraging the public to treat stroke with as much urgency as a heart attack and the ambulance service uses a validated triage such as FAST (the Face Arm Speech Time score) to identify stroke patients for urgent transfer to a specialist stroke service with accurate documentation of the time of onset. Any one of facial asymmetry, arm or leg weakness or speech disturbance suggests a stroke with a sensitivity of 82% and specificity for stroke diagnosis of 37%.

Transient ischaemic attacks

These are isolated or recurrent focal neurological symptoms (usually negative) which resolve within 24 h. They are usually due to platelet emboli from an atheromatous plaque or ulcer in the aorta, the common carotid artery or, most often, the carotid bifurcation or red cell emboli from the heart. Occasionally the pathology is thrombosis or low flow. Monocular loss of vision (amaurosis fugax) hemi- or monoparesis, dysphasia and unilateral sensory disturbance are examples within the internal carotid territory. Most TIAs last less than a couple of hours, usually just a few minutes. The distinction between a TIA and a very small infarct is an anachronism and many older people with no clinical history will have a stroke on a scan.

TIAs also occur within the territory of the vertebrobasilar circulation, although true vertebrobasilar ischaemia or insufficiency is something of a diagnostic dustbin and is very rare. The main features are true vertigo (a sensation of rotary movement of either patient or surroundings), true drop attacks (sudden falls due to total loss of tone without disturbance of consciousness and with rapid and complete recovery) and diplopia, although cortical blindness, tetraparesis, ataxia and dysphagia may also occur. Vertebrobasilar TIAs carry a similar risk of stroke to anterior circulation TIAs and should be treated just as aggressively. TIAs are not a cause of loss of consciousness.

The risk of stroke after a hemispheric TIA is up to 15% in the first month and highest in the first 72 h, so after a probable TIA give aspirin 300 mg (unless on warfarin or contraindicated) and refer to a rapid access TIA clinic according to the degree of risk as assessed by the $ABCD_2$ score (Table 7.4). If confident about the diagnosis some start a statin and antihypertensives at once.

Patients with a high risk of subsequent stroke:

- $ABCD_2$ score of 4 or above,
- two or more TIAs in a week regardless of score (crescendo TIA),
- any patient with neurological symptoms on warfarin,

should have specialist assessment and investigation within 24 h of onset of symptoms.

Patients with a lower risk of subsequent stroke:

- $ABCD_2$ score of 3 or below,
- who present after a week,

should have specialist assessment within 1 week.

The role of a TIA clinic is to:

- Confirm clinical diagnosis.
- Arrange investigations including imaging of the brain, carotids and heart.
- Initiate aggressive secondary prevention.

Patients thought to have had a TIA usually have a brain scan. It is especially important to scan those with isolated aphasia, atypical history or limb jerking as the incidence of space occupying lesions is higher with these presentations.

Management of carotid disease

Doppler duplex imaging or magnetic resonance (MR) angiography is mandatory following anterior circulation TIA or acute non-disabling stroke if the patient would be suitable for carotid endarterectomy (depending on fitness and life expectancy). The standards (with which many stroke services struggle) are that if there is carotid stenosis on the relevant side of between 50 and 99% (according to American criteria) or between 70 and 90%

Table 7.4 $ABCD_2$ score

	Risk factor	Category	Score
A	**A**ge	Age ≥ 60 years	1
B	**B**P at assessment	BP ≥ 140/90	1
C	**C**linical features	Unilateral weakness	2
		Speech disturbance (not weak)	1
D_2	**D**uration	≥ 60 min	2
		10–59 min	1
	Diabetes	Present	1
	Maximum score		7

(according to the more conservative European criteria), the patients should be assessed and referred for carotid endarterectomy within 1 week and have surgery if indicated within 2 weeks of onset. Carotid stenting gives worse outcomes than endarterectomy at 70 + years (due to higher procedural risk) (NICE 2008, 2011).

Data are accumulating favouring endarterectomy for severe **asymptomatic** stenosis for those under 75 if life expectancy is > 10 years. If intracerebral arterial stenosis is found management should be medical as angiographic stenting has been demonstrated to carry a higher risk of harm in Western populations.

The established stroke

Detailed descriptions of the enormous variety of syndromes explicable in terms of the precise anatomy of the damage sustained are beyond the scope of this book. The identification of the major deficits is more important. The classification devised by Bamford (Bamford et al. 1990; Table 7.5) is simple and provides useful prognostic information.

Clinical problems following stroke

- *Dysphagia:* poor swallow is common initially (see Management of hydration and nutrition p. 101).
- *Delirium* occurs in over 10% of patients in the first week, predicted by pre-existing cognitive impairment, right hemisphere stroke, large lesion, post-stroke infection; marker of poor prognosis.

Table 7.5 Brain infarction (Bamford et al. 1990)

Percentage of cases	Clinical	Anatomy/pathology	Outcome
TACI (15%)	All three of: higher cortical dysfunction (e.g. dysphasia, dyscalculia, visuospatial neglect) hemianopia contralateral motor and/or sensory deficit involving two out of three of face, arm or leg	MCA occluded by embolus/spreading thrombus from ICA	Very poor chance of good function and high mortality
PACI (35%)	Two out of three TACI components or higher cerebral dysfunction alone or restricted motor/sensory deficit (e.g. one limb or face, hand, not whole arm)	Branch of MCA or ACA	Fair outcome but very high chance of early recurrence
LacI (25%)	Any one of the following deficits: pure motor pure sensory sensorimotor ataxic hemiparesis clumsy hand-dysarthria higher cortical dysfunction	Occlusion of deep perforating artery (anterior or posterior circulation)	Often good recovery
PoCI (25%)	Any one of: isolated homonymous hemianopia brain stem signs cerebellar ataxia	Brain stem, cerebellum or occipital lobes	High chance of good function but also of recurrence in first year

ICA, internal carotid artery; MCA, middle cerebral artery; ACA, anterior cerebral artery; TACI, total anterior circulation infarct; PACI, partial anterior circulation infarct; LacI, lacunar infarct; PoCI, posterior circulation infarct.

- *Dysphasia:* disorder of language affecting some right-handed patients with left-hemisphere lesions:
  o Anterior dysphasia – non-fluent, impaired naming.
  o Posterior dysphasia – often fluent, jargon type, receptive dysphasia.
  Fluent dysphasia is often confused with acute confusion. In left-handers, two-thirds have left-sided speech dominance; those who have right-sided dominance may/may not develop dysphasia, irrespective of side of lesion.
- *Dysarthria* affects articulation but not the content of the speech. This can be due to unilateral VII palsy but otherwise suggests bilateral disease (or pathology in the cerebellum or basal ganglia).
- *Dyspraxia:* inability to perform purposeful movement despite adequate comprehension and motor function. Varieties include dressing apraxia.

- *Sensory neglect:*
  o Visual – exclude hemianopia first. Test by line bisection or line cancellation (Albert's test).
  o Tactile – if gross, includes loss of body image and denial of problem.
- *Visuospatial perception:* non-dominant hemisphere lesion – besides tests, includes asking the patient to draw simple objects such as a house, face, clock face.
- *Executive function difficulties:* trail-making B timed join the dots test with attentional switching 1 to A to 2 to B, etc. may help predict driving ability.
- *Weakness of limbs:* usually with increased tone; marked 'clasp-knife' spasticity and flaccidity are both adverse signs.
- *Sensory loss:* any modality; gross position sense loss is a very adverse finding.
- *Hemianopia:* major handicap unless patient aware and able to compensate by turning head.

- *Depression:* especially in dominant-hemisphere lesion. Treat with antidepressants.
- *Thalamic pain:* try antidepressant or anticonvulsant.
- *Shoulder pain:* subluxation especially likely following traction on the weak arm, e.g. from poor manual handling.

Multi-infarct disease (dementia)

See vascular dementia in Chapter 4.

Cerebellar infarct or haematoma

Cerebellar strokes can be hard to diagnose. Features include:

- Vertigo.
- Usually reaches maximum intensity at onset.
- Vascular risk factors often present.
- Severe ataxia.
- Great difficulty walking.
- Direction–changing nystagmus (patient looks to right, fast component or 'beats' to the right, when looks to left, 'beats' to left).
- Ninety percent of patients have focal neurological signs.

A study by Kase et al. (1993) suggested that there are two main patterns:

a Posterior inferior cerebellar artery territory infarct: a triad of vertigo, headache and gait imbalance at stroke onset. Mass effect develops in around one-third of cases and may result in brain stem compression or hydrocephalus due to compression of the fourth ventricle. Brain stem may be affected and patients have Wallenberg's lateral medullary syndrome in around one-third of cases with the following symptoms:

  o Dysphagia and dysarthria – lesion to the nucleus ambiguus and vagal nuclei.
  o Ipsilateral Horner's syndrome.
  o Ipsilateral facial sensory loss – pain and temperature.
  o Ipsilateral pharyngeal and laryngeal paralysis – IX and X palsies.
  o Contralateral sensory loss – pain and temperature of the limbs and trunk.

b Superior cerebellar artery infarct: gait disturbance predominates at onset; more benign.

MRI is the investigation of choice as CT scanning is poor for the posterior fossa. If pressure symptoms arise in a biologically fit patient discuss with neurosurgery. Surgical evacuation to decompress the posterior fossa (haematoma or oedema due to infarct) was thought to be beneficial, although recent re-evaluation highlights lack of outcome data.

Differential diagnosis includes the following:

- Benign positional paroxysmal vertigo (BPPV) – brief episodes of intense vertigo, precipitated by a change in position, usually looking up.
- Ménière's disease – simultaneous vertigo, partial hearing loss and tinnitus.
- Migrainous vertigo – features of migraine, normal neurological exam.
- Vestibular neuritis – crescendo onset, marked nausea, unidirectional nystagmus (regardless of where the patient looks) accentuated when looking away from the affected ear; may be unsteady but no ataxia or other neurological signs.
- Labyrinthitis – thought to be the same disease process as vestibular neuritis (viral) with the additional involvement of the auditory system.

Spinal cord infarction

Spinal cord infarction is a stroke within either the spinal cord or the arteries that supply it. It is caused by arteriosclerosis or a compressive lesion. This may cause sudden paraplegia or quadriplegia within minutes or a few hours of the infarction. Other symptoms include intermittent sharp or burning back pain, loss of pain and temperature sensation, and incontinence. Spinal cord ischaemia can cause aching pain down through the legs ('neurogenic claudication') and mimic peripheral vascular disease.

Subarachnoid haemorrhage

Subarachnoid haemorrhage (SAH) is a bleed from a cerebral blood vessel; aneurysm (85% of cases) or vascular malformation, into the subarachnoid space (i.e. the space surrounding the brain where blood vessels lie between the arachnoid and pial layers) and accounts for about 5% of strokes. The patient presents with severe sudden-onset (thunderclap) headache, often with vomiting with or without neurological signs. About half of people die in the first few hours and the overall survival is about 40%, half of whom will have residual disability.

CT scan should be performed urgently if conscious level is impaired, or else within 12 h. If CT is negative, LP should be performed after 12 h to look for xanthochromia. If the diagnosis is confirmed, oral nimodipine 60 mg 4 hourly is started; supportive measures are similar for a stroke, with codeine as analgesia. Discuss the patient urgently with a neurosurgeon. Active management involves CT angiography to delineate the vasculature. A ruptured aneurysm may be clipped or ablated; recent data show better outcomes with endovascular coiling. Treatable complications include secondary hydrocephalus. If there is a family history of SAH or polycystic renal disease, genetic counselling is needed. Long-term BP control must be strict.

Central venous thrombosis

This may present like a stroke, but there is often a history of headache and fits. It is rare but more common if there is a prothrombotic tendency, e.g. disseminated malignancy or sinus infection. The wide range of clinical findings may be a result of highly variable deep venous system drainage. The damage does not follow a typical arterial territory. MR venography is often needed for diagnosis. Although there is often bleeding into the brain, treatment is with heparin.

Investigation of stroke

Typical tests may include: FBC, glucose, renal, clotting studies, liver and bone function, troponin if concomitant MI is possible, cholesterol and thyroid function, ECG, CXR, echocardiogram, 24-h tape if cardiogenic embolus is suspected and carotid Doppler studies (explained above). ESR, CRP and autoantibodies may be useful in infection or if vasculitis is a possibility.

Brain CT scan is now standard, except for moribund patients. Haemorrhage is immediately apparent as a white area (Figure 7.1). The area of low attenuation characteristic of an infarct is often difficult to see in the first 6 h and may not be apparent for 24 h (Figures 7.2 and 7.3). Techniques such as CT perfusion (Figure 7.3) and angiography are being developed for early visualization. Where readily available, MRI is more sensitive than CT early after onset, for small lesions and for imaging the posterior fossa, but is harder for the patient to tolerate.

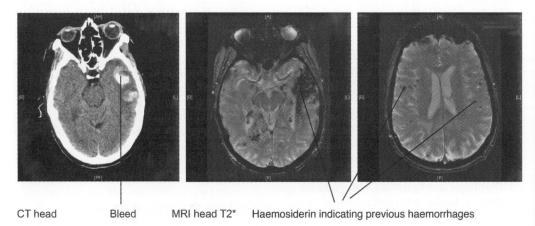

CT head   Bleed   MRI head T2*   Haemosiderin indicating previous haemorrhages

Figure 7.1 CT scan showing a left temporoparietal bleed in March 2011 in a 71-year-old man with prior cognitive decline. MRI head (T2* imaging) 3 months later shows dense haemosiderin deposition (appears black) in the area of the previous bleed and multiple small lesions which look like black holes. These represent multiple small bleeds and are characteristic of cerebral amyloid angiopathy.

Management of the established ischaemic stroke

Where?

With the advent of thrombolysis, the vast majority of patients with suspected stroke are admitted to hospital. Ideally they are fast-tracked through the Emergency Department using the ROSIER scale (Recognition of Stroke in the Emergency Room), triaged for possible thrombolysis, scanned, treated and admitted to a hyperacute stroke unit. Many areas have developed stroke networks to share expertise, and telemedicine is being developed to allow stroke experts to support colleagues in district hospitals with the provision of 24-h thrombolysis. Data from established services, e.g. Finland, show outcomes for telemedicine in stroke similar to bedside evaluation. Diagnosis, with rapid brain imaging, identification of risk factors and initiation of measures for secondary prevention are essential. Even in the early phase, management of a stroke patient is multidisciplinary.

Compared with a general ward, the 'number needed to treat' in a specialist stroke unit is 18

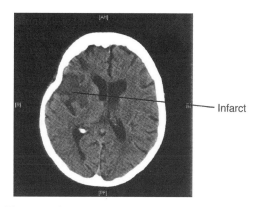

Infarct

Figure 7.2 Imaging in a 92-year-old woman presenting with a left hemiparesis on waking from sleep. Note the irregular area of low attenuation in the right frontal lobe affecting white and grey matter consistent with a recent right MCA infarct.

(95% CI 12–32) to prevent dependency or death. It is unclear which component of stroke unit care leads to the improved outcome, but stroke units have been the most important advance in stroke in the past 15 years. Thereafter, rehabilitation can take place in the patient's own home, in a community hospital or in a day hospital.

ACA

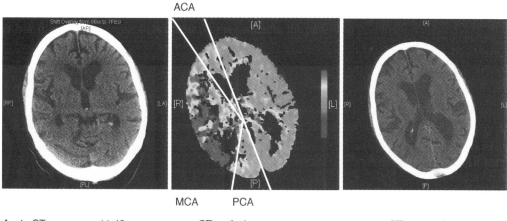

MCA   PCA

Acute CT scan   11.48   CT perfusion scan   CT scan 1 day later

Figure 7.3 Imaging in an 82-year-old man who presented at 09.45 h with sudden-onset left hemiparesis. The initial CT scan shows that it can be difficult to see early infarction whereas the CT perfusion scan shows that more than two-thirds of the right MCA territory is affected: the white lines are drawn on to show the area of cortex supplied by the anterior, middle and cerebral arteries. Although the affected area showed that the contrast time to peak and drain was delayed, only a small area had reduced blood volume, indicating a small infarct within a large penumbra. Thrombolysis IV produced an excellent clinical response and minimal long-term damage was sustained, as can be seen from the CT scan the next day.

General care of acute stroke patients

Arterial oxygen, temperature, hydration and blood glucose should be maintained within normal limits, although evidence is weak. Limited data support the use of antipyretic medication lowering the temperature to 37 °C, but the largest RCT of blood glucose reduction in stroke reported no benefit from insulin infusion. Complications such as pressure sores and chest infection (consider aspiration) may be present on admission and are treated in the usual way. Prevention of further complications is essential. The unconscious patient will need full nursing care, with particular attention to airway, pressure areas and bladder drainage. Correct positioning and chest physiotherapy are needed.

Thromboembolic-deterrent stockings (TEDS) are not beneficial and are associated with skin problems (CLOTS, or Clots in Legs Or sTockings after Stroke, trials) (Kearon and O'Donnell 2011).

Although subcutaneous heparin reduces deaths from PE, haemorrhagic deaths are increased, so heparin is not routinely used. Untargeted use of nutritional supplements is not associated with benefit. High BP should only be treated acutely if it is likely to produce its own complications, e.g. hypertensive encephalopathy (> 220/120 mmHg for infarct, > 180 systolic for haemorrhage). A recent trial of careful BP lowering with the angiotensin-receptor blocker candesartan in patients with acute stroke and raised BP showed a trend to harm. Aspirin (300 mg) should be given as soon as primary haemorrhage is ruled out and then 75 mg is given daily (guidelines state 300 mg for the first 2 weeks but the evidence for this is not strong) via an NG tube or rectally if the patient is dysphagic.

Dispersing the thrombus

By 2004, 19 trials carried out over 15 years showed that thrombolytic therapy resulted in benefit in stroke. Intravenous rt-PA (recombinant tissue-type plasminogen) activator (alteplase) did better than streptokinase which had initially been used in heart attack. More patients suffered intracranial haemorrhage but overall fewer had severe disability at 3 months. Alteplase was approved by the US Food and Drug Administration (1996) and the UK Medicines Agency (2002) for treating acute ischaemic

Table 7.6 Outcome data in clinical practice (stroke register 14 countries n = 6,483) compared to intervention data from RCTs (*Lancet* 2007)

	SITS-MOST (% of cases)	RCTs (% of cases)
ICH at 7 days	7.3	8.6
3-month mortality	11.3	17.3
3-month complete recovery	38.9	42.3

SITS-MOST, Safe Implementation of Treatments in Stroke Monitoring Study; RCTs, randomized controlled trials.

stroke within 3 h of onset of symptoms. By 2005 there had been little uptake of thrombolysis in the UK because of practical problems including getting patients to hospital rapidly, performing a CT scan within the time frame, interpreting early scans and anxiety amongst physicians about the risk of poor outcomes. However, the 2008 guidelines (NICE 2008; RCP 2008), the development of stroke networks and making stroke targets a national priority have led to a dramatic increase in the availability of the treatment. A licensing condition for rt-PA was that all patients were put into a register and these data have been very useful. The SITS-MOST (Safe Implementation of Treatments in Stroke Monitoring Study) findings in 2007 were reassuring that the benefits seen in RCTs did translate into protocol-based clinical practice (Table 7.6). The time-window has been increased to within 4.5 h (but ideally as soon as possible).

Major criteria are:

- Age 18–80.
- Within 4.5 h of stroke onset.
- Haemorrhagic stroke excluded on CT.
- National Institutes of Health Stroke Scale (NIHSS) score 5–25 (very minor and very major strokes excluded).
- No stroke within preceding 3 months.
- No previous stroke with long-term damage.
- BP < 185/110.
- Not on anticoagulation (prior aspirin and clopidogrel OK).
- Consent/assent/best interests.

At an individual level, for 100 patients treated: 3 will have a worse outcome, 32 will benefit, i.e. rt-PA is 10× more likely to help than harm.

Give rt-PA in ED after CT (0.9 mg/kg up to a maximum of 90 mg, 10% as a bolus IV in 1–2 min and the rest infused over 1 h). Watch patient for at least 20 min as there is a risk of anaphylaxis. Aspirin is delayed for 24 h after thrombolysis.

Results in the over 80s

Although 80 is the upper age limit recommended for thrombolysis, a number of patients above this age have received rt-PA and the SITS data have been published. In this group (likely to have been offered treatment because of 'biological fitness') there was no increase in intracranial haemorrhage, but the outcomes were not as good as in younger patients.

Decompressive hemicraniectomy for severe middle cerebral artery (MCA) infarction is only offered to those under 60 years.

Vasodilatation and cerebral oedema

No convincing advantage has emerged from various trials of vasodilators, partly because the vessels in the infarcted zone are already maximally dilated. The same applies to various agents designed to relieve cerebral oedema. Trials of haemodilution have also been unsuccessful.

Neuroprotection

In a stroke there is a central zone of irreversibly damaged cells surrounded by a penumbra of ischaemic but potentially salvageable cells. These face a number of threats including oedema, the release of glutamate, aspartate and lactate, and an influx of calcium ions. The penumbral tissue increases its oxygen extraction (normally about 40%) from the available blood supply for a day or two after the event, indicating the time scale available for intervention. Trials of N-methyl-D-aspartate (NMDA) receptor blockers, which prevent the released glutamate from causing a toxic influx of calcium ions into the neurons, have been disappointing. This may be an example of poor extrapolation from animal work to the clinical situation: glutamate does kill neurons immediately after brain injury but preserves endangered neurons in the long term. The only way to provide neuroprotection with NMDA antagonists would be to administer them before the insult and for a very short period (minutes) after the injury, which is impossible in a clinical stroke, as opposed to an experimental model.

Management of haemorrhagic stroke

Intracerebral haemorrhage (ICH) commonly affects cerebral lobes, the basal ganglia, the thalamus, the brain stem (predominantly the pons) and the cerebellum. Vessels damaged by hypertension (at or near the bifurcation of small penetrating arteries) or cerebral amyloid angiopathy rupture. Oedema, inflammation, apoptosis and necrosis develop around the haematoma. Oedema increases in volume by about 75% in the first 24 h, peaks at around 5 days and lasts up to 14 days. There has been little improvement in outcomes. Trials of treatment have focused on:

- reducing the volume of the clot by
  - o improving haemostasis – vitamin K and prothrombin complex concentrate (Beriplex) if on warfarin, otherwise recombinant factor VII;
  - o lowering blood pressure < 180 mmHg systolic;
- attempting to maintaining cerebral perfusion, e.g. with mannitol;
- surgery to remove clots.

Unfortunately trial evidence of benefit is lacking and management remains supportive. Secondary prevention is similar to that for ischaemic stroke, but aspirin, warfarin and statins are generally avoided.

Hydration and nutrition

Post-stroke dysphagia is common (up to half of patients) and is associated with increased risk of aspiration pneumonia and poor outcomes related to disability, increased length of stay and death.

There are four situations in which taking fluid and nutrition becomes a problem:

1 The unconscious or drowsy patient (transient).
2 Pseudobulbar palsy due to bilateral stroke (often prolonged).
3 Brain stem stroke with bulbar involvement (sometimes prolonged).
4 The common hemisphere infarct (usually transient) (about 40% of cases).

The patient is usually 'nil-by-mouth' until their swallow has been assessed by a trained stroke nurse or speech and language therapist. Inadequate airway protection does not equate with an absent gag reflex, nor is the reverse true. The ability to swallow fluids is assessed by sitting the patient up and observing ability to swallow a teaspoon (5 mL), a tablespoon (15 mL) and then 50–100 mL of water. If the patient is unable to swallow, pooling occurs in the mouth. Choking and obvious aspiration may ensue, but some patients aspirate 'silently', which is where monitoring the oxygen saturation is helpful. Fluid and electrolytes are given intravenously. In a patient who is clearly doing very badly, artificial hydration may not be relevant. Fluid (usually about 1 L/day) may be given subcutaneously.

The decision must be taken whether to feed as well as to hydrate the persistently dysphagic patient. The usual practice is to give nutrition via a fine-bore NG tube at around 36 h after the stroke. The FOOD trial (Feed or Ordinary Diet Trials to assess Feeding Policy for Patients with Stroke) supported early NG tube feeding, but at the risk of increasing the proportion of survivors with poor outcome. NG tubes are easily dislodged; consider 'bridling'. If the swallow still fails to recover by 14 days a percutaneous endoscopic gastrostomy (PEG) tube may be considered. This procedure should not be undertaken lightly. Remember, the purpose of feeding tubes is to nourish and hydrate, not to protect the airway; they do not prevent aspiration of contaminated oral secretions or regurgitated gastric contents. This needs to be explained to many nurses as well as the family. Decisions about hydration and feeding are difficult ethically, particularly after a stroke. Always seek senior advice.

Information for the family and patient

Depending on the severity of the stroke the patient and/or the family need appropriate information. Their information needs will change with the clinical situation and the passage of time. Leaflets from a patient-based society such as the Stroke Association are very helpful.

Palliative care

If the patient is not doing well, the team should make a decision about whether to attempt cardiopulmonary resuscitation (CPR) in the event of cardiorespiratory arrest. This is a clinical decision based on the patient's condition. It may be possible to discuss this with the patient or find out from the family what they feel the patient would have wanted. In the context of a major stroke, CPR is most unlikely to be successful. If recovery is very poor, end-of-life decisions, such as the futility of repeated antibiotic treatment, should be discussed. If a patient continues to deteriorate, move to a palliative approach, e.g. Liverpool Care Pathway. See Chapter 17.

Rehabilitation

The first week of stabilization of the stroke is followed by 2–3 weeks of rapid recovery and then a further 6 months of slow but continuing improvement. The patient may only achieve a further 10% of recovery during this phase. The multidisciplinary aspects of rehabilitation are discussed in Chapter 3. Late rehabilitation also improves function.

The sequence of sitting, transferring, standing and walking may take a couple of months if the initial hemiparesis is severe. In general, proximal movements recover better than distal, and lower limbs more than upper. Visual problems may be helped by referral to an orthoptist. Prisms may be helpful for persistent diplopia and hemianopia and advice may be given about compensatory strategies. Depression is common after stroke, both initially and after discharge home when the elation at making it home is tempered with the reality of the residual handicap.

Primary and secondary prevention

This overlaps with prevention in IHD and is detailed in Table 7.1.

Indicators of poor outcome

- Significant preceding cognitive impairment.
- Severity of stroke, e.g. TACI.
- Admitted comatose.
- Delirium.
- Paralysis of conjugate gaze.
- Neglect, persistent visuospatial perceptual disorder.
- Homonymous hemianopia.
- Depression and other reasons for poor motivation.
- Persistent incontinence.
- Persistent dysphagia/needing PEG feeding at 1 month.
- No grip at 3 weeks – useful hand function unlikely.
- Significant associated pathology.

Driving after a stroke

After a TIA or stroke of any severity the patient must not drive for a month and should inform their insurance company. Driving may be resumed after 1 month if there is no residual deficit; if there is a deficit, the Driver and Vehicle Licensing Authority (DVLA) must be informed and formal assessment may be required. Cognitive and visual problems are more of a challenge than physical limitations which can be managed by adapting the car.

Information on discharge from hospital

Despite the fact that simple lifestyle changes can significantly cut the risk of a second stroke, the Healthcare Commission (2005) found that nearly half of stroke patients were not given any information about dietary changes and a third were not given advice about physical exercise. The risk of a recurrent stroke is around 35% within 5 years. Even moderate physical activity can reduce the risk of stroke by up to 27% and eating five portions of fruit and vegetables a day can cut the risk of stroke by

25%. Patients also need full information about their medication, out-of-hospital services, equipment including assistive technology, benefits, carers' services and local support groups.

 REFERENCES

Bamford J, Sandercock P, Dennis M, Burn J, Warlow C (1990) Classification and natural history of clinically identifiable subtypes of cerebral infarction. *Lancet* 337: 1521–1526.

Healthcare Commission (2005) *Survey of Patients; Stroke.* http://www.rsucardiff.org.uk/resource/HC.StrokePatientSurvery.2005.pdf.

Kase CS, Norrving B, Levine SR, et al. (1993) Cerebellar infarction. Clinical and anatomic observations in 66 cases. *Stroke* 24: 76–83.

Kearon C, O'Donnell M (2011) Should patients with stroke wear compression stockings to prevent venous thromboembolism? *Annals of Internal Medicine* 154: 506–507. http://www.annals.org/content/154/7/506.2.full.

NHS HTA (2011) Systematic review and economic evaluation of clopidogrel and modified-release dipyridamole for the prevention of occlusive vascular events (review of NICE TA 90). *Health Technology Assessment* 15 (31): 1–178.

NICE (2008) *Diagnosis and Initial Management of Acute Stroke and Transient Ischaemic Attack (TIA).* http://www.nice.org.uk/CG068.

NICE (2011) *Carotid Artery Stent Placement for Symptomatic Extracranial Carotid Stenosis.* http://www.nice.org.uk/guidance/IPG389/Guidance/pdf.

RCP (2008) *Royal College of Physicians National Clinical Guidelines for Stroke*, 3rd edn. http://bookshop.rcplondon.ac.uk/contents/6ad05aab-8400-494c-8cf4-9772d1d5301b.pdf.

 FURTHER INFORMATION

Cochrane Library: http://www2.cochrane.org/reviews/en/topics/93.html. For regularly updated stroke reviews.

Ford GA, Ahmed N, Azevedo E, et al. (2010) Intravenous alteplase for stroke in those older than 80 years old. *Stroke* 41: 2568–2574.

Langhorne P, Bernhardt J, Kwakkel G (2011) Stroke rehabilitation. *Lancet* 377: 1693–1702, doi: 10.1016/S0140-6736(11)60325-5.

Mant J, Hobbs FDR, Fletcher K, et al., on behalf of the BAFTA Investigators (2007) Warfarin versus aspirin for stroke prevention in an elderly community population with atrial fibrillation (the Birmingham Atrial Fibrillation Treatment of the Aged Study, BAFTA): a randomised controlled trial. *Lancet* 370 (9586): 493–503, doi: 10.1016/S0140-6736(07)61233-1.

Massachusetts medical students' website written with the American Stroke Association: http://www.umassmed.edu/strokestop.

McArthur KS, Quinn TJ, Dawson J, Walters MR (2011) Diagnosis and management of transient ischaemic attack and ischaemic stroke in the acute phase. *BMJ* 342, doi: 10.1136/bmj.d1938.

McArthur KS, Quinn TJ, Higgins P, Langhorne P (2011) Post-acute care and secondary prevention after ischaemic stroke. *BMJ* 342, doi: 10.1136/bmj.d2083.

Qureshi AI, Mendelow AD, Hanley DF (2009) Intracerebral haemorrhage. *Lancet* 373: 1632–1644, doi: 10.1016/S0140-6736(09)60371-8.

Rothwell PM, Algra A, Amarenco P (2011) Medical treatment in acute and long-term secondary prevention after transient ischaemic attack and ischaemic stroke. *Lancet* 377: 1681–1692, doi: 10.1016/S0140-6736(11)60516-3.

Stroke Association: http://www.stroke.org.uk/.

Stroke Association summary of the FOOD trials: http://www.stroke.org.uk/research/stroke_research_information/key_achievements/the_food_trial_.html.

Washington University School of Medicine: http://www.strokecenter.org/trials/. This has a record of trials in progress so you can see which drugs may make a clinical impact shortly.

8

Other diseases of the nervous system

Age changes and clinical examination

1 A full neurological examination can be an ordeal for both a frail elderly patient and their doctor. Patience and understanding are required by both and compromise will often be needed.
2 Much can be gained by simply observation. The patient's memory and speech during history taking and their ability to walk to and get on to the examination couch may give you clues to underlying pathology.
3 Ageing changes and co-morbidities, e.g. arthritis, may confuse the clinical picture. Gait becomes slower and less regular in pattern, with feet closer together, less firm heel strike and more time with both feet on the ground. The older the patient, the more difficult are the problems. One-third of 'normal' over 80 year olds have a shuffling gait and almost half have a flexed posture but most do not have PD.
4 Muscle wasting is common (usually proximal) due to disuse, especially in very elderly women, who may find it very difficult to rise from a chair without assistance. Thus chairs in out-patient clinics should have arms. Wasting of the small muscles of the hand does not automatically have the sinister connotations of the same finding in young subjects.
5 Reflexes may be difficult to elicit because of other pathologies, e.g. osteoarthritis, and ankle jerks in particular are difficult to elicit in almost 1/3 elderly people. Abdominal reflexes are almost universally absent.
6 Pupils are often small and react sluggishly, plus cataracts are common, so that examination of the fundi is often difficult (even after mydriasis).
7 Fine changes in sensation may be difficult to determine – moving from abnormal to normal is generally easier for patients to detect. Vibration sense is often lost or not understood, so position sense is usually a better test to employ (but fixed joints may make even this difficult).
8 Do be gentle with your patients if you want their cooperation. If necessary, break the CNS examination down into stages and do not expect perfection from yourself or your patient.

Symptomatic classification of neurological disease in the elderly

1 Headache:
  - Raised intracranial pressure, but fewer than 10% of patients with brain tumour present with headache alone.
  - Pain radiating from cervical spondylosis.
  - Giant-cell arteritis – tender temporal arteries, tenderness over proximal muscles, high ESR/CRP.

Lecture Notes Elderly Care Medicine, Eighth Edition. Claire G. Nicholl and K. Jane Wilson.
© 2012 John Wiley & Sons, Ltd. Published 2012 by John Wiley & Sons, Ltd.

- Psychological – but the prevalence of 'tension' headaches declines with age, consider depression.
- Paget's disease of the skull is occasionally painful when active – often obvious.
- Migraine, but new-onset is unusual over 50 years.

2 Pain in face:
- Trigeminal neuralgia – mean age of onset is around 50 years; it rarely starts in old age.
- Dental problems.
- Sinusitis.
- Giant-cell arteritis (pain on chewing).
- Post-herpetic neuralgia (look for post-inflammatory pigmentary change in a trigeminal dermatome).

3 Hemiparesis:
- Vascular disease.
- Space-occupying lesion.
- Unilateral PD.

4 Paraparesis:
- Cord compression – either vascular or space-occupying lesion.
- CSF infection.
- Guillain–Barré syndrome.
- Pressure from disc, bone or collection of pus.

5 Unsteadiness:
- Neuropathy.
- Proximal myopathy.
- Cerebellar disease.
- Drug-induced.
- Cerebrovascular disease.
- Middle-ear disease.
- Myxoedema.

6 Rigidity/immobility:
- PD.
- Drugs – especially phenothiazines.
- Disuse.
- Joint/bone problems.
- Spasticity of multi-infarct dementia.

7 Asymmetrical weakness:
- Nerve entrapment.
- Motor neurone disease (MND).
- Diabetes – mononeuritis.

8 Clouding of consciousness:
- Meningitis, encephalitis or sepsis at any site.
- Raised intracranial pressure.
- Drugs (sedatives, hypnotics).
- Biochemical disturbances.
- Delirium.
- Lewy body dementia.

9 Coma:
- Stroke (large lesions in the cerebral hemispheres, small lesions in the brain stem).
- Space-occupying lesion.
- Fits.
- Drugs (sedatives, hypnotics, alcohol).
- Poisoning (accidental – remember carbon monoxide, self-harm and iatrogenic).
- Biochemical disturbance (do not miss hypoglycaemia).

10 Involuntary movement:
- PD.
- Drugs (anti-Parkinsonian treatment, neuroleptics).
- Essential tremor.
- Vascular disease (in old age choreiform movements and hemiballismus are usually due to stroke).
- Epilepsy.
- Cerebellar disease.

Aetiological classification

Vascular disease

See Chapter 7 for stroke and multi-infarct disease.

Trauma

Fractured skull

Depressed fractures are important: pieces of bone may damage underlying cortex. Diplopia may indicate a fractured orbit. Fractures through a sinus or the ear may allow entry of organisms and lead to meningitis (prophylactic antibiotics are no longer recommended). Fracture through the temporal bone can result in an extradural haemorrhage. However, a routine X-ray of the skull after an uncomplicated fall is not justified. If an X-ray is done, fractures are hard to spot, but always look for a horizontal line indicating an air/fluid (blood) level.

Subdural haematoma

This is more common in old age because of increased frequency of falls and it is said that cerebral atrophy allows continued oozing of blood into the subdural space. A subdural may be asymptomatic, cause mild unilateral weakness, intellectual impairment, fits or loss of consciousness. A fluctuating course or disproportionate drowsiness in a patient with a hemiparesis may alert the clinician to this diagnosis. Increased use of anticoagulants in old age (e.g. AF) exposes more patients to the risk of subdural bleeding, especially if prone to fall or drinking to excess, or INR control is poor due to frequent changes in drug regime or poor compliance.

Diagnosis is confirmed by head CT. The hardest decision is whether to operate, and although the appearance of the blood alters with time, it can be hard to be precise about when the subdural haematoma developed. It is difficult to predict whether drainage will improve the clinical state, particularly in dementia. Find out as much as possible about the patient's prior functional performance from carers or relatives and discuss with a neurosurgeon.

Cord compression

Cord compression may be secondary to a prolapsed disc, pressure from tumour, osteophytes (especially cervical spondylosis) or collapsed vertebra (usually metastatic disease especially prostate cancer rather than osteoporosis), discitis (vertebral osteomyelitis) or an epidural abscess. A fall may be the precipitating event in a patient who had asymptomatic pathology. Plain X-rays are sometimes difficult to interpret, especially in the cervical spine, where degenerative changes are very common.

The motor effect of a cord lesion depends on the level. A very high neck lesion gives upper motor-neuron (UMN) signs in the arms and legs (spastic quadriparesis). Lower in the neck, compression leads to nerve root or lower motor-neuron (LMN) symptoms and signs in the arms but UMN changes in legs. A thoracic lesion will lead to a spastic paraparesis with UMN signs in the legs. A sensory level, if present, will help identify the region for further investigation; it is usually several segments below the level of cord compression. Patients with cervical and thoracic lesions often have an irritable bladder due to loss of supraspinal inhibition. Remember that the cord ends at L1/2 and the spinal roots (cauda equina) then continue down the spinal canal to their exit foramina. Lumbo-sacral lesions present with LMN signs and sensory loss. Urinary retention is common as the bladder does not empty. Check for anal tone and saddle anaesthesia (use a neurotip in the perianal area).

Sudden onset of compression of the cord or cauda equina is an emergency and rapid investigation is essential if active intervention (surgery or radiotherapy) is to avoid permanent damage. MRI is better than CT, but the latter may be more available.

Lumbar canal stenosis

This is usually due to a congenitally narrow spinal canal but presents in middle or old age when osteophytes or a disc encroach on the cauda equina. It may present with weak legs or intermittent pain in the buttocks and legs on walking. It can be distinguished from intermittent claudication (peripheral vascular disease) as patients find climbing stairs easier than walking on the flat (the spine is flexed), the discomfort takes longer – around 10 min – to improve with rest and there may be sensorimotor signs.

Normal pressure hydrocephalus (NPH)

NPH is exclusive to later life. Its cause is unknown, but it is assumed that when the condition is developing, abnormal CSF flow must at least sporadically increase the pressure. Its presentation is insidious, with a triad of intellectual failure, unsteadiness (with broad-based gait or gait apraxia) and early urinary incontinence. Diagnosis is made by CT, which will show enlarged ventricles without widened sulci. However, variation in the relative amounts of ventricular enlargement to cerebral atrophy in normal ageing and dementia make this a difficult diagnosis. By the time of diagnosis, the CSF pressure is 'normal'. Treatment by shunting may be successful. In specialist centres, external lumbar CSF drainage and flow studies are used to try to improve prediction of outcome.

The likelihood of identifying treatable NPH is low. Of 560 cases of dementia seen at the Mayo Clinic from 1990 to 1994, 1% had suspected NPH, but none of the 3/5 treated with ventriculoperitoneal shunting improved. In a small series with functional MRI before and after CSF drainage, motor function improved but cognition did not. Where there is benefit, subjects with short duration gait problems do best. A meta-analysis found that the mean rate of shunt complications (including death, infection, seizures, shunt malfunction and subdural haemorrhage) was 38%. Enthusiastic neurosurgeons continue to offer shunting and report good outcome data, but there is only one trial identified in PubMed and it is not clear if patients were randomized. Cochrane concludes that there is no evidence to support shunting.

Hydrocephalus may also be secondary to previous cerebral damage from episodes of bleeding (especially SAH) or meningitis. A strategically placed space-occupying lesion in the mid-brain may also lead to hydrocephalus.

Degenerative or idiopathic disease

Parkinson's disease (PD)

This is an idiopathic degenerative condition with progressive death of the dopaminergic neurons of the substantia nigra (SN) in the basal ganglia. Symptoms appear when around 80% of the dopamine has been lost and are due to a lack of dopamine and a relative excess of acetylcholine. PD is thought to occur in the genetically susceptible exposed to an environmental trigger, but the nature of both components remains unknown (chronic low-dose pesticide exposure remains an environmental favourite). Rare young-onset PD has a clearer genetic component and some of the gene defects are characterized. The post mortem finding of Lewy bodies (intracytoplasmic inclusion bodies containing alpha synuclein) restricted to the SN is pathognomonic (Figure 8.1). Many cases diagnosed in life, even by experts (perhaps 10%), are not confirmed as PD on post-mortem examination. The incidence increases with age (250 in 10^5 aged 60–69 to 2,000 in 10^5 aged over 80). Patients can be encouraged to donate their brain to the PD brain bank.

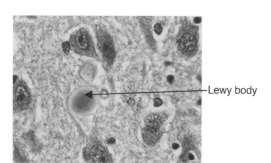

Figure 8.1 Immunohistochemistry for alpha-synuclein showing positive staining of an intraneuronal Lewy-body in the substantia nigra in Parkinson's disease (Marvin, http://commons.wikimedia.org/wiki/File: Lewy_Body_alphaSynuclein.jpg.)

Diagnosis

PD is always a difficult diagnosis in the early stages, especially in the very old, who may 'normally' have some features of extrapyramidal rigidity. The triad of classical symptoms and signs are poverty of movement (akinesia, bradykinesia), regular tremor at rest (5/sec, 'pill rolling') and rigidity of extrapyramidal type ('lead pipe') or cogwheel rigidity in the presence of tremor.

The tremor may be obvious, is usually a rest tremor and may be unilateral. It disappears in sleep. The bradykinesia may be apparent as paucity of facial expression (Parkinsonian facies) and fine movements are difficult, typically doing up buttons. Handwriting may get smaller during the course of a sentence (micrographia). Speech is soft (dysphonic), monotonous and becomes dysarthric. The stiffness may be misinterpreted as arthritis, and although PD does not affect the sensory system, the joint stiffness, particularly in bed at night, may be painful. The gait is characteristic with a flexed posture, tendency to shuffle, loss of arm swing and impaired postural reflexes, which make the patient likely to fall. Stopping, starting and turning pose most difficulty, and if a walking frame is needed, the wheeled type is usually recommended. As the disease progresses, constipation, bladder instability and drooling may be troublesome.

Documented response to therapy may be helpful in confirming the diagnosis, e.g. measuring the time to walk a set distance (10 m) or to carry out a tap test – the number of pronations and supinations the patient can achieve in a minute, tapping on a desk, or inspection of handwriting (micrographia should be seen to improve). Diagnosis is clinical, but a ^{123}I-FP-CIT-SPECT [single-photon emission computed tomography (SPECT) scan, which uses a cocaine analogue to image dopamine transporter receptors on the presynaptic nigrostriatal terminals, can distinguish PD (where the cells die so the amount of receptor falls) from essential tremor (appearance resembles healthy controls).

Management

All patients with PD benefit from a multidisciplinary package of care of which drug treatment is only one component. As the disease progresses, the relative emphasis of the components will change. Learn the following list – suitably modified, it will provide an outline of how to manage most chronic conditions at any age, from MS to COPD!

Management options include:

1 *Education and support* – encourage all patients and carers to join the Parkinson's Disease Society.
2 *Continuity of care* – chronic progressive diseases are best managed in settings promoting continuity of care to enable the patient and clinician to develop a working relationship and to assess the benefits and side-effects of treatment. In many areas there is a PD clinic run by a geriatrician, neurologist or both, often with a nurse specialist. The nurse may visit the patient at home and provide telephone advice between appointments.
3 *Therapy* – assessment and treatment:
   • Physiotherapy: work on posture, gait and falls prevention.
   • Occupational therapy: maintaining skills, home modification, etc.
   • Speech and language therapy: speech, facial expression, swallowing.
4 *Dietitian* – advice on maintaining nutrition and protein spacing (see Table 8.1).
5 *Assessment for benefits.*
6 *Legal advice* – lasting power of attorney, driving regulations and living will, etc.
7 *Maintenance of general health and fitness.*
8 *Treat other problems* – cataracts and in-growing toenails impair gait, refer appropriately.
9 Maintenance of *morale and mood* (consider complementary medicine, antidepressants; support from a clinical psychologist if available).

Drugs

Research is aimed at finding 'neuroprotective' drugs that prevent cell death. Increasing evidence suggests that in PD neurons die by apoptosis, which may be triggered by mitochondrial impairment and oxidative stress. Selegiline was thought to be neuroprotective but this is not the case. Several drugs now in trials have looked promising in animal studies. There is some evidence for benefit of co-enzyme Q10, a supplement available in health shops, but larger trials are needed.

Current drug treatment aims to restore transmitter balance in the basal ganglia. Whilst the classes of drugs available are logical (Figure 8.2), the order in which they are used varies not only with the patient but also with the prescriber, i.e. the weight of evidence does not clearly support one course of action. Details of drugs used in the management of PD are given in Table 8.1. Assuming the diagnosis is correct, levodopa preparations usually provide excellent benefits initially, but over a few years the 'long-term levodopa syndrome' emerges. Problems may be predictable at first. For example, soon after a dose there may be involuntary movements (peak-dose dyskinesia), and as the next dose becomes due, the effect of the previous dose may wear off so that the patient becomes rigid, immobile and frozen or 'off'. These effects can be ameliorated by careful juggling of doses and timing, but eventually the fluctuations can become severe, apparently random and the patient may alternate between being 'on' for short periods only, with 'offs' and disabling dyskinesias. There is some evidence that the duration or dose × years of levodopa treatment affects the development of this syndrome, perhaps because of pulsatile stimulation of the receptors. Long-acting agonists are another option for initial treatment and may be favoured in younger patients. There are two groups of agonists, ergot and non-ergot derived, but a range of emerging and serious idiosyncratic reactions have almost stopped new prescriptions of the ergot family. In frail older people, if PD is already impacting on function, many doctors start with levodopa. In this group, the dose of levodopa is often limited by neuropsychiatric problems (confusion, hallucinations). Younger patients tolerate bigger doses without confusion, but dyskinesias tend to become more troublesome with time. The development of a transdermal drug delivery system is an attractive option. However, local skin reactions are common with rotigotine, the first patch to be available.

Notes on drug management

Treat nausea with domperidone. Combination preparations may help compliance, e.g. levodopa and carbidopa plus entacapone (Stalevo). If a neuroleptic is needed use quetiapine; clozapine appears best but has restricted prescription. Whenever any other dopaminergic agent is added to levodopa, reduce the dose of levodopa. If a PD patient is nil by mouth for any reason other than 'gut failure' use a nasogastric tube to keep giving the drugs. After abdominal surgery a rotigotine patch may be useful until the gut can be used. All dopaminergic drugs should be withdrawn gradually to avoid neuroleptic malignant syndrome (life-threatening fever, unstable BP and rigidity).

Table 8.1 Drug management of Parkinson's disease

Mechanism	Name	Prescription tips (see BNF section 4.9)
Replenish striatal dopamine	Levodopa with peripheral dopa-decarboxylase inhibitor as Sinemet® (co-careldopa) or Madopar® (co-beneldopa)	Start low, increase slowly balancing response with side-effects, with meals initially to reduce nausea, later before meals as drug competes for absorption with amino acids from a protein meal. Can use slow-release preparation from the start (but little benefit) or to cover the night; dispersible preparation if swallowing a problem. About 85% of patients respond to levodopa
	Duodopa®	Direct duodenal infusion of levodopa (see text)
Catechol-O-methyltransferase inhibitor (COMTI)	Entacapone, tolcapone	Entacapone, used with levodopa to reduce end of dose deterioration, may colour the urine red. Tolcapone only used if entacapone unsuitable as tolcapone occasionally causes severe hepatotoxicity
Monoamine-oxidase-B inhibitor (MAO-BI)	Selegiline, rasagiline	Used as early monotherapy or with levodopa to reduce end of dose deterioration. Concern (inconclusive) that selegiline increased mortality led to sublingual preparation to avoid first-pass, reducing amphetamine-related metabolites. Give in the morning as a mild stimulant. Rasagiline, once a day, may be better as metabolites are not amphetamines
Dopamine agonists	Increase dose slowly as hypotension can occur in the first few days. The therapeutic effect is mediated via the D2 receptor; other effects depend partly on their activity at other dopaminergic receptors and whether they are derived from ergot	
	Ergoline family: • lisuride • pergolide • cabergoline	Rarely used in new patients
	Non-ergoline: • ropinerole • pramipexole • rotigotine • apomorphine	Ropinerole and pramipexole licensed for monotherapy or with levodopa. Eye checks recommended with pramipexole so ropinerole gaining market share. Rotigotine patch for monotherapy in early PD. Apomorphine used subcutaneously; via a pen or pump under specialist supervision for intractable fluctuations
Antimuscarinic drugs	Orphenadrine, benzatropine, procyclidine, trihexphenidyl	Little to choose between drugs. Rarely used in elderly as worsen cognition, GI side-effects and urine retention. Used for drug-induced PD, tremor and may help drooling

All dopaminergic drugs and advanced PD itself can cause sudden sleepiness, so warn drivers. A minority of PD patients develop compulsive behaviours while receiving dopamine-replacement therapy, including pathological gambling, binge eating, hyperlibidinous behaviour and punding (aimless repetitive behaviour) and may need to have the dose reduced at the expense of motor function.

Non-motor features of PD

Associated problems relating to bladder, bowels, digestion, sleep and mood often complicate PD. These features were thought to be secondary to

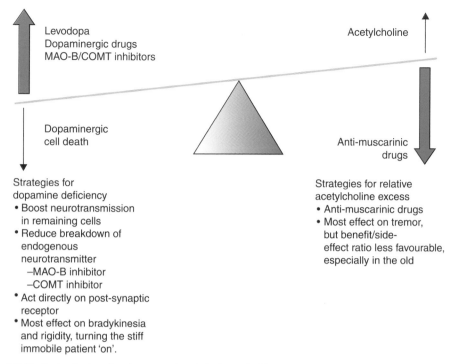

Figure 8.2 Strategies for treating the transmitter imbalance in PD.

chronic disability but several studies have shown that the paravertebral sympathetic ganglia, the enteric system and the epicardium are affected by synuclein pathological changes in early PD; i.e. these are non-motor features of PD.

- Olfactory dysfunction.
- Neuropsychiatric – the most significant complication of PD is the associated dementia, which is common in elderly patients. Depression is also common and psychosis may result from the dementia, depression or the drugs. Rivastigmine may be helpful. Confusion may limit the patient's ability to continue with levodopa treatment.
- Autonomic disturbance is common with dysphagia, drooling, bowel dysfunction (including constipation), weight loss, bladder dysfunction, sexual dysfunction, postural hypotension and excessive sweating.
- Sleep disturbance (hypersomnolence) is not just a consequence of difficulty turning over in bed due to nocturnal akinesia. Other factors include rapid eye movement sleep behaviour disorder, restless legs syndrome and inverted sleep–wake cycle.

Pain is secondary to immobility and dystonia. Falls, osteomalacia and osteoporosis add to the disability.

The life expectancy of people with PD has improved but the terminal stages are distressing, the patient being robbed of mobility, cognitive function, swallowing and sphincter control. Enormous amounts of support to both carers and patients are required at this distressing stage.

Trials continue apace, to evaluate non-drug management (e.g. the use of Wii-fit), to compare currently available drugs and look at new therapies. Promising drugs include:

- Droxidopa, an orally active synthetic precursor of norepinephrine for the treatment of orthostatic hypotension.
- Preladenant, an adenosine A2A receptor agonist.
- Pimavanserin, a 5-HT(2A) inverse agonist for L-dopa-induced psychosis.
- Smilagenin (Cogane), an orally active, non-peptide neurotrophic factor inducer that crosses the blood–brain barrier.

Invasive treatment in PD

More invasive forms of treatment are offered in specialist centres but are not usually recommended for/available to frail older patients.

- **Intra-duodenal infusion.** When motor fluctuations become disabling deliver levodopa/carbidopa gel (Duodopa) directly into the duodenum over 24 h via a PEG with a long tube into the duodenum and a portable pump. This is relatively easy to insert but prone to problems with the delivery system and is very expensive.

- **Neurosurgery.** Pallidotomy saw a resurgence in the 1990s but has largely been replaced by deep brain stimulation (DBS).
- **Deep brain stimulation.** DBS, particularly of the subthalamic nuclei, is useful for biologically fit patients with disabling motor fluctuations or intractable tremor refractory to optimal medical treatment. (NB: Patients with electrodes in situ must have bipolar not unipolar diathermy during surgery to avoid heat trauma to the brain.)
- **Transplantation** with foetal adrenal tissue did not fulfil expectations but may eventually become a reality with cultured cells, once fundamental issues such as how to 'turn off' dopamine production from transplanted cells have been solved; initial trials where the grafts 'took' produced ghastly results due to dopamine excess.
- **Nerve growth factor infusions.** Trials infusing glial cell-line derived nerve growth factor (GDNF) were stopped amid controversy as to whether brain damage resulted.
- **Gene therapy.** Early studies of the glial cell-derived neurotrophic factor analogue neurturin were encouraging but benefit was not confirmed in larger trials. However, the randomized controlled trial of bilateral delivery of AAV2-GAD (glutamic acid decarboxylase, which makes GABA inserted into an adeno-associated virus that readily infects humans but does not cause disease) in the subthalamic nucleus compared with sham surgery in patients with advanced PD shows promise in terms of safety and efficacy. ProSavin, another gene therapy approach, is designed to deliver three key enzymes directly into the brain – AADC (aromatic amino acid decarboxylase), TH (tyrosine hydroxylase) and CH1 (GTP-cyclohydrolase 1) – to trigger cells to produce dopamine.

Parkinsonian syndromes

Causes of Parkinsonian syndromes are as follows:

1 *Drugs* – the most frequent being the neuroleptics, the saddest of which is prochloperazine; Parkinsonism is a devastating sequel to a usually ineffectual prescription for 'dizziness'. Some patients with drug-induced Parkinsonism have subclinical nigral pathology which becomes clinically evident when dopamine blockers are prescribed. Imaging of dopamine transporter receptors with SPECT can help to identify such patient; if the SPECT scan is abnormal the patient will respond to levodopa therapy.

2 *Virus* – post-encephalitic.

3 *Toxins* – contaminated illegal drugs – MPTP (1-methyl-4-phenyl-1,2,3,4-tetrahydropyridine) and, more worryingly, case reports associated with Ecstasy.

4 *Trauma* – as in ex-boxers.

5 *Vascular disease* – the final stage of multi-infarct dementia, i.e. rigidity with dementia. The gait is shuffling (*marche à petits pas*) but without the forward shift of the centre of gravity seen in PD, sometimes referred to as 'lower body Parkinsonism'.

Parkinsonism often responds badly to standard PD treatments, which may cause adverse effects, e.g. increased confusion and falls secondary to postural hypotension.

Conditions allied to PD

Essential tremor (ET)

ET is one of the most common neurological disorders (seen in about 5% of over 65 s). It is characterized by postural tremor, which worsens with movement and stress. It can be mistaken for the pill-rolling tremor of PD but other Parkinsonian features are absent. It used to be tagged 'benign' to distinguish it from the progressive course of PD, but it can be disabling and embarrassing. Some cases are familial. It may respond to small doses of alcohol, beta-blockers (non-selective, e.g. propranolol, are best), low dose primidone or topiramate. LINGO1 is a candidate gene and has reopened the historical debate as to whether there is an overlap between ET and PD (there probably is as both are probably heterogeneous syndromes).

Restless legs (Ekbom's syndrome)

This is characterized by a profound desire to move the legs and motor restlessness, which is worse at night. There is a familial trend. The dopamine agonists ropinirole and pramipexole taken before bed are now licensed for severe cases; there is also some evidence of efficacy for pregabalin.

Dementia with Lewy bodies

This is a syndrome in which Parkinsonism overlaps with features of AD and psychiatric phenomena (see Chapter 4). Brain pathology shows Lewy bodies identical to those in PD but scattered throughout the cortex.

Progressive supranuclear palsy (PSP)

PSP (Steele–Richardson–Olszewki syndrome) is extrapyramidal rigidity of rapid onset, with paralysis of eye movement (initially upward gaze but not specific until other eye movements are involved). There is marked instability and frequent falls, pseudobulbar swallowing and speech difficulties and dementia.

Multiple-system atrophy (MSA)

MSA (formerly Shy–Drager syndrome) can be misdiagnosed as PD but at onset rigidity and autonomic features are more prominent, tremor is rare and response to levodopa is very poor. The only intervention is to maintain postural BP (avoid diuretics and hypotensives, keep hydrated, try TEDS, head-up tilt in bed, caffeine, fludrocortisone and midodrine).

Corticobasal degeneration (CBD)

CBD is characterized by progressive nerve cell loss and atrophy of multiple areas of the brain including the cerebral cortex and the basal ganglia and typically presents in the 60s. Symptoms may be unilateral at first and include poor coordination, akinesia, rigidity and dystonia. It can cause an alien limb, usually the arm, which feels 'foreign' to its owner and has observable involuntary movement. Cognitive and visio–spatial impairments, apraxia, hesitant speech, myoclonus and dysphagia develop and the patient becomes bed bound.

Motor neuron disease (MND)

MND is a rapidly progressive fatal neurological disease of unknown aetiology producing paralysis of limb, swallowing and breathing muscles. The average time to diagnosis is around 17 months and from diagnosis to death 14 months. It usually presents in 6th and 7th disease and may be misdiagnosed initially in older people who more commonly have MND mimics:

- benign fasciculation (cramps) increase with age,
- UMN lesions can be commonly due to vascular disease,
- cervical radiculomyelopathy gives UMN and LMN signs (but sensory signs too),
- cervical myelopathy and unrelated peripheral neuropathy (but sensory signs too).

Most cases are sporadic, but around 5% are familial. In about a fifth of those the gene defect is in the superoxidase dismutase 1 gene. In MND, cognition usually remains normal, sensory changes are absent and sphincter control is retained. However, a small group develops a frontotemporal dementia (FTD). Identification of the same cytoplasmic inclusions in FTLD and some cases of familial and sporadic amyotrophic lateral sclerosis (ALS), with mutations in a pair of DNA/RNA-binding proteins called TDP-43 and FUS/TLS, make this the most promising area for a breakthrough in understanding the pathogenesis (see p. 59).

MND tends to be focal in onset affecting:

- Limb muscles (70%):
  - ALS is commonest form with mixed UMN and LMN
  - pure UMN presentation, primary lateral sclerosis.
  - pure LMN presentation, progressive muscular atrophy.
- Bulbar muscles (25%): speech deteriorates before swallow, bulbar and pseudobulbar (emotional lability) features.
- Respiratory muscles (5%).

There is no specific diagnostic test, but findings on electromyogram/nerve conduction studies (EMG/NCS) may be very suggestive. Muscle CK can be elevated (muscle damage from denervation), but this is too non-specific to be diagnostic.

Patients usually present with asymmetrical weakness of the hands or foot drop and examination reveals brisk reflexes in a wasted fasciculating limb. Those with predominantly distal signs affecting legs and mobility tend to have slower progression of their disease.

The management is supportive and multidisciplinary and advance planning is important. Two interventions have proven benefit. Patients with good quality of life and bulbar function should be referred for:

- Non-invasive ventilation, which has been shown to improve quality of life measures and give a median survival benefit of 7 months.

- Riluzole (a glutamate release inhibitor) which decreases firing of the motor neurons and prolongs the time to ventilation but is of limited benefit (improves median survival by 2–3 months).

Those with a bulbar presentation fare much less well, especially with the onset of speech and swallowing problems, of which the patient is only too aware. Such patients should be considered for early PEG to maintain nutrition and hydration. The patient will normally be able to be fully involved in deciding on such a course of management. Many areas have specialist nurses who can greatly improve symptom control and provide education and support. The MND website has excellent information sheets for professionals, e.g. tackling excess saliva (sialorrhoea) and for the patient covering difficult areas such as 'How will I die?'

Epilepsy in old age

Epilepsy has a bimodal age curve, with a high incidence in infants and then a sustained rise from middle age, exceeding that in children (children and adolescents up to 100 in 10^5 a year; aged 30–55 about 30 in 10^5; rising to 150 in 10^5 aged over 70 years).

Causes of fits in the elderly include:

- Stroke disease – commonest cause (up to 50%), usually 3–12 months after the event, higher risk after haemorrhagic stroke.
- Tumours (5%), primary brain tumours, metastases – in > 40% the first presentation of the cancer.
- Trauma following head injury, contusion or subdural haematoma.
- Primary dementias, e.g. AD.
- Drugs or alcohol (excess or withdrawal).
- Other causes: sepsis, pyrexia, biochemical disturbance.

Fits occurring in old age are usually partial seizures with a single focus of activity due to scar tissue following a stroke, and may be simple partial (no impairment of consciousness), most commonly, complex partial (in which consciousness is impaired) or a partial seizure which proceeds to generalized tonic clonic seizures. A temporal lobe focus and hence features such as olfactory auras and automatisms are less common.

Management

Investigate for an underlying cause. An EEG can support a diagnosis of epilepsy but cannot rule it out as the yield of specific epileptiform activity is less than half that in a younger population. MRI scanning is preferred to CT where available. In younger adults it is usual to treat only after a second fit. Treatment is usually started after a single unprovoked fit in an elderly person as underlying brain damage is likely. Care is needed with antiepileptic drugs (AEDs); monotherapy is preferred, as elderly patients are more susceptible to adverse effects (including cognitive impairment and ataxia). Carbamazepine or sodium valproate were the traditional first-line drugs, but levetiracetam (Keppra) and lamotrigine both have better continuation rates at 1 year and the patient is more likely to be fit free. Check the rest of the patient's medication; some drugs increase the chances of a fit and the older AEDs have many interactions. Avoid ciprofloxacin for a post-fit chest infection because it is epileptogenic, as is tramadol, and care is needed with antidepressants. Rectal diazepam or buccal midazolam are recommended for urgent treatment of prolonged or recurrent fits in the community.

Fits may result in injury such as fractures because of underlying osteoporosis, and recovery may be prolonged by postictal symptoms especially confusion and focal weakness lasting for 24 h and occasionally days (Todd's paresis). The psychological and social consequences are at least as great as in younger patients. Patients and their families need a full explanation and education; this is best managed by an epilepsy specialist nurse as part of a team. Think about safety at home – open fires should be guarded. Check whether advice on driving is relevant – do not assume that your patient is a non-driver.

Status epilepticus (SE)

SE is a medical emergency with significant morbidity and mortality (> 80 years mortality of at least 50% of cases). The definition of SE is more than 30 min of either continuous seizure activity or intermittent seizures without full recovery of consciousness between seizures. SE has a twofold increased incidence in the elderly and co-morbidity may complicate therapy and worsen prognosis. Acute or previous stroke is the most common aetiology. Non-convulsive SE (NCSE) has a wide range of clinical presentations, ranging from confusion to obtundation. It occurs commonly in elderly patients who are critically ill and in the setting of coma. EEG is the only reliable method of diagnosing NCSE. The goal is to stop the fit activity as soon as possible. Usual treatment is intravenous lorazepam, followed by phenytoin, but if treatment fails, refer to intensive care for consideration of a general anaesthetic agent.

Infective diseases of the CNS

Meningitis

Less than 10% of cases but over 50% of deaths occur in the elderly. Delay in diagnosis occurs because the symptoms are more vague, and signs, especially neck stiffness, are difficult to interpret because of the frequency of cervical spondylosis. Examination of the CSF is essential, but only perform a lumbar puncture after CT scan (papilloedema is frequently absent in elderly patients with raised intracranial pressure, and fundoscopy is often difficult because of eye pathology).

Pneumococcus and listeria are common in old age and other atypical organisms must always be considered. In the White population in the UK, tuberculous meningitis is more common in the elderly than in the middle aged. Ceftriaxone plus amoxicillin (to cover listeria) with dexamethasone is appropriate empirical treatment for bacterial meningitis until culture or PCR results are available. Steroids should not be given in septic shock and should be stopped if the LP suggests viral meningitis, when aciclovir should be started.

Encephalitis

Headache, fever and malaise are followed by focal signs, fits and coma. Herpes simplex and zoster (particularly when a cranial dermatome is involved in shingles) are the most common causes. Consider the possibility early, as acyclovir is most effective when used without delay. EEG is helpful if it shows focal abnormalities particularly in the temporal lobes.

Guillain–Barré syndrome (GBS)

This often occurs 1–3 weeks after a viral infection (respiratory or gut, especially *Campylobacter jejuni*) and usually takes the form of a rapidly ascending polyneuropathy. Although it is relatively rare it was the first condition where carbohydrate mimicry between the human ganglioside GM1 and the *C. jejuni* lipo-oligosaccharide was shown to induce the production of pathogenic autoantibodies and the development of GBS.

The commonest pattern in Europe and North America is acute inflammatory demyelinating polyradiculoneuropathy (AIDP). In other areas, an axonal neuropathy is most common. Motor features (flaccid paralysis with reduced reflexes) dominate but there may be some sensory involvement. By the third week of the illness, 90% of patients are at their weakest. Investigations include LP (CSF is usually cellular with high protein) and NCS. Treatment consists of support, intravenous immunoglobulin, and plasma exchange and ventilation if respiratory muscles are involved. The Miller Fisher variant is characterized by paralysis of the eye muscles, areflexia and ataxia; a characteristic antibody anti-GQ1b IgG is present. If the initial progressive phase lasts longer than 6 weeks, this is termed 'chronic', i.e. chronic inflammatory demyelinating polyradioculoneuropathy (CIDP). Steroids may be useful.

Poliomyelitis

New cases are very rare in the UK because of the polio vaccination programme but you will see older people with the sequelae – usually a flaccid wasted weak leg with absent reflexes (pathology is damage to the anterior horn cells). If the damage occurred in the teens or younger the limb may be small and an ankle-foot orthosis (AFO) is often worn for foot drop. About half the survivors (now mainly from the epidemics in the 1940s and 1950s) will develop the post-polio syndrome (PPS), which begins 30–40 years after the acute illness and is slowly progressive. Common problems include fatigue, cold intolerance, joint deterioration with pain, new weakness, muscle pain and atrophy, dysphagia and dysphonia, sleep apnoea and respiratory failure. The aetiology is unclear, but premature exhaustion of the new sprouts that developed after acute poliomyelitis appears most likely. Treatment is primarily supportive, although non-fatiguing strengthening exercise may improve strength over the short term. Drugs have not been beneficial in controlled trials.

Herpes zoster

Herpes zoster (shingles) is a reactivation of the varicella virus, which has lain dormant in the dorsal root ganglia since an earlier attack of chicken pox. Patients do not catch shingles from other people with varicella or shingles, but a susceptible person can catch chicken pox from someone with active shingles. Patients with shingles are isolated in hospital to protect care staff. Shingles is said to afflict the debilitated and immunosuppressed and may involve a dermatome where there is spinal disease. By the age of 85 years, 50% of people will have had shingles.

Clinical features

- Pain in the distribution of the dorsal root with paraesthesia and hyperaesthesia usually preceding the rash by a couple of days, although the illness may be painless.
- The characteristic rash, like that of varicella, follows the sequence papules–vesicles–pustules–crusts, and then ceases to be infectious. The dermatome affected is thoracic in over 50% of cases but is trigeminal in 10–15% and, less commonly, the geniculate ganglion (Ramsay–Hunt syndrome), where a Bell's palsy may be the first manifestation.
- Anteriorly, the rash does not cross the mid-line, but posteriorly it follows the posterior primary ramus a few centimetres across the spinous processes. Sometimes more than one adjacent dermatome is involved but it is very seldom bilateral.
- Less common complications include muscle wasting in the relevant segment, an internal rash in the same segment (e.g. the bladder), a mixed varicella–zoster eruption, meningoencephalitis and eye involvement.

Management

Management involves attention to hydration and general health, plus aciclovir 800 mg five times daily by mouth or, particularly in the immuno-compromised, intravenously, in the weakly evidence-based hope of minimizing the likelihood of post-herpetic neuralgia. Prednisolone 40 mg may be given, again with weak evidence. The advantage of famciclovir is that it can be given once daily. The pain may be severe and appropriate analgesia should be given.

Ophthalmic zoster

This requires urgent ophthalmological referral in case of corneal ulceration and with a view to local atropine, idoxuridine and/or aciclovir.

Post-herpetic neuralgia

Continued burning neuropathic pain for months or years afflicts more than half of elderly patients following an attack of shingles. It is often severe, debilitating and intractable. It responds better to tricyclic antidepressants, gabapentin, pregabalin, topical capsaicin or lidocaine patches than to conventional analgesics.

Malignant disease

Intracranial neoplasms

Metastases are more common than cerebral primaries. In 50% of cases, cerebral metastases are solitary. Primary lesions may be amenable to surgery, radiotherapy or chemotherapy, depending on site and nature – advice will be needed from the neuro-oncology multidisciplinary team.

Cerebral metastases are most commonly from lung or breast. Palliative treatment with dexamethasone will often be beneficial in both untreatable primaries and secondaries. The window of symptom relief will be of value to both the patient and their families and help them come to terms with the prognosis.

Non-metastatic disease of the CNS

This is important in older patients (see further information at end of chapter) and may take the form of:

1 Cerebellar syndrome.
2 Peripheral neuropathy.
3 Myasthenic syndrome.

Deficiency/toxicity states

The B group of vitamins maintains neurological integrity. Deficiencies can have central effects, e.g. dementia, and peripheral effects, e.g. neuropathy. Neurological complications may arise before other systems are affected, e.g. subacute combined degeneration of the cord may precede a macrocytic anaemia. In B_{12} deficiency, the findings depend on whether the spinal cord degeneration (pyramidal tracts and dorsal columns 'combined') or neuropathy dominates.

Always consider deficiency states (including myxoedema) as they can be easily confirmed and treated. The 'tea and toast' diet may produce a normal weight but is short of vitamins and minerals. Toxicity and deficiencies may occur together, as in alcohol abuse. Alcohol is a neurotoxin (central and peripheral) and many alcoholics have a poor diet and malabsorption with multiple nutritional deficiencies including vitamins B_1 (thiamine), B_2 (riboflavin), B_3 (niacin), B_6 (pyridoxine) and C, magnesium, zinc and folate.

Diabetes can be included in this section as a cause of peripheral neuropathy, either symmetrical or in the form of mononeuritis multiplex.

Drugs should also be included as a cause for many neurological conditions, e.g.:

o Parkinsonism – secondary to neuroleptics.
o Ataxia – secondary to anticonvulsant toxicity.
o Tardive dyskinesia – secondary to neuroleptics.
o Peripheral neuropathy – especially antineoplastic drugs, occasionally statins, nitrofurantoin, colchicine, amiodarone.
o Fits – drugs that lower the fit threshold include ciprofloxacin, tramadol, antidepressants.

Previous surgery may also be relevant, e.g. thyroidectomy, gastrectomy or ileal resection, the latter two leading to B_{12} malabsorption.

Neuropathies

Neuropathies can be axonal or demyelinating and affect motor or sensory function or both (see Figure 8.3). Axonal degeneration is a dying-back process affecting longest large diameter fibres first (hence glove and stocking) whereas demyelination can occur anywhere along the nerve and is more patchy. Small fibre neuropathies affect pain, temperature and autonomic function.

The list of possible causes of a neuropathy is very long but more common causes include:

• Diabetes:
   o Diabetic sensorimotor polyneuropathy (DSPN) is chronic, symmetrical, length-dependent and caused by microvascular damage reflecting total hyperglycaemic exposure. It occurs with retinopathy and nephropathy.
   o Diabetic autonomic neuropathy (DAN) can occur in impaired glucose tolerance and may affect the cardiovascular, gastrointestinal and urogenital systems. Impaired sweating with dry feet is a factor in foot ulceration.
• Alcohol.
• Paraneoplastic
• Vitamin deficiencies.
• Drugs.
• Paraprotein-associated
• Hypothyroidism.
• Vasculitis.
• Post-inflammatory:
   o acute – GBS (commonest acute onset)
   o chronic – CIDP
• Hereditary motor and sensory neuropathy (HSMN) (Charcot–Marie–Tooth disease) is an inherited peripheral neuropathy with two forms:
   o Type 1 – demyelinating, affecting the glia-derived myelin.
   o Type 2 – axonal. Type 2 D is caused by mutations in glycyl–tRNA synthetase (GARS), the first tRNA synthetase gene to be linked to a disease.
The two forms can be distinguished by means of electrophysiological or neuropathological studies. Inheritance can be autosomal dominant, recessive or X-linked. HSMN is characterized by distal symmetrical polyneuropathy, with slowly progressive weakness and atrophy (particularly peroneal muscular atrophy) resulting in foot drop, secondary steppage gait and pes cavus. The presentation and course are variable.

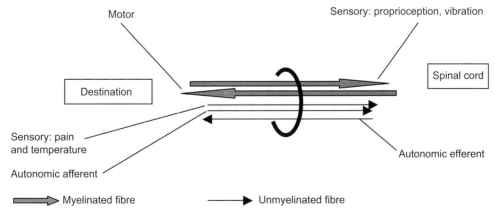

Figure 8.3 Peripheral nerve.

Entrapment neuropathies

Carpal tunnel syndrome

This is due to compression of the median nerve in the wrist. Look for reduced sensation over the lateral palm splitting the ring finger, wasting of the thenar eminence and weakness of abductor pollicis brevis. Steroid injections may give temporary relief, but if there are signs of nerve damage, refer for NCS and then surgery.

Meralgia paraesthetica

This is not serious, but if you recognize it, the patient will be grateful for the reassurance! It is entrapment of the lateral cutaneous nerve of the thigh under the inguinal ligament, commonly in the obese, resulting in numbness and tingling in the anterolateral thigh.

➡ FURTHER INFORMATION

Arain AM, Abou-Khali BW (2009) Management of new-onset epilepsy in the elderly. *Nature Reviews Neurology* 5: 363–371, doi: 10.1038/nrneurol.2009.74.

British Epilepsy Association website – Epilepsy Action: http://www.epilepsy.org.uk/. Clinical trials in PD: http://www.clinicaltrials.gov/ct2/home.

Esmonde T, Cooke S (2002) *Shunting for Normal Pressure Hydrocephalus (NPH) (Cochrane Review)*. The Cochrane Library, Issue 3. Update Software Ltd, Oxford. DOI: 10.1002/14651858. CD003157. Still considered current in 2008 – there is still no further review.

Johnston A, Smith PEM (2010) Epilepsy in the elderly. *Expert Review Neurotherapy* 10: 1899–1910. http://www.medscape.com/viewarticle/733423

Ferrara JM, Stacy M (2008) Impulse-control disorders in Parkinson's disease. *CNS Spectrum* 13: 690–698.

Guillain–Barré Society website: http://www.gbs.org.uk/index2.shtml.

Kiernan MC, Vucic S, Cheah BC, et al. (2011) Amyotrophic lateral sclerosis. *Lancet* 377: 942–955, doi: 10.1016/S0140-6736(10)61156-7.

Lagier-Tourenne C, Polymenidou M, Cleveland DW (2010) TDP-43 and FUS/TLS: emerging roles in RNA processing and neurodegeneration. *Human Molecular Genetics* 19 (R1): R46–R64, doi: 10.1093/hmg/ddq137.

LeWitt PA, Rezai AR, Leehey MA, et al. (2011) AAV2-*GAD* gene therapy for advanced Parkinson's disease: a double-blind, sham-surgery controlled, randomised trial. *Lancet Neurology* 10: 309–319.

Louis ED (2009) The essential tremors: a family of neurodegenerative disorders? *Archives of Neurology* 66: 1202–1208, doi: 10.1001/archneurol.2009.217.

Morley JF, Hurtig HI (2010) Current understanding and management of Parkinson disease: five new things. *Neurology* 75 (18 Suppl 1): S9–15.

Motor Neurone Disease Association website: http://www.mndassociation.org/index.html, http://www.mndassociation.org/for_professionals/for_gps/index.html.

National Institute of Neurological Disorders and Stroke website: http://www.ninds.nih.gov/. A fantastic website with patient-friendly (hence student-friendly) material on a whole variety of neurological diseases you didn't know existed as well as the standard topics.

NICE Guidelines for Epilepsy in Adults 2004: http://www.nice.org.uk/CG020adultsquickrefguide.

NICE Guidelines (RCP) for PD 2006: http://www.nice.org.uk/guidance/CG35/guidance/pdf/English.

Schmader KE, Baron R, Haanpää ML, et al. (2010) Treatment considerations for elderly and frail patients with neuropathic pain. *Mayo Clinic Proceedings* 85 (3 Suppl): S26–32. A good review of the problems of evidence-based prescribing in the aged.

Shprecher D, Schwalb J, Kurlan R (2008) Normal pressure hydrocephalus: diagnosis and treatment. *Current Neurological Neuroscience Report* 8: 371–376.

Wu Y, Le W, Jankovic J (2011) Preclinical biomarkers of Parkinson disease. *Archives of Neurology* 68: 22–30, doi: 10.1001/archneurol.2010.321.

9

Cardiovascular disorders

Age changes

1 Loss of cardiac myocytes secondary to apoptosis, with compensatory hypertrophy of remaining cells.
2 Accumulation of intracellular lipofuscin and extracellular amyloid.
3 Increased intercellular collagen, leading to reduced LV diastolic compliance.
4 Loss of pacemaker cells in the sino-atrial node, causing sinus bradycardia and predisposing to sick sinus syndrome.
5 Patchy fibrosis of the conduction system leading to increased incidence of first degree heart block and bundle branch block.
6 Reduced responsiveness of arteries to β adrenergic stimulation, which reduces the capacity for vasodilatation, plus reduced responsiveness of the myocardium impairing relaxation.
7 Variable decline in stroke volume, cardiac output, maximum heart rate and maximal oxygen consumption. Many of these changes can be reversed by regular exercise (for the average women aged 70–75 in the UK, walking at 5 km/h represents maximal aerobic exercise).
8 Diastolic dysfunction secondary to prolonged left ventricular (LV) relaxation means that filling pressure depends on atrial contraction.
9 Lateral displacement of the apex beat is a common finding and the cardiothoracic ratio on chest X-ray (CXR) is greater than 50% in 70% of women aged over 70, partly owing to chest distortion, e.g. kyphoscoliosis.
10 Calcification of aortic valve cusps and the mitral ring.
11 After years of pulsatile stretching, the arteries increase in length and diameter leading to tortuosity of the aorta.
12 Reduced baroreceptor sensitivity leads to increased risk of orthostatic hypotension.

> **Heart disease is extremely common in old age:**
>
> 40% of > 65 year old men and 50% of > 65 year old women have hypertension.
> 15% of > 65 year olds have chronic stable angina.
> 10% of > 70 year olds have heart failure.
> 10% of > 70 year olds have atrial fibrillation.

Manifestations (Figure 9.1)

Coronary artery disease (CAD)

CAD is the most common cause of death in the UK and the USA. Over 80% of all cardiac deaths in the UK occur in those aged over 65. The sex incidence is equal, unlike in younger age groups. The risk factors are the same as for cerebrovascular disease; see Table 7.2, Chapter 7.

Managing cardiovascular disease in older people

There is a huge body of research and guidelines on managing cardiovascular disease. Some of the guidance regarding the management of older

Lecture Notes Elderly Care Medicine, Eighth Edition. Claire G. Nicholl and K. Jane Wilson.
© 2012 John Wiley & Sons, Ltd. Published 2012 by John Wiley & Sons, Ltd.

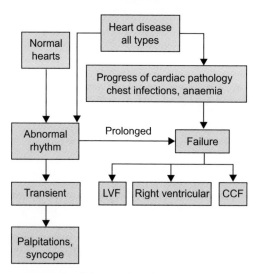

Figure 9.1 Possible sequelae of heart disease.

people is contradictory. This is because older people are hugely under-represented in trials and registries of heart disease. Many studies looking at older people count over 75 year olds as being representative of the 'very' old! In addition, these 75 year olds have been screened to exclude many co-morbidities. Thus much of the advice is extrapolated to older people without considering other problems, functional and cognitive abilities, not to mention pharmacological considerations. The cardiovascular community is finally beginning to recognize this, so future guidance will be more age-appropriate.

Presentations

- Angina.
- Acute coronary syndromes (ACS): unstable angina and myocardial infarction (MI).
- Sudden death.
- Heart failure.
- Arrhythmias.

Chronic stable angina

Angina is pain secondary to ischaemia caused by reduced blood flow to the heart muscle secondary to atherosclerotic plaques. Stable angina suggests stable plaque disease.

- The classical presentation is retrosternal pain radiating to the left arm and throat on exertion.
- The pain is reproducible by increased oxygen demand, e.g. on exertion and stress.

- The pain is not affected by inspiration, coughing or changing position.
- It is relieved by rest or glyceryl trinitrate (GTN) spray, usually in less than 5 min.
- Patients may deny pain but describe a heaviness or feeling of pressure across the chest.
- They may describe breathlessness on exertion, fatigue or even faintness.
- If the chest pain becomes more frequent, lasts longer or is more severe, this is suggestive of plaque rupture, i.e. an ACS.
- In older people, atherosclerosis is often diffuse throughout the coronary arteries and co-existent left ventricular failure (LVF) is more likely.

Investigations

- ECG: may be normal at this point or show signs of LV hypertrophy or features of ischaemia, e.g. Q waves, ST and T wave flattening or inversion or left bundle branch block (LBBB) from previous ischaemic events.
- CXR: likely to be normal, but may show cardiomegaly or signs of LVF.

Management

- Patient education: stop smoking, increase exercise.
- Aspirin, 75 mg daily; clopidogrel, 75 mg if allergic or intolerant.
- Advise GTN prior to exercise as it is fast acting and lasts for 30–45 min.
- Commence anti-anginal treatment, for example:
  o Long-acting nitrates (ensure nitrate-free period by giving isosorbide mononitrate modified release once daily or remind patient to take the patch off at night).
  o Beta-blockers, e.g. bisoprolol, slow the heart rate and give more time for coronary perfusion.
  o Calcium antagonists, e.g. diltiazem, amlodipine (but watch out for ankle oedema).
  o Nicorandil, a potassium channel opener, is a good choice for patients with low BP and symptoms of orthostatic hypotension secondary to other anti-anginal therapy. Avoid doses greater than 30 mg bd in older people because of the risk of large, painful mouth ulcers and occasionally anal ulcers which may bleed.
  o Ranolazine is an add-on therapy for refractory angina. It inhibits the sodium current which occurs late in systole in ischaemic myocytes. It does not reduce the heart rate or BP during

exercise. It does prolong the QT interval, but does not seem to be pro-arrhythmogenic. It may also improve HbA1c in diabetics.

o Ivabradine is a selective and specific blocker of the I_f channel of the sino-atrial node cells. Thus heart rate is reduced without lowering BP. It is most beneficial where patients cannot tolerate enough beta-blocker to slow the heart; use reduces hospital admissions.

- In fit older people, consider lowering cholesterol, usually with simvastatin 40 mg.
- Address all risk factors (optimize diabetic control; treat anaemia, hypertension and aortic valve disease).
- Stratification of fit older people for angiography and revascularization can be difficult. Exercise testing has a lower specificity and sensitivity in women and is not useful in LBBB. Older people are likely to have background calcification in CT calcium scoring. Therefore a MIBI scan (technetium 99 2-methoxy isobutyl isonitrile) is likely to be most useful.
- Angiography is appropriate for patients with severe symptoms or being considered for vascular surgery including aortic repair, femoral bypass and carotid surgery.
- Angioplasty, bare metal stents and drug eluting stents are currently being evaluated in older people.

Acute coronary syndromes (ACS)

Definition

ACS can be divided into two broad groups: ST elevation myocardial infarcts (STEMI) and unstable angina/non-ST elevation myocardial infarcts (NSTEMI). This is because they are managed differently and they have a different prognosis.

ST-elevation myocardial infarction

Increasing evidence shows that older people with acute STEMI respond just as well to primary percutaneous coronary angiography and intervention (PCI) and thrombolysis as younger patients.

Examination

- The patient is usually severely unwell, clammy and peripherally shut down.
- Monitor the pulse rate and rhythm and blood pressure frequently.

Reasons for under-use of reperfusion strategies in older people

- Atypical presentation (see box entitled 'Presenting clinical features of MI').
- Late presentation to medical help.
- Delay to first ECG.
- Increased incidence of pre-existing bundle branch block.
- Increased incidence of NSTEMI.
- Multiplicity of co-morbidities and contraindications.
- Older people are more likely to be managed by non-cardiologists.

Investigations

- ECG changes: by definition, ST elevation (see Figure 9.2), new left bundle branch block.
- Serial troponin I measurements to demonstrate myocyte damage.
- The CXR may show cardiomegaly or signs of pulmonary oedema (see Figure 9.3).

Management

Pre-hospital:

- Give oxygen 2–4 litres via nasal prongs.
- Treat pain with intravenous (IV) opiates to reduce sympathomimetic drive on heart.
- Stat dose of 300 mg aspirin. Continue 75 mg on daily basis if no contraindication.
- Best practice is to admit to specialist centre offering PCI. Angiography will demonstrate the nature of the lesion causing the ECG changes and will lead to appropriate intervention including angioplasty or stenting. Evidence suggests that older people do better with primary PCI because of the lower risk of cerebral haemorrhage compared with thrombolysis.
- If PCI is not locally available and there no contraindications thrombolyse with IV streptokinase. Tissue plasminogen activator (tPA) is associated with increased risk of cerebral haemorrhage in older people.
- Give low-molecular-weight heparin (LMWH), e.g. enoxaparin.
- Treatment with oral beta-blockers, again to be continued if no contraindications; this has been proven to be of benefit to older people.
- ACE inhibitors in patients with evidence of LV failure (to reduce LV remodelling).

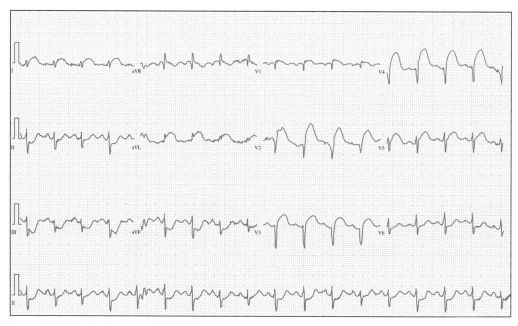

Figure 9.2 ECG showing acute STEMI. Note hyperacute 'tombstone' elevation of the anterior leads and tachycardia. From Wikimedia Commons (public domain).

- Consider cholesterol-lowering treatment.
- Older people should have equal access to cardiac rehabilitation facilities post MI.

Unstable angina and NSTEMI

This is chest pain secondary to enlargement or rupture of atherosclerotic plaque. The unstable plaque is profoundly thrombogenic so treatment is aimed at reducing this. Features include:

1 Chest pain at rest or minimal exertion.
2 The pain is not relieved by GTN.
3 The pain lasts for more than 15 min.
4 Crescendo angina on chronic background.
5 Angina of new onset on minimal exertion.

Investigations

- Serial troponin I measurements to assess myocyte damage.
- The ECG may show signs of ischaemic heart disease: LVH, Q waves from previous MI, ST depression.
- The CXR may show cardiomegaly or signs of pulmonary oedema (see Figure 9.3).

Management

- Admit to a monitored bed if possible.
- Bed rest.
- Aspirin 300 mg stat.
- $P2Y_{12}$ inhibitors including clopidogrel. Of the newer agents, ticagrelor may have a role in older people with chronic kidney disease (CKD), but prasugrel has been associated with a higher risk of bleeding.
- GTN spray/tablet.
- IV GTN or buccal nitrate.

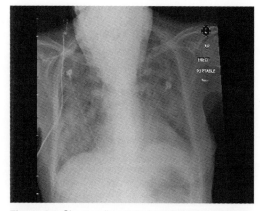

Figure 9.3 Chest radiograph demonstrating acute pulmonary oedema. Note: (1) portable film with head obscuring part of chest suggesting the patient is sick; (2) cardiomegaly even allowing for portable film; and (3) extensive pulmonary fluid.

- Low-molecular-weight heparin (LMWH).
- Beta-blockers (metoprolol is short acting and can be stopped if side-effects develop), unless contraindicated.
- If the pain does not improve, add calcium antagonist (diltiazem).
- The use of IV glycoprotein IIa/IIIb blockers (e.g. tirofiban and abciximab, which prevent platelets from cross-linking and therefore prevent platelet aggregation) has not been fully established in older people. There seems to be increased risk of intracranial haemorrhage.
- Caution – watch for bradycardia and hypotension.
- Following successful management, reduce all possible risk factors and establish an oral medication regime.
- If the patient is biologically fit, they should be considered for revascularization, either angioplasty or coronary bypass grafting. If no intervention is planned/appropriate, then a 12-month course of clopidogrel is associated with a reduced risk of further events.

Presenting clinical features of MI

- 'Typical' chest pain (20%).
- Sudden death.
- Mild chest discomfort sometimes attributed to indigestion.
- Abdominal pain.
- 'Silent', i.e. ECG changes or rise in troponin levels with no chest pain (up to 45% in the longitudinal Framingham Heart Study 2004), found in a patient admitted after a fall or 'off legs'.
- Heart failure, shortness of breath.
- Arrhythmias.
- Functional decline or confusion.
- A fall, found lying on floor unconscious, hypotension.
- Stroke.
- Peripheral gangrene.
- Post-operative fever, tachycardia, hypotension.

Heart failure

Heart failure is an extremely common cause of hospital admissions, readmissions, reduced function and institutionalization. Although usually biventricular, it is conventionally divided into acute LV failure and congestive cardiac failure.

Acute left ventricular failure

Clinical features

- Severe breathlessness, orthopnoea, paroxysmal nocturnal dyspnoea.
- Frothy pink sputum.
- On examination, there may be tachycardia, a third heart sound, crackles at the lung bases and, sometimes, pleural effusions.

Investigations

- ECG may show evidence of an acute infarction, LV hypertrophy, tachycardia or LBBB. Also look for AF and other arrhythmias.
- Blood tests may show a troponin rise.
- In early failure, the CXR may show upper lobe blood diversion and fluid in the horizontal fissure or septal lines. With increasing pulmonary oedema, there may be perihilar shadowing and bilateral pleural effusions. If the effusion is unilateral, it is more likely to be on the right. See Figure 9.3.

Management

- The patient is likely to be sitting bolt upright already, but be sure to check as frail older patients slide down modern hospital beds!
- Give oxygen via a face mask.
- Urinary catheter to monitor urine output.
- GTN infusion to offload right heart and reduce angina if present. Aim to keep systolic BP above 90 mmHg.
- IV loop diuretics, i.e. furosemide.
- Opiates (with an anti-emetic) are very useful in this situation, as they not only reduce anxiety and pain therefore reducing oxygen demand, but also reduce pre-load.
- Treat precipitant, e.g. fast AF.
- If there is evidence of an acute MI, treat as above.
- Treat co-existing pneumonia with IV antibiotics.

Chronic heart failure

- In the UK 900,000 patients have heart failure.
- Average age at diagnosis is 76.
- The prevalence will rise with the ageing population and owing to better management of CAD.
- Prognosis of heart failure is poor: 30–40% die within 1 year of diagnosis.
- The annual mortality after that ranges from 10–50% depending on severity.
- Frequent features include fatigue, functional decline, confusion, falls and cachexia.

Note: Ankle oedema is often non-cardiac: e.g. chair-bound immobility increases venous pressure, due to gravity, loss of muscle-pump activity and pressure on thigh veins by the chair.

Causes include:

- Coronary artery disease (most common).
- Hypertension.
- Valvular heart disease.
- Cor pulmonale including secondary to pulmonary emboli.
- Thyrotoxicosis.
- Severe anaemia.
- Arrhythmias, especially fast AF.
- Drugs, including non-steroidal anti-inflammatory drugs (NSAIDs) leading to fluid overload.
- Cardiomyopthies.

Investigations

NICE guidelines on heart failure recommend:

- Early transthoracic echo.
- Measure brain natriuretic peptide (BNP) or N terminal pro-B-type natriuretic peptide (NTpro BNP).
- High BNPs confer poor prognosis. (NB: Also high in other conditions including PE and may be low in obese patients and those on beta blockers.)
- Baseline urea, electrolytes, eGFR, TSH, LFTs, fasting lipids and glucose, FBC.
- CXR.
- Peak expiratory flow rate (PEFR) to exclude COPD.

Treatment

1 Advise the patient to reduce salt and fluid intake.
2 Stop smoking.
3 Control any abnormal rhythm.
4 Diuretics to reduce overload.
5 ACE inhibitor, unless contraindicated by poor renal function, hypotension or aortic valve disease (initiate in hospital in high-risk cases). If not tolerated, try a nitrate infusion.
6 Angiotensin II blockers can be used in patients who cannot tolerate ACE inhibitors.
7 Increase diuretics and ACE inhibitors as required/tolerated.
8 There is an increasing role for beta-blockers such as carvedilol and bisoprolol. They are now indicated for most grades of heart failure. They should be started at very low doses and titrated up as tolerated.

9 There is evidence that spironolactone reduces morbidity and mortality in heart failure and is often well tolerated in older people. Check potassium frequently.
10 Treat causative or precipitating factors, e.g. valve surgery if indicated, hypertension, anaemia.
11 Anticoagulation is only indicated if there is a risk of thromboembolic disease or echo suggests LV aneurysm or intracardiac thrombus.
12 Add metolazone to diuretic regime for massive oedema, but check urea and electrolytes (U&E) daily. Start with 2.5mg alternate days.
13 The criteria for cardiac resynchronization include symptoms of moderate heart failure, ejection fraction of 35% or less, QRS of 150 or more and optimal pharmacological treatment.
14 Terminal stage: opiates and oxygen as required.

Diastolic heart failure

- This is thought to account for up to 50% of cases with symptoms and signs of heart failure with a normal LV ejection fraction on echo.
- Estimated annual mortality rate of 7%.
- Risk factors include:
  o Aged over 75.
  o Female.
  o Overweight.
  o History of hypertension (leads to stiff arteries).
  o Diabetes.
  o CAD.
  o AF.
- The cause is thought to be impaired LV relaxation (especially during exercise) owing to changes in cytoskeletal proteins of the myocardium and increased LV diastolic stiffness secondary to increased myocardial fibrosis. This leads to incomplete LV filling in diastole, which in turn increases diastolic pressures causing pulmonary congestion and poor ability to increase cardiac output.
- It can cause flash pulmonary oedema precipitated by AF or fluid overload.
- The ECG may show LVH secondary to hypertension or a large left atrium (p mitrale).
- Echocardiography is essential for diagnosis: the LV ejection fraction should be above 50%, the LV volumes should be normal with no valvular lesions.
- Management involves lifestyle changes such as losing weight and reducing salt intake.

- Treat contributing disease such as respiratory problems and anaemia.
- Treat fluid overload with furosemide or spironolactone. Aldosterone antagonists reduce fibrosis. Their role in diastolic heart failure is being investigated by the TOPCAT study (ongoing).
- Treat hypertension with an ACEi.
- Drug treatment has been shown to improve symptoms of diastolic heart failure, but not improve mortality.

Hypertension

Definition

The definition of hypertension is constantly being updated. Current NICE/British Hypertension Guidelines suggest a clinic BP of <140/90 under 80y and <150/90 over 80y. This is in line with the European guidelines. Isolated systolic hypertension implies that only systolic pressure is elevated.

The American College of Cardiology and American Heart Association are now advocating a systolic measurement of 140–145 and a diastolic of less than 90 for older people.

Prevalence

Among people aged 65–74, prevalence ranges from 45% to 64% according to different surveys.

Effects of hypertension

Hypertension is a major risk factor for atherosclerosis and thus stroke, coronary artery disease, diastolic heart failure and peripheral vascular disease.

Effects of treatment

Up to age 80, treatment produces considerable benefit (more than in younger subjects) in total mortality and cardiovascular morbidity and mortality, but sometimes at the expense of making the patient feel worse. The Hypertension in the Very Elderly Trial (HYVET) now shows definite advantages of treating relatively fit elderly patients. However, remember to consider risk of falls and symptoms of dizziness in each individual patient before treating.

Treatment

1 Try non-pharmacological therapies first: low-salt, low-calorie, low-alcohol, high-exercise regime.
2 Drugs can be matched to other co-morbidities:

- Thiazide or loop diuretics/ACEi/ARBs for patients with heart failure.
- Beta-blockers/calcium antagonists for patients with angina.
- Alpha-blockers for men with BPH.

Atrial fibrillation (AF)

- AF is the most common arrhythmia.
- The prevalence increases with advancing age.
- Rates are 5–15% of patients over 80.
- The incidence increases markedly in those with biventricular heart failure and valvular heart disease.
- Fibrotic changes to the myocardium of the left atrium predispose older people to AF.
- Ventricular rates are often (1/3 cases) less than 100 bpm because of fibrosis of the conducting pathway.
- AF increases the risk of thromboembolic stroke because the reduced contraction of the atria leads to reduced blood flow allowing development of mural thrombi specifically around the left atrial appendage.
- AF is more common in patients with vascular dementia and Alzheimer's disease; thought to be related to silent cerebral emboli causing ischaemia and leukoariosis.
- Treatment aims are to reduce the risk of thromboembolic complications, reduce symptoms of AF by rate and/or rhythm control and manage concomitant heart disease.

Common causes of AF

- Coronary artery disease.
- Biventricular heart failure.
- Valvular heart disease, especially mitral (30% of cases).
- Long-standing hypertension.
- Thyroid disease.
- PE.
- Pneumonia.
- Chronic alcohol excess.

Management

History

- Establish whether AF is new onset.
- Duration.

Adverse outcomes associated with AF

- Stroke: risk increased threefold in non-valvular AF and 17-fold in AF associated with mitral valve disease.
- Thromboembolic events.
- Increased mortality 1.5–2 times greater than age-matched controls not in AF.
- Heart failure.
- Increased risk of hospitalization.
- Reduced quality of life.
- Reduced exercise capacity.

Factors to be taken into consideration

- Duration of the AF.
- Symptom severity:
  o Dizziness, syncope, presyncope
  o Chest pain
  o Breathlessness.
- Existence of coexisting structural and valvular heart disease.
- Risk of stroke, e.g. CHA_2DS_2 VASc (see box below).
- Risk of bleeding, e.g. HAS-BLED (see box below).
- Falls risk.
- Dementia.

- Frequency of episodes.
- Severity of symptoms.
- Risk factors for AF: CAD, history of rheumatic fever.
- Complications of AF: heart failure, stroke.
- Ask about symptoms suggestive of hyperthyroidism, pneumonia, pulmonary embolus.
- Alcohol intake, other drug abuse.

Examination

- Is the patient ill or well?
- Assess radial and apical rate.
- Confirm pulse is irregularly irregular.
- Check blood pressure.
- Look for signs of heart failure.
- Listen for murmurs.
- Listen for signs of pneumonia.
- Look for signs of thyrotoxicosis.

Investigations

- 12-lead ECG: confirm whether paroxysmal AF or continuing in AF, ventricular response rate, signs of acute or chronic ischaemia; LV hypertrophy tachycardia and RV strain (S1Q3T3 is rare) are suggestive of new PE.
- CXR: cardiac size, evidence of heart failure, pneumonia.
- Transthoracic echocardiogram: assess the valves, size of left atrium, LV ejection fraction.
- Consider Holter monitor if symptoms occur 3–4 times per day, are paroxysmal or exercise related.
- Consider event recorder if symptoms 24 h apart.
- Transoesophageal echo may be useful to exclude left atrial appendage or left atrial thrombus prior to cardioversion after 48 h of symptoms.
- Ventilation/perfusion scan or CT pulmonary angiogram (CTPA) if high suspicion of PE.
- Check TSH, FBC, U&Es, LFTs.

Treatment

Rate control versus rhythm control
- Elderly people often have factors making cardioversion unlikely to work:
  o Longstanding AF.
  o Enlarged left atrium.
  o Previously failed cardioversion.
  o Mitral stenosis.
- Thus, for the majority of elderly people with multiple co-morbidities and the very elderly, rate control is the most appropriate option.
- May revert spontaneously, especially if due to pneumonia, PE or MI.
- There is evidence that 50% of older people revert to atrial fibrillation 1 year post cardioversion anyway.
- Rate control can be achieved with verapamil (avoid in heart failure) or a beta-blocker which will be faster and more effective.
- If these agents do not control the rate sufficiently, digoxin can be added.
- If this is still inadequate, consider oral amiodarone.
- Digoxin is mainly only used as monotherapy in sedentary patients or those with heart failure (positive inotropic effect).
- The European Society of Cardiology Guidelines (2010) now suggest aiming for a resting heart rate of < 110 bpm.
- If aiming for tighter rate control (because of symptoms) it is important to repeat a Holter test

to exclude bradyarrhythmias, AV block and long pauses.

- Paroxysmal AF: digoxin is potentially harmful. Sotalol or amiodarone reduce frequency of attacks and ventricular rate during them. The risk of stroke is high, so consider anticoagulation as above.

Options for achieving sinus rhythm

New onset (less than 48 h):

- If the patient is shocked, DC cardioversion is the most appropriate management.
- In the rare case of an elderly patient who is biologically fit with no history of ischaemic heart disease or echo evidence of failure, give flecainide or propafenone. Flecainide is contraindicated in patients with CAD because of risk of sudden cardiac death.
- Consider amiodarone via a central line.
- If the patient is not anticoagulated, they should be given heparin, and if they are suitable for anticoagulation, the heparin should be continued until the INR is therapeutic.

Beyond 48 h:

- If the plan is chemical or electrical cardioversion, arrange transoesophageal echo as above. If there are thrombi, the patient must be anticoagulated for 1 month prior to cardioversion,
- If sinus rhythm is achieved, continue with maintenance sotalol or amiodarone to prevent recurrence, remembering that older people are susceptible to the side-effects of both these drugs.
- Fit older people who revert back to AF can be considered for pacemaker insertion plus AV ablation.

Oral anticoagulation

- The target INR is 2.5 (range 2.0–3.0).
- Valvular heart disease confers very high risk and therefore anticoagulate unless there is a profound contraindication.
- For non-valvular AF, the CHA_2DS_2 VASc score may be useful.

Balance the risk of thromboembolic stroke against the risk of bleeding using, for example, the acronym HAS-BLED:

Clearly, risks such as age and hypertension cancel each other out.

The BAFTA trial (Mant et al. 2007) demonstrated that anticoagulation in older people is safe and effective.

CHA_2DS_2 VASc score

Congestive heart disease = 1 point
Hypertension = 1 point
Age > 75 = 2 points
Age between 65 and 74 = 1 point
Diabetes = 1 point
Vascular disease, previous MI, PVD = 1 point
Stroke or TIA = 2 points
Female = 1 point
0 = low risk
1 = low risk
> 2 = high risk, consider oral anticoagulation

HAS-BLED

Hypertension
Abnormal renal/liver function
Stroke
Bleeding history
Labile INR
Elderly
Drugs/alcohol
  Score 1 for each positive; a score of ≥ 3 confers a high risk of bleeding with warfarin.

Examples of use of aspirin versus warfarin

Aspirin for patients with:	Warfarin (INR 2–3) for patients with:
• High risk of bleeding	
• Frequent changes of medication	• Previous stroke
• Dementia plus poor social support	• Mitral valve disease
• Recurrent falls (risk of subdural haematoma)	• Enlarged left atrium
• Uncontrolled hypertension	• Poor LV function
• Non-compliance with monitoring of INR	• Controlled hypertension
Consider clopidogrel for those intolerant of aspirin	

New developments

1 Oral anticoagulants
   - Dabigitran, a direct thrombin inhibitor; the RE-LY studies (Connolly et al. 2009) show that a dose of 110 mg bd gives the same reduction

in thromboembolic risk as warfarin with less bleeding risk. The benefit is not as marked in locations where the INR is well controlled. However, the current cost is extremely high even taking into account the cost of monitoring INRs with warfarin. Rivaroxaban, an oral Xa inhibitor already being used as thromboprophylaxis post orthopaedic surgery in some centres, may also have a role in AF.

2 Antiarrhythmic
  • Dronedarone is similar to amiodarone but without the iodine moiety, and was eagerly awaited as a 'less-toxic amiodarone'. It may be useful in treating AF and flutter in older people without heart failure, but its efficacy is disappointing.

Atrial flutter

• Similar risk of stroke as with AF, so it is important to consider anticoagulation.
• Responds to cardioversion, but often reverts back because of a large left atrium and structural heart disease.
• Rate control can be achieved with amiodarone.

Pacing indications

Ageing leads to fibrosis of the conduction pathways in the heart; therefore bradycardia and bradyarrhythmias are more common. Bradycardia is exacerbated by medications such as digoxin, beta-blockers, amiodarone and calcium channel blockers, which should be stopped. Patients may present with recurrent unexplained falls, syncope, increasing angina and heart failure, or be asymptomatic.

Dual chamber pacemakers are indicated for most conditions except patients with chronic AF and who are very frail and elderly.

Indications for pacemakers include:

• Complete heart block.
• Sick sinus syndrome.
• Tri-fasicular block.
• Cardio-inhibitory carotid sinus hypersensitivity and cardio-inhibitory vasodepression on tilting.
• Synchronous pacing for heart failure (as above).

Valvular heart disease

Systolic murmurs are audible in 30–60% of elderly patients and when significant arise from the mitral valve in 50%, the aortic valve in 25% and both in 25% of cases.

> **Common causes of mitral regurgitation in elderly people**
>
> • Calcification of mitral ring.
> • Dilatation of LV and mitral ring.
> • Mucoid (myxomatous) degeneration of cusps.
> • Floppy mitral valve with prolapse of posterior cusp.
> • Papillary-muscle dysfunction – usually ischaemic.
> • Rupture of chordae tendineae (often partial).
> • Infective endocarditis.
> • Rheumatic heart disease.

Mitral regurgitation

This condition is thought to be associated with some cases of transient cerebral or retinal ischaemia.

Calcific aortic stenosis

• Aortic stenosis (AS) is the most common cardiovascular disease after hypertension and CAD.
• Common mechanisms are degenerative calcification of a tri-leaflet valve or stenosis of a congenital bicuspid valve.
• Rheumatic heart disease is much less common in the Western world.
• Stenosis is slowly progressive with time which leads to concentric hypertrophy of the left ventricle, which eventually starts to fail.
• Risk factors are diabetes, hypertension, smoking and raised cholesterol.
• AF is poorly tolerated because the loss of atrial contraction plus rapid ventricular response reduces diastolic filling of the left ventricle.
• The triad of symptoms is angina (30%), breathlessness (50%) and syncope or presyncope (15%).
• The murmur may be unimpressive.
• The slow rising pulse may be absent because of reduced elasticity of the carotid artery.
• ECG may show LV hypertrophy. There may be conduction abnormalities including RBBB and LBBB secondary to calcification of the conduction pathway.
• Once gradient across the valve is over 60 mm on echo, if symptoms present and LV function is good, the patient should be considered for an aortic valve repair or replacement.
• Average life expectancy without treatment is 2–3 years.

- Options for treatment include open valve replacement.
- Transcatheter aortic valve insertion (TAVI) is useful for frailer patients. A balloon is fed via a catheter through the femoral vein into the heart and is used to crush the native valve and a new valve is inserted in its root. This procedure seems to have a lower risk of haemorrhage but possibly a higher risk of vascular complications including stroke.

Infective endocarditis

- This is an infection of the endocardial surface of the heart. Pathogens such as *Staphylococcus aureus*, *Streptococcus* spp and *Enterococcus* spp adhere to proteins present on damaged valves and produce vegetations to hide in.
- Despite advances, the mortality remains 15–30%, with about 200 deaths in England and Wales each year.
- The mortality is higher in older people because of co-morbidities and less likelihood of being fit enough for surgical correction of the diseased valve.
- Most patients are aged 60 or over.
- Risk factors include atheromatous and calcific valve disease, intra-cardiac devices including prosthetic valves and pacemakers, exposure to nosocomial infections and reduced host immunity.
- Some published series of cases show that older people may be more often affected by gastrointestinal bacteria including Group D *Streptococcus* (*S. bovis*) and *Enterococcus faecalis* compared with younger people who tend to have underlying *Staphylococcus aureus* and Gram negative organisms.
- This suggests that the portal of entry for the bacteria is more often colonic or urogenital than in younger people.
- Some authorities recommend full antimicrobial prophylaxis when undergoing gastrointestinal and urological invasive tests as well as the universally accepted dental procedures.
- Also, patients with prosthetic heart valves merit scrupulous protection from nosocomial infections.

Clinical features

A clinical suspicion of infectious endocarditis can be supported by using Duke's criteria, as in the box below. Have a high index of suspicion in older people as the response to infection may be attenuated, so that there may not be a fever or a leucocytosis. Consider infectious endocarditis in patients presenting with the following:

- Chronic, unexplained fever.
- Anorexia and weight loss.
- Malaise.
- Intermittent confusion.
- New or changing murmurs help clinch the diagnosis, but absence of a murmur does not exclude it.
- Splinter haemorrhages at the nail base.
- Classical signs such as Janeway lesions and Osler's nodes are rare.

Modified Duke's criteria for diagnosis of infective endocarditis

Major criteria
  Positive blood cultures
  Positive finds on echocardiogram: vegetations, abscess and damage to seating of prosthetic valve
  New valvular regurgitation
Minor criteria
  Predisposing heart disease
  Fever > 38 °C
  Vascular phenomenon: arterial emboli, septic infarcts, Janeway lesions (non-tender maculae on palms and soles)
  Immunological phenomenon: Roth's spots (retinal haemorrhages), Osler's nodes (tender subcutaneous nodules on distal pads of fingers)
  Definite diagnosis: 2 major or 1 major and 3 minor or 5 minor criteria
  Likely diagnosis: 1 major and 1 minor or 3 minor criteria

Investigations

- Raised ESR and CRP.
- Mild–moderate normocytic normochromic anaemia.
- Three sets of blood cultures should be taken at least an hour apart from different sites. *Streptococcus viridans* is the organism most commonly isolated.
- Urine dipstix may show haematuria and/or proteinuria.

- Transthoracic echocardiography: can miss endocarditis in older people because the vegetations are sometimes smaller.
- Transoesophageal echocardiography (TOE) can increase the diagnostic yield to 45%. It may also detect local complications such as valve ring abscesses.

Management

- Empirical IV antibiotics as guided by the local microbiology guidelines, until blood culture results are available. IV antibiotics should be continued for at least the first 2 weeks.
- Oral antibiotics for a further 2–4 weeks. The patient will have to remain on IV antibiotics longer if the organism is only sensitive to vancomycin or gentamicin. In this situation, consider longer-term IV access such as a peripherally inserted central catheter (PICC) line.
- If the valve is badly damaged, the organism is resistant or if the patient is in refractory heart failure, the valve may need to be replaced.
- Advise the patient about the need for antibiotic prophylaxis for procedures in the future.
- If the patient makes a good recovery, it may now be appropriate to look for the underlying colonic or urological tumour which allowed entry of the bacteria in the first place.

Syncope, transient loss of consciousness (T-LOC)

Definition

Syncope is now defined as 'a transient loss of consciousness due to transient global cerebral hypoperfusion characterized by rapid onset, short duration and spontaneous and complete recovery'.

- The incidence of syncope in over 60 year olds is 6% (probably a gross underestimate owing to under-diagnosis).
- Two-year recurrence rate is 30%.
- It must be considered in patients with recurrent unexplained falls.
- Cerebral blood flow is about 50 mL/100 g/min in older people but is lower in those with hypertension or atherosclerosis.
- Symptoms of cerebral ischaemia occur when the blood flow is reduced to 25–30 mL/100 g/min.
- Neurally mediated/reflex syncope is the most common type.

- It is important to differentiate neurally mediated syncope from cardiac syncope because it has a better prognosis and the patients need not be admitted for urgent investigations.

History

A careful history is often the key to the diagnosis. See syncope in Chapter 5 and epilepsy in Chapter 8.

Causes of a single episode

Any acute episode that causes a dramatic drop in blood pressure, e.g.:

- MI.
- PE.
- GI bleed.

Causes of recurrent episodes (Table 9.1)

The following are red flag features in history and examination:

- LOC during exercise is suggestive of an arrhythmia or strucutral heart disease.
- Chest pain prior to syncope is suggestive of cardiac syncope.
- Family history of sudden cardiac death is less relevent in older people, but should be considered if family members black out on the ward! Think of Brugada syndrome (RBBB, ST elevation and T wave inversion in V1-3), long QT syndrome or hypertrophic obstuctive cardiomyopathy (HCM).

Carotid sinus massage

- The patient is lying down with their head in a neutral position.
- The carotid sinus is massaged longitudinally for 5 s on the right side first as this has a higher yield, then repeat on the left if necessary, allowing 30 s in between.
- The test should be repeated with the patient tilted up to 70°.
- Contraindications: recent MI, ventricular tachycardia.
- If there is a suspicion of carotid disease, this should be excluded by carotid doppler before starting.

Indications for permanent pacemaker

- Symptomatic bradycardia, pulse less than 40 b.p.m.
- Complete heart block.

Table 9.1 Causes, investigations and management of different types of syncope

Cause	Subtypes	Results of investigation	Management
Neurally mediated			
Carotid sinus hypersensitivity	Cardio-inhibitory	CSM causes asystolic pause	Pacemaker
	Vasodepressor	CSM causes drop in BP	Lifestyle advice
	Mixed	CSM causes both	Pacemaker and lifestyle advice
Recurrent vasovagal syncope	Cardio-inhibitory	Bradycardia provoked by HUT	Pacemaker
	Vasodepressor	Hypotension on HUT	Advice about optimum fluid intake, consider extra salt, caffeine; if symptoms of presyncope, recruit muscles
	Mixed	Bradycardia and hypotension on HUT	Pacemaker and above advice
Situational	Cough	Good history	Avoid situation where practical
	Micturition/ Defaecation	Good history	Suggest men sit to urinate, avoid constipation
	Swallowing	Good history	Suggest small mouthfuls
	Post-prandial	Good history	Eat, little and often
Orthostatic hypotension	Primary/ Secondary	Drop in blood pressure provoked by standing associated with symptoms	See main text
Cardiac syncope			
Cardiac ischaemia		ECG changes, troponin rise	See main text
Arrhythmias	Bradycardia/pauses	24 h tape, external or internal loop recorder	Pacemaker
	Tachycardia		Antiarrhythmic drugs
	Tachybrady syndrome		'Pace and block'
Structural heart disease	Aortic stenosis	Echocardiogram	TAVI or valve replacement
	HCM	Echocardiogram	ACEi
Subclavian steal syndrome			

CSM, carotid sinus massage; HUT, head-up tilt; HCM, hypertrophic cardiomyopathy.

- Asystolic pauses lasting 3 or more seconds.
- Persistent failure, lethargy and poor exercise tolerance are indications for pacing in patients with atrioventricular (AV) block, especially if trifasicular or bifasicular.
- AF with partial block and a slow ventricular response.
- Tachy-brady syndrome.
- Chronotropic incompetence (a failure to speed up to cope with exercise – elderly people are unable to compensate for this with a rise in the stroke volume).
- Cardio-inhibitory response to head-up tilt, or asystole demonstrated on carotid sinus massage secondary to carotid hypersensitivity.

Orthostatic (postural) hypotension

- Orthostatic hypotension occurs in about 20% of community dwelling older people.
- Increased incidence in patients living in long-term care homes, up to 50% in some series.
- Increased risk secondary to reduced baroreceptor responsiveness and reduced arterial compliance.
- It is more common among people with coexisting disorders, especially hypertension.
- Any drop in BP on standing up is poorly tolerated in older people because cerebral autoregulation is often defective, especially those with a history of hypertension.

- Orthostatic hypotension is defined as a drop of 20 mm or more in systolic BP or 10 mm diastolic BP provoked by standing up and accompanied by symptoms.
- It may be an incidental finding, and is only clinically relevant if there is good correlation with symptoms or distress caused by standing up.
- Symptoms include dizziness, presyncope, syncope, falls and visual disturbance.
- Dizziness when getting out of bed first thing in the morning or standing after sitting for some time is common.
- Ask whether symptoms are related to meal times.
- Ask about Parkinsonian symptoms.
- Take a careful drug history.

Causes of orthostatic hypotension

Autonomic failure:

- Primary autonomic failure syndromes, e.g. pure autonomic failure, multiple system atrophy, Parkinsonism plus syndromes

Secondary:

- Diabetic neuropathy, amyloid neuropathy
- Drugs: diuretics, alpha-blockers, calcium channel blockers, phenothiazines, antidepressants, levodopa, vasodilators including alcohol, narcotic analgesia, verapamil, disopyramide
- Post-prandial
- Post-exercise

Volume depletion:

- GI bleed
- Diarrhoea
- Addison's disease

Investigations

- Measure lying and standing BP with heart rate, especially first thing in the morning and after meals. Use a manual sphygmomanometer. Document standing BP immediately on standing and ideally every 30s for 3 min.
- If the heart rate goes up, this suggests volume loss. Absence of compensatory tachycardia is suggestive of autonomic failure.
- Twenty-four hour BP monitoring.
- U&E.
- Short Synacthen test (synthetic ACTH).
- Blood sugars and glycosylated haemoglobin level.

Treatment

- Correct any cause identified.
- Stop any drugs that may be contributing and consider alternatives, e.g. choose nicorandil for angina instead of nitrates which cause more venous vasodilatation.
- Advise concerning sensible precautions ('have a bath with a friend').
- Compression stockings, preferably full-length. Abdominal bands are less well tolerated.
- Medication: fludrocortisone (a mineralocorticoid) can be helpful, but its use is limited by leg oedema and hypokalaemia.
- Midodrine is a peripheral alpha-agonist which causes arterial and venous constriction. It is not licensed in the UK but is very useful at treating orthostatic hypotension with minimal side-effects. Avoid in patients with CAD.
- Head-up tilt to bed (20°) to promote salt retention and to reduce nocturnal diuresis.

Vascular disease

Abdominal aortic aneurysm

- The incidence is 78 per 100,000 in over 70 year olds.
- Cause 6,000–10,000 deaths annually in England and Wales.
- Most are discovered by chance when patients are having scans for other reasons.
- If up to 4 cm, regular ultrasound screening is advised; over 5.0–5.5 cm, advise surgery (if patient suitable).
- Of those not operated on, 5% rupture per annum if the diameter is 5–6 cm; the rate rises exponentially if the aneurysm is larger.
- Affects 3× as many men as women.
- The risk is increased in hypertension and COPD and patients who smoke or have a positive family history.
- Symptoms of impending rupture include a pulsating sensation in the abdomen, severe abdominal pain or back pain which radiates into the abdomen.
- The mortality associated with rupture is 80%.
- Aneurysm repair can be via open surgery or laparoscopically aided. Open surgery involves a long general anaesthetic and post-operative care is best managed on a high-dependency unit.
- Aortic aneurysms that are below the kidneys and have not ruptured can be repaired endovascularly by endovascular aneurysm repair (EVAR).

A stent-graft is inserted via a catheter in the femoral arteries. The stent-graft is activated under X-ray guidance and positioned across the aneurysm. Further procedures may be necessary, including insertion of stents into the iliac arteries and femoro-femoral bypass grafts.

- The advantages of the EVAR are: shorter procedure and shorter anaesthetic, less risk of major haemorrhage and reduced post-operative pain. The disadvantage is the risk of small leaks at the edges of the stent-graft which are not always clinically obvious.

Peripheral vascular disease

Clinical features

- Intermittent claudication: pain usually in the back of both calves which occurs during exercise and is relieved by rest.
- Critical ischaemia may present as pain at rest, painful ulcers, and necrotic or septic skin lesions. This sometimes follows trauma or a haemodynamic crisis. Those of limited mobility may not give a history of previous claudication.

Diagnosis

Affected extremities may be discoloured, with trophic changes in skin and nails (loss of hair on the legs is sensitive but extremely non-specific), cool and pulseless feet, and bruits over femoral, superficial femoral (frequent site of obstruction) or popliteal arteries. Elicit blanching on elevation and delayed hyperaemia and venous filling on dependency. Measure ankle systolic pressure with Doppler probe: should be 0.8 of the brachial pressure. Check for ulcers and gangrene. See Figure 9.4.

Management (Figure 9.5)

Education is an extremely important component of the management of peripheral vascular disease. The patient needs to be supported with smoking cessation advice, compliance with exercise regimes to improve the distance walked and development of collateral vessels.

Giant-cell arteritis

- This affects the elastic lamina of large and medium sized arteries.
- Temporal biopsy reveals transmural inflammation of the intima, media and adventitia with patchy infiltration by lymphocytes, macrophages and multinucleate giant cells.

Symptoms and signs of giant-cell arteritis

- Headache, usually over the temples, sometimes worse at night.
- Scalp tenderness, e.g. when combing hair.
- Tender, thickened superficial temporal arteries.
- Constitutional – fever, weight loss.
- Occlusion of short posterior ciliary artery causes blindness: amaurosis fugax.
- Jaw claudication.
- Pain in tongue.
- Functional decline.
- If not treated, risk of complications:
  - Stroke.
  - Coronary artery involvement.
  - Peripheral arterial involvement.

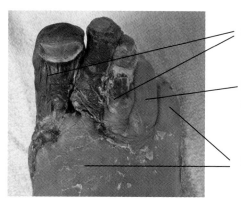

Dry gangrene - these toes would probably mummify

Blue / purple discoloration and swelling, more suggestive of wet gangrene that will spread

Red hyperaemic skin of just viable tissue

Figure 9.4 Gangrene of the toes in a diabetic. From James Heilman, Wikimedia Commons: http://commons.wikimedia.org/wiki/File:GangreneFoot.JPG.

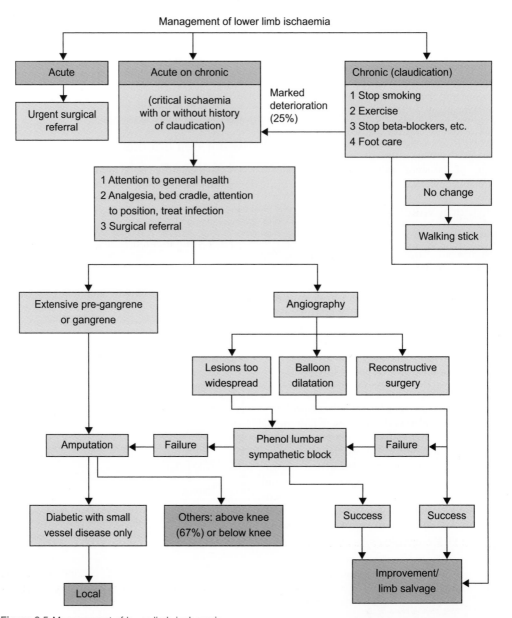

Figure 9.5 Management of lower limb ischaemia.

- Thickening of the arterial wall leads to distal ischaemia.
- The incidence is 10–50 per 100,000.
- Women are more frequently affected than men.
- Mean age of onset is 70 years old.
- There is overlap with polymyalgia rheumatica (see Chapter 6).

The features of this disease are given in the box below.

Investigation

- ESR is typically very high, often above 100.
- CRP is also raised. It tends to fall more rapidly than ESR after treatment is commenced.
- There may be a normochromic normocytic anaemia
- LFTs may also be abnormal.
- Temporal artery biopsy is the gold standard investigation. However, it may be negative because

the artery is affected in a patchy distribution; if symptoms are highly suggestive, treat anyway. Ultrasound improves the yield.

Treatment

- Initially 1 mg/kg oral prednisolone to prevent irreversible visual complications.
- Give aspirin 75 mg for the first month to reduce strokes.
- Wean the steroid guided by symptoms and reduction in CRP and ESR.
- Usually burns out in 1–2 years.
- Remember gastric protection and osteoporosis prevention.

Venous and pulmonary thromboembolic disease

Diagnosis of deep vein thrombosis (DVT) requires confirmation by ultrasound scan of thigh veins and, if negative but strongly suspected, venography. Patients with DVT who are otherwise well can now be treated as an out-patient with treatment doses of LMWH for at least 4 days, together with warfarin. LMWH prevents further thrombosis and allow endogenous fibrinolysis to occur. Warfarin is a vitamin K antagonist and takes several days to become effective. In cancer patients, lifelong LMWH gives better results than warfarinisation.

Prevention is always preferable to cure: prophylactic LMWH is given to high-risk hospitalized patients, which includes all elderly patients, those with underlying carcinoma and those with reduced mobility.

Risk factors for pulmonary embolism

- Increasing age.
- Immobility.
- DVT.
- Surgery especially abdominal.
- Fractures especially lower limb.
- Malignant disease.
- Obesity.
- Procoagulant states.

Pulmonary embolism

- Often underdiagnosed in older people because presentation may be atypical.
- Forty percent of PEs found at post-mortem were not suspected in life.
- Increasingly common with increasing age.
- High morbidity and mortality.

Presenting features of pulmonary embolism

- Breathlessness (60%).
- Pleuritic chest pain (40%).
- Haemoptysis (10%).
- Syncope (8–20%).
- Sudden death.
- Feeling of impending doom.
- Fever.
- Arrhythmia.
- Cough, 'pneumonia'.
- Bronchospasm.
- Right heart failure.
- Pulmonary oedema.
- Increasing exertional dyspnoea.
- Confusion.
- Falls.
- Functional decline.
- Hypotension.

Investigation

- Have a high index of suspicion.
- ECG most commonly shows sinus tachycardia. Rarely, signs of right heart strain, or new AF.
- CXR is often normal but may show segmental collapse, a raised hemidiaphragm or pleural effusion.
- Blood gases may be normal early on, but hypoxaemia and hypocapnoea (secondary to hyperventilation) are suggestive of PE.
- A negative d-dimer in a patient with low clinical probability reliably excludes DVT/PE.
- D-dimer may give a false positive in inflammation.
- Isotope V/Q scan can be used for diagnosis except where the CXR is abnormal secondary to coexisting COPD, heart failure, pneumonia, etc.
- If there is co-existent cardiorespiratory disease CT pulmonary angiography is extremely useful in detecting PEs. It has the additional advantage of demonstrating the alternative diagnosis if no PE is present.

Treatment of venous thromboembolism (VTE)

- Commence LMWH whilst confirming the diagnosis.
- Load with warfarin, aiming for an INR of 2–3. Remember, 'start low and go slow', and that antibiotics such as ciprofloxacin inhibit warfarin metabolism and thus raise the INR significantly.
- Once INR is within range, stop LMWH.

- In the case of massive PE, especially where cardiac arrest is pending, consider thrombolysis with IV alteplase.

Duration of anticoagulation

- First idiopathic PE: 3 months.
- Older patients are at increased risk of haemorrhage with anticoagulation. Avoid concomitant use of aspirin. Those with a history of GI bleeding are most at risk.
- The risk–benefit of treating ongoing risk of VTE versus bleeding must be assessed on an individual basis for those with recurrent PEs.

📖 REFERENCES

Connolly SJ, Ezekowitz MD, Yusuf S, et al. (2009) The randomized evaluation of long-term anticoagulation therapy (RE-LY). *New England Journal of Medicine* 361: 1139–1151. www.nejm.org/doi/full/10.1056/NEJMoa0905561.

European Society of Cardiology (2010) *Clinical Guidelines on the Management of Atrial Fibrillation.* http://www.escardio.org/guidelines-surveys/esc-guidelines/Pages/atrial-fibrillation.aspx.

Framingham Heart Study (2004) *Longitudinal Data Documentation.* https://biolincc.nhlbi.nih.gov/static/studies/teaching/framdoc.pdf.

HYVET (2008) *Hypertension in the Very Elderly Trial.* http://www.hyvet.com/.

Mant J, Hobbs FDR, Fletcher K, et al. (2007) Warfarin versus aspirin for stroke prevention in an elderly community population with atrial fibrillation (the Birmingham Atrial Fibrillation Treatment of the Aged Study, BAFTA): a randomised controlled trial. *Lancet* 370: 493–503.

TOPCAT study (ongoing) *Treatment of Preserved Cardiac Function Heart Failure with an Aldosterone Antagonist.* http://www.topcatstudy.com/.

➡️ FURTHER INFORMATION

American College of Rheumatology – giant-cell arteritis: www.rheumatology.org/practice/clinical/patients/diseases_and_conditions/giant-cellarteritis.asp.

Beever G, Lip G, O'Brien E (2007) *ABC of Hypertension,* 5th edn. Blackwell BMJ Books, Birmingham; Conway Institute of Biomolecular and Biomedical Research, University College Dublin.

British Thoracic Society Guidelines on Management of Pulmonary Embolism: www.brit-thoracic.org.uk/c2/uploads/PulmonaryEmbolismJUN03.pdf.

Lip GHY, Blann AD (2003) *ABC of Antithrombotic Therapy.* Blackwell BMJ Books, Birmingham.

Medscape Education Cardiology: antiplatelet therapy in the elderly: a very useful review: www.medscape.org/viewarticle/749325?src=0_mp_ cmenl_0.

NICE Guidelines for Management of Hypertension 2011: http:\\www.niceorg.uk\CG127\QuickRefGuide\pdf\English.

NHS Improvement. Guidance on Risk Assessment and Stroke Prevention for Atrial Fibrillation (GRASP-AF): www.improvement.nhs.uk/graspaf.

NICE Guidelines for Management of Atrial Fibrillation: http://guidance.nice.org.uk/CG36/QuickRefGuide/pdf/English.

NICE Guidelines for Management of Stroke: http://www.nice.org.uk/nicemedia/live/10982/30054/30054.pdf.

Ouzounian M, Lee DS, Liu PP, et al. (2009) Diastolic heart failure: mechanisms and controversies. *Nature Clinical Practice Cardiovascular Medicine* 5 (7): 375–386.

Pisters R, Lane DA, Nieuwlaat R, et al. (2010) A novel user-friendly score (HAS-BLED) to assess one-year risk of major bleeding in atrial fibrillation patients: The Euro Heart Survey. *Chest* chestjournal.chestpubs.org/content/early/2010/03/18/chest.10-0134.full.pdf + html.

10

Respiratory disease

Respiratory disease causes approximately 20% of all deaths if lung cancer is included. It is the second most common reason (13%) for emergency hospital admission, after injury and poisoning. More people die from respiratory disease than from coronary artery disease in the UK. In Europe, five countries of the former USSR together with Ireland and Malta are the only seven countries that had higher death rates from respiratory disease than the UK in 2001. Social inequality causes a higher proportion of respiratory deaths than for any other disease. Death rates increase steeply with age, and 87% occur among people 65 years or older. The three main respiratory killers are respiratory cancers, pneumonia and chronic obstructive pulmonary disease (COPD). Lung cancer now kills more women in the UK than breast cancer.

COPD causes about 90% of respiratory disability; 900,000 people have a formal diagnosis of COPD in the UK, but the Department of Health estimates that the true figure is closer to 3 million. Respiratory disease is a common reason to visit the GP; in 2004, nearly 1 in 5 males and 1 in 4 females consulted the GP for a respiratory complaint.

Age changes

Physiology

Age-related changes affect virtually all aspects of the respiratory system. Structural and functional changes occur, decreasing efficiency of gas transfer. However, because the lungs have huge reserve capacity, significant clinical issues only arise when an elderly person becomes sick unless lung function has been progressively damaged by smoking or air pollution. Older people may have difficulty performing many lung function tests, but spirometry is usually possible.

- Reduced lung elasticity and chest wall compliance lead to air trapping, a rise in residual volume and a fall in the forced vital capacity (FVC), forced expiratory volume in 1 s (FEV_1) and peak expiratory flow as shown in Figures 10.1 and 10.2. Some normal old people will have an FEV_1/FVC ratio of < 0.7. Do not treat (beyond smoking cessation advice) unless they are symptomatic.
- An increase in airway size and loss of alveolar surface decrease the lung volume available for gas exchange and increase dead space, reducing efficiency of gas exchange. Premature closure of small airways results in ventilation–perfusion mismatching, contributing to an increase in the alveolar-arterial oxygen gradient. Arterial oxygen tension (PaO_2) falls from 12.7 kPa at age 30 to 10 kPa at age 60.
- Oxygen delivery to tissues (VO_2 max) decreases due to age-related decreases in cardiac output and body muscle mass, as well as ventilation–perfusion mismatching and decreased alveolar volume.
- Mucociliary protection of the lower airway is impaired.

Examination

Check the rate and pattern of respiration. Tachypnoea suggests a cardiorespiratory problem, which can be very useful if the patient cannot give much history. Cheyne–Stokes respiration, in which the breathing becomes progressively shallower, sometimes culminating in an apnoeic episode before becoming progressively deeper again in a cyclical pattern, is more common in the elderly. It is often seen in stroke but may occur in

Lecture Notes Elderly Care Medicine, Eighth Edition. Claire G. Nicholl and K. Jane Wilson.
© 2012 John Wiley & Sons, Ltd. Published 2012 by John Wiley & Sons, Ltd.

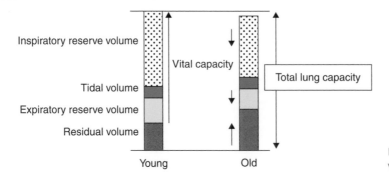

Figure 10.1 Changes in lung volumes with age.

apparently normal individuals. Note the chest shape. Significant kyphosis is usually now due to osteoporosis (previously TB). Look for thyroid and thoracotomy scars. The normal trachea may deviate slightly to the right around an unfolded aorta. Many older patients have basal crackles that clear on coughing and have no significance. Conversely, if the patient has poor air entry, an area of consolidation may appear silent. A silent chest is a danger sign in airway obstruction.

After a fall, check for bruising of the chest wall and 'spring' the ribcage for fractures (pneumonia usually follows). Remember other systems associated with chest problems, e.g. aspiration in PD, and check for heart failure. Oxygen saturation measured by a fingertip probe is a useful bedside

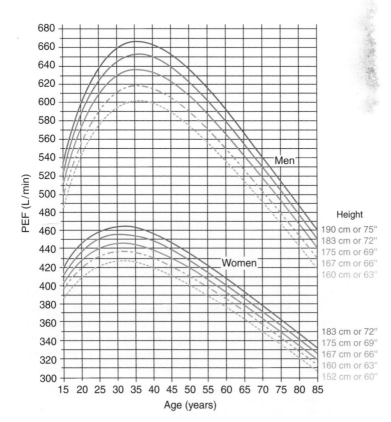

Figure 10.2 Normal values for peak expiratory flow (PEF) with age.

test. The admission CXR in an ill old patient is often difficult to interpret; usually taken AP or even supine (check for scapular lines), often with rotation (check relation of heads of clavicles to spinous processes), sometimes with the head in the chest and with poor inspiration. A subtle diagnosis may require a repeat film when the patient is improving.

Upper respiratory tract infection

Rhinoviruses (species of the genus *Enterovirus* from the *Picorna* virus family) and corona viruses cause coryza, the common cold. This is a mild systemic upset with nasal symptoms, but older people, particularly smokers and those with pre-existing chronic illness, may develop lower respiratory complications.

Influenza is usually debilitating in the elderly, particularly in the presence of chronic heart, chest or renal disease, or diabetes and may be complicated by pneumonia, especially due to *Staphylococcus aureus*. Everyone aged over 65 years should be offered immunization in October/November. The influenza viruses are constantly altering their antigenic structure, so every year WHO recommends which strains should be included in the flu vaccine. The vaccine may cause a mild local reaction and hypersensitivity to egg products is a contraindication. Immunity takes 2–4 weeks to develop and lasts 6–8 months. There is evidence that immunization of staff is the best way to protect residents of institutions, and some hospitals offer free vaccination to their staff. The prevalence of influenza A/H1N1 (pandemic swine flu) increased in 2010 but unlike seasonal flu is more common and severe in the young and pregnant. Oseltamivir (a neuraminidase inhibitor) is given if H1N1 is suspected.

Acute breathlessness

The acutely dyspnoeic elderly patient is a very common medical emergency.

Common causes of acute respiratory distress

- Left ventricular failure.
- Pneumonia.

- Exacerbation of COPD.
- Exacerbation of asthma.
- Pulmonary embolism.
- Pneumothorax.
- Inhaled foreign body (stridor, choking).

Airway obstruction

Most cases are due to COPD but a number of patients have long-standing asthma and late-onset asthma may be increasing. COPD includes chronic bronchitis, defined clinically as sputum production on most days for 3 months of two successive years, and emphysema, defined histologically as air space dilatation due to destruction of alveolar walls. There may be a reversible component especially in asthmatics who have smoked. COPD causes progressive breathlessness and reduction in exercise capacity. The presence of airflow obstruction should be confirmed by *post-bronchodilator* spirometry. The death rate for COPD has increased in recent years whilst rates of other causes of mortality (heart, neoplasm and cerebrovascular diseases) are falling. About 15% of those dying from COPD have never smoked and air pollution is thought to be a significant factor.

Features of severe attack of airways obstruction requiring admission

- Unable to cope at home.
- Already receiving long-term oxygen therapy (LTOT).
- Cannot complete sentences.
- Respiratory rate > 25/min.
- Pulse rate > 110 b.p.m. (unreliable in AF).
- Peak flow < 50% of patient's normal or predicted.
- SaO_2 < 90%.
- PO_2 < 7 kPa, PCO_2 > 6.7 kPa on air.

Management of acute exacerbation of airway obstruction

1 Humidified oxygen: 24% or 28% to keep the SaO_2 within an individualized target range (usually 88–92% for an elderly COPD patient). Oxygen must be prescribed on the drug chart. If the patient is very ill or becomes drowsy check arterial blood gases (ABGs) for pCO_2 and pH.

2 $\beta 2$-agonist (2.5 mg salbutamol) by nebulizer using humidified air not oxygen as the carrier.

3 Antimuscarinic (ipratropium bromide 500 μg) by nebulizer.

4 Antibiotics if evidence of infection (amoxicillin 500 mg t.d.s.; clarithromycin 500 mg b.d. if penicillin allergic). Treat as pneumonia (see below) if sputum purulent, patient ill or febrile, high WBC or CRP, or CXR suggestive.

5 Prednisolone 30 mg (20 mg if low weight) daily for 7–14 days (100 mg IV hydrocortisone if unable to take tablets). Elderly patients may have problems with short courses of steroids including steroid psychosis, CCF precipitated by fluid overload and unmasking of diabetes (as well as the well-known long-term complications).

6 Intravenous fluids.

7 Monitor temperature, pulse rate and respiration, oxygen saturation and peak flow.

8 Chest physiotherapy if secretions retained.

9 DVT prophylaxis unless contraindicated, e.g. enoxaparin 40 mg o.d.

10 Aminophylline infusion if obstruction remains severe (not if on oral theophylline unless levels are available).

11 If the patient is beginning to tire, CO_2 is rising and pH < 7.35 consider:

- Non-invasive ventilation (NIV) has replaced doxapram and is a good option for patients who are poor candidates for intubation because extubation may be difficult.
- Intensive care for ventilation if above measures ineffective. Find out about the patient's functional status prior to this illness before contacting ITU to discuss admission. Patients with COPD may do better than anticipated in this situation.

Post-acute/chronic phase

1 Unless the patient is very disabled, stopping smoking is still worthwhile. Patients need advice and information and results are better with nicotine replacement therapy, bupropion or the selective nicotine receptor partial agonist varenicline; refer to a 'stop-smoking clinic'.

2 Inhaled drugs used include:
SABA (short-acting beta$_2$ agonists) – salbutamol, terbutaline.
SAMA (short-acting muscarinic antagonists) – ipratropium.
LABA (long-acting beta$_2$ agonists) – salmeterol, formoterol.
LAMA (long-acting muscarinic antagonists) – tiotropium.

ICS (inhaled corticosteroids) and LABA/ICS combinations – budesonide/formoterol = Symbicort; fluticasone/salmeterol = Seretide. Patients with mild COPD need a SAMA or SABA.

If the patient remains breathless or has exacerbations and $FEV_1 \geq 50\%$ predicted, offer a LAMA **or** a LABA. If $FEV_1 < 50\%$ predicted, offer a LAMA **or** LABA/ICS.

Tiotropium and the combination inhalers are expensive but persistent breathlessness or frequent exacerbations warrant a LAMA **and** a LABA/ICS regardless of FEV_1. This is common in frail older people with recurrent admissions with COPD. ICS have been shown to increase pneumonia but the benefit in terms of reducing exacerbations is worth it. Recurrent exacerbations are associated with increasing morbidity and a strong predictor of mortality (see also 3 below).

Different types of inhaler are available requiring different levels of manual dexterity, cognition and inspiratory flow. Ensure inhaler and spacer device are understood by the patient. Prescribe SABA as 'rescue medication'.

3 Consider supplying antibiotics and oral steroids for the patient to initiate self-treatment of an exacerbation (with clear instructions).

4 Pulmonary rehabilitation programme for those with respiratory disability (exercise and nutrition).

5 Depression is common – consider an SSRI.

6 Pneumococcal vaccine and annual flu vaccine should be offered.

7 Mucolytics, e.g. carbocysteine, may be useful if sputum production is marked.

8 Long-term corticosteroids should be avoided if possible – if frequent courses are given remember osteoporosis prophylaxis.

9 Theophylline (phosphodiesterase inhibitor) is usually only given once inhaled therapy is maximal because of its narrow therapeutic index; caution with macrolides and fluoroquinolones which increase levels.

10 Domiciliary oxygen can be provided as short burst oxygen therapy (SBOT) for symptomatic relief of episodic severe breathlessness (cylinder) or as long-term oxygen therapy (LTOT) if the patient meets the criteria listed in the BNF (PaO_2 on air when stable < 7.3 kPa) and will use oxygen for at least 15 h a day; then LTOT via a concentrator improves life expectancy. The Home Oxygen Order

Form (HOOF) can be completed by the hospital or GP.

11 Palliative care for end-stage chronic lung disease. In addition to oxygen, an opiate or benzodiazepine can relieve respiratory distress.

Pneumonia

As in younger adults, the commonest organism is *Streptococcus pneumoniae*, followed by *Haemophilus influenza*. Other organisms include *Mycoplasma* in epidemic years (every third year), viruses, *Branhamella*, *Legionella*, *Chlamydia pneumoniae* and *Staph. aureus*, especially during outbreaks of influenza. Prevalent pathogens and their sensitivities vary from one locality to another. It is often difficult to identify the organism, as elderly patients tend to swallow their sputum, but blood culture is sometimes positive. Presentation may be typical or atypical, with tachypnoea and functional decline. Pre-existing airway disease is almost certain to deteriorate.

Aspiration pneumonia is common in older patients with swallowing disorders or following an episode of unconsciousness.

Pneumococcal pneumonia has a mortality rate approaching 35% in elderly subjects. In addition to splenectomized patients where it is mandatory, frail patients with chronic heart, lung, renal, liver disease and diabetes should be offered pneumococcal vaccine, which usually provides immunity for 5–10 years.

Antibiotics are traditionally given intravenously in the first instance to those with life-threatening features, as well as those unable to swallow, although there is little evidence of greater effectiveness by this route. Most hospitals have an antibiotics policy – be familiar with yours. The regime often included a second-generation cephalosporin, such as cefotaxime, but many hospitals discourage cephalosporin use in older people, as they are strongly associated with the often serious (for the patient) and always disruptive (for the hospital ward) complication of *Clostridium difficile* colitis.

The CURB-65 score predicts the likely outcome of pneumonia in adults at all ages:

- Confusion of new onset (AMT of 8 or less).
- Urea > 7 mol/L.
- Respiratory rate of 30 breaths a minute or more.

- Blood pressure < 90 mmHg systolic or < 60 mmHg diastolic.
- Age 65 or older.

Other features indicating life-threatening pneumonia include arterial PO_2 < 8 kPa, WBC > 20,000 × 109/L or < 4000 × 109/L, multiple lobes affected on CXR, serum albumin < 35 g/L or co-morbidity, e.g. diabetes, heart disease.

In older people, a recommended regime for severe community-acquired pneumonia is co-amoxiclav 1.2 g t.d.s. IV and clarithromycin 500 mg IV b.d. If co-amoxiclav is used, there is no need to add flucloxacillin after influenza or metronidazole for aspiration. Vancomycin plus ciprofloxacin can be used in penicillin allergy and for MRSA.

Other measures include oxygen (same precautions as in airway obstruction), IV fluids, physiotherapy for retained secretions, relief of bronchospasm if prominent and nutritional supplements if cachectic.

A follow-up CXR is recommended at 6 weeks to check that the consolidation has resolved fully; persistent shadowing should prompt chest CT scan to exclude a cancer.

Pulmonary tuberculosis

A resurgence of pulmonary TB has been anticipated when patients who had contracted TB in the pre-drug era (before the 1950s) reached old age and their immune systems became less effective; there may be a little evidence that this is occurring. The number of TB cases in England has increased steadily since 2000, reaching over 8,000 in 2009. Most cases are in young adults, 73% of whom were born outside the UK. In the non UK-born, the case rate is bimodal with a second peak occurring in people in their eighth decade. Rates are much lower in the UK-born but the highest rates do occur in the elderly, in their ninth decade (7/100,000). See Figures 10.3 and 10.4.

Remain alert to the possibility of TB (especially in elderly immigrants from the Indian subcontinent and in conurbations especially London). Look out for the signs and X-ray findings of TB from the pre-drug era [chest deformity from thoracoplasty, scars in neck from TB node removal, phrenic crush or artificial pneumothorax, the common findings of apical calcification, granuloma and calcified lymph nodes or, rarely now, 'balls' (plombage) on the CXR]. Haemoptysis may

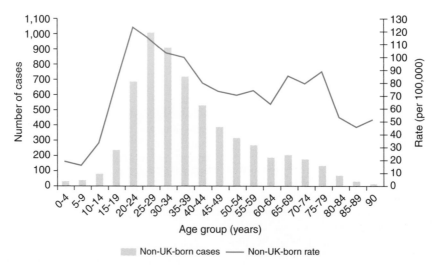

Figure 10.3 Non UK-born TB case reports and rates by age (UK 2009 HPA data).

indicate recrudescence of TB or a complication, such as the development of a fungus ball (aspergilloma) in an old cavity. Infections with atypical mycobacteria occur in damaged lung and immunosuppressed patients.

Isolate patients with suspected TB and productive cough until the sputum smear microscopy has been found negative for acid-fast bacilli (AFB). Send three sputum samples for AFB and request a chest opinion if TB is possible. Bronchoscopy and lavage may be needed to obtain sputum. Start treatment without waiting for culture results if the patient has clinical signs and symptoms of TB and complete treatment even if culture results are negative. The standard regimen is a '6-month,

four-drug initial regimen' of 2 months of isoniazid, rifampicin, pyrazinamide and ethambutol, followed by 4 months of isoniazid and rifampicin. If your patient dies, warn the pathologist and send autopsy samples for culture if respiratory TB was a possibility.

Pleural effusion

Common causes

- Left ventricular failure (LVF) (transudate, but closer to an exudate after prolonged diuretics).

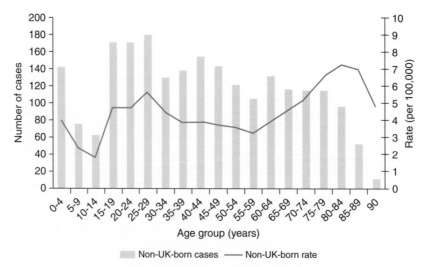

Figure 10.4 UK-born TB case reports and rates by age (UK 2009 HPA data).

- Parapneumonic – empyema often presents atypically (exudate).
- Pulmonary embolism (exudate – can be contralateral to the embolus).
- Malignancy (1° or 2°) especially if 'white-out' on CXR (exudate, often bloody).

Management

If LVF is likely, monitor the response to diuretics and only tap if features are atypical or treatment fails. Effusions are classified as an exudate (protein > 30 g/L) or transudate, but this is often less clear-cut in an elderly patient with a low serum albumin, so measure total protein and lactate dehydrogenase (LDH) in blood and pleural fluid. Diagnostic aspiration should be done with ultrasound guidance, a 21-G needle and 50-ml syringe and pleural fluid sent for:

- Protein (pleural fluid protein divided by serum protein is > 0.5 = exudate).
- LDH (pleural fluid LDH divided by serum LDH is > 0.6 = exudate).
- Gram stain.
- Microbiological culture (in blood culture bottles).
- Cytology (all the remaining sample).
- Additional tests only if specific indication.

If the diagnosis is still unclear, request contrast enhanced CT chest and a specialist opinion.

Therapeutic aspiration may be needed to relieve breathlessness from a huge effusion. Advice should be sought from the respiratory team for the management of symptomatic malignant pleural effusion. For example, a talc slurry pleurodesis may be performed: fluid is removed to 'dryness' with a small-bore tube, and lidocaine and graded talc are introduced. Patients with mesothelioma need prophylactic radiotherapy to prevent seeding if a large-bore chest drain is used, but this is not a complication of diagnostic aspiration.

Bronchiectasis

Bronchiectasis, abnormal irreversible thickening and dilatation of the muscular and elastic walls of the bronchi resulting in chronic infection, is usually post-infectious (measles, whooping cough or TB in this age group). The initial insult impairs mucociliary clearance and initiates an inflammatory cycle. High resolution CT (HRCT) scan is the diagnostic investigation of choice. The features and treatment overlap with recurrent chest infections and COPD; physiotherapy with airway clearance techniques and postural drainage are particularly important. Saline and bronchodilator nebulizers and then LAMA and LABA may be used but avoid inhaled corticosteroids unless there is coexisting asthma. As with all lung disease causing breathlessness, pulmonary rehabilitation is useful. Prognosis is worse once *Pseudomonas aeruginosa* colonization occurs. Local guidelines and preferably sputum samples should guide antibiotic use.

Chest trauma

- Rib fracture – common after mild trauma, e.g. coughing fit.
- Diagnosis – local tenderness and pain on springing chest.
- Complications – shallow breathing and reluctance to cough may cause sputum retention and segmental collapse. Pneumo- or haemothorax: refer for usual treatment.
- Treatment – adequate regular analgesia (e.g. paracetamol, an NSAID with gut protection if renal function is good, or tramadol/meptazinol), usually with physiotherapy, is essential to avoid infection. If associated with minor trauma, treat long term for osteoporosis.

Carcinoma of the bronchus

This is the commonest life-threatening cancer in the West. In the UK, between 1993 and 2008 male lung cancer incidence rates decreased by almost a third (32%) but over the same period there was an increase in the female rate (11%). It has become mainly a disease of older people (87% of cases occur in those aged over 60) as shown in Figure 10.5 and, in the UK, of social disadvantage.

Lung cancers are classified into two main categories: small-cell lung cancers (SCLC), which account for approximately 20% of cases, and non-small-cell lung cancers (NSCLC), which account for the other 80%. NSCLC include squamous-cell carcinomas (35%), adenocarcinomas

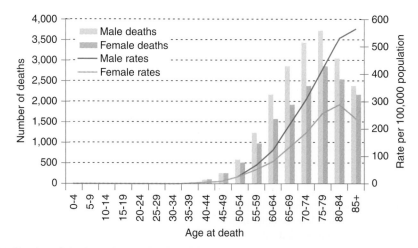

Figure 10.5 Number of deaths and age-specific mortality.

(27%) and large-cell carcinomas (10%). Adeno-carcinomas are less clearly smoking-related.

Presentation may be cough, haemoptysis, dyspnoea or slowly resolving infection but is often late, with symptoms relating to distant spread or non-metastatic, metabolic complications. Patients are managed by a multidisciplinary team. After CXR, a contrast CT scan including the liver and adrenals is usually done before bronchoscopy for central lesions or transcutaneous biopsy for peripheral lesions. PET CT scanning with ^{18}F deoxyglucose is very helpful in staging patients.

In early NSCLC, pneumonectomy or lobectomy remain the most effective treatment offering the possibility of cure: 70% 5-year survival for $T_1N_0M_0$ if the patient is fit enough and lung function is adequate ($FEV_1 > 1.5\,L$). Surgical outcomes have improved, peri-operative mortality of pneumonectomy is around 6% (right pneumonectomy is riskier) but there is major morbidity in 30% of cases. Carefully selected older patients do as well as younger ones. Radical radiotherapy (CHART – continuous hyperfractionated accelerated radio therapy) produces a few long-term cures. Chemotherapy sometimes offers worthwhile life extension (a few months). Radiotherapy offers useful palliation for superior mediastinal obstruction, chest pain, painful bony metastases and haemoptysis. Involve palliative care services early.

SCLC has usually metastasized at presentation and is staged as limited or extensive disease. Unless the patient is too frail, multi-drug platinum-based chemotherapy is offered and continued for 4–6 cycles if there is response. Limited stage disease has a life expectancy of 12 weeks with no treatment

and 12 months after chemotherapy, with a 5-year survival of 5–10%.

Pleural plaques

Pleural plaques are discrete circumscribed areas of hyaline fibrosis usually of the parietal pleura. They are benign and usually asymptomatic but are the commonest manifestation of past exposure to asbestos. Patients may be anxious if they know they are present. Reassure that they are at no more risk of developing serious lung disease than other individuals with the same asbestos exposure. They should stop smoking and like anyone they should report breathlessness or chest pain, as there is a link with lung cancer.

Malignant mesothelioma

This arises in the pleura and presents with chest pain, dyspnoea and bloody pleural effusion, as a result of asbestos exposure. Check for a history of industrial exposure – builders, shipyard workers and the person who washed the overalls may also be at risk. The initial course may be indolent and high-resolution CT scan may be helpful but diagnosis requires pleural biopsy. Because of the association with asbestos exposure and the long interval between exposure and presentation the effect of strict industrial regulation will not be apparent for years. Mesothelioma is increasing rapidly in prevalence, with an expected peak in 2015. It is important to diagnose; although management is palliative, compensation may be available – seek specialist advice.

Interstitial lung disease

Interstitial lung disease (ILD) or diffuse parenchymal lung disease (DPLD) is a heterogeneous group of non-infectious non-malignant processes of the lower respiratory tract characterized by the abnormal accumulation of cells and/or non-cellular material within the walls of the alveoli. This results in thickening and stiffness of the elastic tissues of the lung, so that patients breathe in a rapid and shallow manner. Alveolar thickening decreases the efficiency of oxygen transfer. It is assumed that a variety of triggers, e.g. viruses, smoking and pollution, with some genetic component lead to alveolar damage and then an inflammatory and fibrotic cycle. The conditions are loosely referred to as 'pulmonary fibrosis' but the relative amounts of fibrosis and inflammation depend on the aetiology. In general, inflammation is more amenable to treatment than fibrosis. Alveolar filling diseases present with similar symptoms and X-ray findings and are included as ILDs.

ILD is poorly understood (by most doctors as well as students):

- 'Rag bag' of conditions, many of which are very rare.
- Classification, particularly of the 'idiopathic' types, keeps changing.
- Names are cumbersome and overlap.
- Pathogenesis is poorly understood.

BUT

- Incidence is increasing in the UK/USA.
- The commonest idiopathic subgroup, pulmonary fibrosis (see below), causes more deaths each year than ovarian cancer, lymphoma or leukaemia.

Causes

- Granulomatous disease, e.g. sarcoid.
- Inhalational, e.g. asbestosis; hypersensitivity pneumonitis (extrinsic allergic alveolitis), e.g. pigeon fancier's lung, farmer's lung due to the mould *Thermoactinomyces vulgaris*; silicosis in stone masons; pneumoconiosis due to coal dust

berylliosis in aerospace industry workers (histology is granulomatous and looks like sarcoid).
- Connective tissue disease associated ILD, e.g. rheumatoid and scleroderma.
- Systemic vasculitis associated ILD, e.g. Wegener's and Churg–Strauss.
- Drug induced, e.g. amiodarone, bleomycin.
- Post radiotherapy.
- Idiopathic interstitial pneumonias around 40% of cases:
  o Idiopathic pulmonary fibrosis (IPF), previously 'cryptogenic fibrosing alveolitis'.
  o Non-IPF interstitial pneumonias:
    ▪ Non-specific interstitial pneumonia (NSIP).
    ▪ Acute interstitial pneumonia (AIP) idiopathic acute respiratory distress syndrome – mortality > 50%.
    ▪ Cryptogenic organizing pneumonia (COP).
- Alveolar filling diseases, e.g. alveolar proteinosis.

Features

Most patients present with insidious progressive breathlessness and some have a troublesome dry cough, but other cases have an acute or episodic presentation. Widespread or bibasal fine crackles and sometimes clubbing may be found. Look for the features of any associated disease. The course is generally progressive but the rate is very variable depending on the aetiology and this was a major factor driving the new classification.

Investigations include lung function tests – typically a restrictive defect with reduced lung volumes and increased transfer factor, ABGs showing widened $AaPO_2$ and oxygen desaturation on walking, HRCT and sometimes bronchoalveolar lavage and lung biopsy.

Idiopathic pulmonary fibrosis (IPF)

IPF, the most common form of ILD, had a mean age at diagnosis of 74 years (SD 64–84 years) in a recent English study. It is more common in males and with a smoking history. It is rapidly progressive with median survival from diagnosis around 3 years. Pulmonary hypertension is frequent. Steroids, azathioprine and N-acetyl cysteine are used but results are poor so patients should be enrolled in drug trials if feasible; lung transplantation is offered in younger patients. Interferon gamma-1 beta was unhelpful. Pirfenidone, which inhibits fibroblast growth factor, has recently been licensed in the EU but evidence is slight. Histology, described as **UIP** ('usual interstitial pneumonia') shows destruction of lung architecture and dense areas of fibrosis with an advancing front.

Non-specific interstitial pneumonia (NSIP)

NSIP is clinically indistinguishable from IPF but has a median survival of around 6 years. The histology, intra-alveolar septal fibrosis, is more homogeneous and is seen in a number of ILDs including connective tissue disorders, drug-induced fibrosis and as a sequel of ARDS and COP.

Cyrptogenic organizing pneumonia (COP)

COP, previously known as bronchiolitis obliterans organizing pneumonia (BOOP), presents with breathlessness developing over a few weeks, cough with clear sputum and constitutional symptoms. CXR often shows multifocal consolidation that cannot be distinguished from infection or malignancy. Bronchoscopy is often needed to exclude the former and for transbronchial biopsy. Unlike many ILDs, COP responds well to corticosteroids. Acute histology shows budding of fibro-proliferative tissue into alveolar spaces and chronically resembles NSIP.

Some elderly patients will have had documented pulmonary fibrosis for a number of years, usually NSIP.

Carbon monoxide poisoning

Incidence

- Accounts for 50,000 emergency room attendances in the USA per year.
- Causes the death of 50 people per year in the UK.

Clinical features and sequelae

- Carbon monoxide (CO) reduces oxygen delivery to tissues by two effects: it has an affinity for haemoglobin 220 times greater than that of oxygen, and it shifts the oxyhaemoglobin dissociation curve to the left.
- CO also binds to intracellular proteins, causes activation of neutrophils leading to lipid peroxidation and may cause apoptosis in the brain.

- Think about this if an elderly couple present together with confusion.
- Patients are hypoxic but not cyanosed. The skin and mucous membranes may appear 'cherry red' but this is very rare unless on the post-mortem slab.
- Mild exposure carboxyhaemoglobin (COHb) < 30%: headache, lethargy, nausea and vomiting.
- Moderate exposure COHb 50–60%: tachycardia, tachypnoea, syncope and fits.
- High exposure HbCO > 60%: cardiorespiratory failure and death.
- CNS tissue damage can progress for up to 80 days after exposure (lipid peroxidation causes delayed reversible demyelination) causing neuropsychiatric problems including Parkinsonism, akinetic mutism, as well as acute confusion.

Causes

CO is produced by incomplete combustion of carbon-containing compounds in an inadequate supply of oxygen:

- Smoke inhalation, e.g. house fire.
- Faulty heating and cooking appliances especially solid fuel, but oil, paraffin and gas too.
- Poor ventilation of such appliances.
- Deliberate inhalation of car exhaust fumes; less common in older people.

Management and prevention

- The key is to think about the possibility of CO poisoning and to take an arterial sample to check the level of COHb.
- Give 100% oxygen via a face mask for up to 24 h.
- Do not be misled by pulse oximeter readings: the oximeter cannot distinguish between COHb and HbO_2.
- Hyperbaric oxygen is not recommended in the UK.
- Treat fits with IV diazepam.
- Prevention is obviously important. CO alarms are readily available. In the UK, landlords are legally required to have all domestic gas appliances checked annually by an approved engineer.

➔ FURTHER INFORMATION

American Lung Association website:www.lungusa. org/lung-disease/finder.html. Large number of lung conditions described in detail for patients and clear for students.

British Lung Foundation website: www.lunguk.org/ you-and-your-lungs/conditions-and-diseases.

British Thoracic Society: management guidelines: www.brit-thoracic.org.uk/library-guidelines. aspx.

British Thoracic Society (2006) *The Burden of Lung Disease*, 2nd edn. www.brit-thoracic.org.uk/ Portals/0/Library/BTS%20Publications/burdeon_ of_lung_disease2007.pdf.

Chambers A, Routledge T, Pilling J, Scarci M (2010) In elderly patients with lung cancer is resection justified in terms of morbidity, mortality and residual quality of life? *Interactive CardioVascular Thoracic Surgery* 10: 1015–1021, doi: 10.1510/ icvts.2010.233189.

ESC Guidelines on Pulmonary Embolism 2008: www.escardio.org/guidelines-surveys/esc-guidelines/GuidelinesDocuments/guidelines-APE-FT.pdf.

McGill, Virtual stethoscope: http://sprojects.mmi. mcgill.ca/mvs/mvsteth.htm.

NICE website: www.nice.org.uk/. Type in 'respiratory' for all relevant guidelines.

Omni medical search engine: www.omnimedical-search.com/medproindex.html.

Tuberculosis in the UK: Annual report on tuberculosis surveillance in the UK, 2010: Health Protection Agency Centre for Infections, October 2010 – www.hpa.org.uk/web/HPAwebFile/HPAweb_ C/1287143594275.

UK Cancer Statistics 2010: http://info.cancerresearchuk.org/cancerstats/types/lung/incidence/.

11

Gastrointestinal disease and nutrition

Gastrointestinal (GI) symptoms are common throughout life. Structural changes, e.g. hiatus hernia and diverticular disease, and functional changes, e.g. bowel dysmotility, become more common with age. Almost one-fifth of patients presenting at a geriatric outpatient clinic have GI problems.

Age changes

1 Impairment of smell and taste can further reduce poor appetite.
2 Older people cannot open their mouths as wide and chew with less power than younger people.
3 Loss of teeth (see Chapter 15) and/or poorly fitting dentures secondary to alveolar margin atrophy impair mastication.
4 Tongue atrophy means older people can only manage smaller boluses of food.
5 Impaired coordination of swallowing and uncoordinated or reduced oesophageal peristalsis (presbyoesophagus).
6 Reduced pressure of the upper oesophageal sphincter plus delayed relaxation after swallowing lead to problems with the oeosophageal phase of swallowing.
7 Slower gastric emptying of fluids, but not solids.
8 Reduced pancreatic function due to duct and parenchymatous changes.
9 Reduced splanchnic blood flow.
10 Reduced small bowel surface area.
11 Changes in intestinal microflora including a decrease in anaerobes and bifidobacteria and an increase in enterobacteria reduce immunity to *Clostridium difficile*.
12 Diverticula develop in the bowel.
13 Reduced large bowel motility predisposes to constipation.
14 Reduced rectal wall elasticity increases the risk of faecal incontinence.

Unintentional weight loss

Loss of > 5 kg of weight in 6–12 months is clinically significant, associated with increased morbidity and mortality, and affects:

- 20% of over 65s living in the community
- 50% of those in nursing homes.

1 *Ageing changes*: account for only 0.1–0.2 kg weight loss per year. There is a tendency to weight loss in old age (in contrast to the weight gain common in middle age) due to reduced body-water content, bone loss (osteoporosis), thinning of connective tissue and the conversion of muscle to fat. Those who maintain their lean body mass into old age have a better life expectancy than their shrinking peers.
2 *Oral and dental disease:* see Chapter 15.
3 *Systemic disease:* weight loss is associated with all chronic disorders, e.g. COPD, cardiac failure, kidney disease, poorly controlled diabetes mellitus, thyrotoxicosis and Addison's disease.

Lecture Notes Elderly Care Medicine, Eighth Edition. Claire G. Nicholl and K. Jane Wilson.
© 2012 John Wiley & Sons, Ltd. Published 2012 by John Wiley & Sons, Ltd.

4 *Malignancy*: GI malignancy accounts for 50% of cancers presenting with severe weight loss.

5 *Psychiatric disease*: the apathy of depression and self-neglect in some people with dementia lead to weight loss. The paranoia of a psychosis may make food unacceptable. The hyperactivity of some demented and hypomanic patients may result in weight loss. Alcohol abuse should also be considered.

6 *Iatrogenic disease*: impaired appetite may be due to unpalatable treatments, side-effects, e.g. antibiotics (especially metronidazole and erythromycin), opiates, antidepressants, metformin, levodopa or toxicity, e.g. digoxin. ACE inhibitors may cause loss of taste or an unpleasant taste. Diarrhoea may be due to proton pump inhibitors, anti-cholinesterase inhibitors, misoprostol or antibiotics. The burden of too many tablets may suppress appetite. Do not forget how unpleasant it is for patients in hospital to have to eat where they sleep, open their bowels, etc. and their proximity to others performing the same functions.

7 *GI disease*:
   • Dysphagia.
   • Dyspepsia.
   • Malabsorption.

Diagnosing weight loss

• History: diet, appetite, taste, nausea, vomiting, dysphagia, abdominal pain, diarrhoea, change in bowel habit.
• Examination: cachexia, anaemia, teeth, tongue, jaundice, lymphadenopathy, goitre, gross oedema, severe heart failure, obvious masses, organomegaly, rectal examination.
• Assess mood and cognitive function.
• Baseline tests:
  o FBC: micro- or macrocytic anaemia.
  o LFTs: high alkaline phosphatase (ALP) may represent bone or liver metastases.
  o TSH suppressed in hyperthyroidism.
  o CRP and ESR: if normal, the cause is unlikely to be organic.
  o CXR: may demonstrate unexpected primary or secondary tumours.
  o Other tests as indicated by the features above.
• Refer to the dietician.
• Treat underlying causes where possible.
• Explain to patient and family if this is an end of life event (see Chapter 17).

Dysphagia

• Dysphagia is increasingly common in older age affecting:
  o 10% of over 60s
  o 30–60% of nursing home residents
  o Up to 60% of post-stroke patients.
• Patients with dysphagia have a worse 6-month mortality than those without.
• There are three stages of swallowing and dysfunction results from a combination of age-related problems and pathology.
• Dysphagia can affect the oropharynx or oesophagus and be due to structural changes or neuromuscular disease (Table 11.1).

Assessing dysphagia

History

• Is it difficult to swallow liquids (suggests neurological problem), solids (suggests obstruction) or both?
• Is there evidence of inflammation – indigestion, acid burn?
• Does the food stick at one level?
• Is there a sensation of fatigue? 'Yes' suggests myasthenia gravis.

Examination

Check dentition and fit of dentures and look for candidiasis. Are there tongue fasiculations suggestive of MND?

Investigation

If there is concern that endoscopy may perforate the oesophagus, arrange a barium swallow first. This will demonstrate a pharyngeal pouch, corkscrew contractions secondary to achalasia or shouldering characteristic of oesophageal carcinoma. Gastroscopy allows direct visualization and biopsy of abnormal tissue. Active bleeding can be treated, a benign stricture can be dilated and a malignant stricture can be stented.

Management

Specific management depends on the cause, but is often multidisciplinary involving dieticians and speech and language therapists.

Table 11.1 Causes of dysphagia

	Oropharyngeal	Oesophageal
Structural	Zenker's diverticulum, pharyngeal pouch	Peptic stricture, rings or webs
		Severe oesophagitis
	Carcinoma of palate or tongue	Intrinsic oesophageal carcinoma
	Infection, abscess	Severe candidiasis
		Compression from extrinsic carcinoma, e.g. bronchial
		Vascular compression, e.g. aortic aneurysm
		Foreign body
Neuromuscular	Stroke	Achalasia
	Bulbar palsy, e.g. MND, pseudobulbar palsy	Diffuse muscle spasms of presbyoesophagus
	Brain stem lesion including tumour	Motility disorder secondary to GORD
	Polymyositis, dermatomyositis	Motility disorder secondary to systemic diseases such as diabetes, CREST
	Myasthenia gravis	

GORD, gastro-oesophageal reflux disease.

Neuromuscular dysphagia

1 Presbyoesophagus.
2 Pseudobulbar palsy is bilateral upper motor neuron spastic weakness of muscles supplied by V, VII, X, XI and XII secondary to lesions of the corticobulbar tracts in the mid-pons, e.g. bilateral internal capsule strokes or MS.
3 Bulbar palsy is the impairment of function of the cranial nerves due to a lower motor lesion. A posterior inferior cerebellar artery infarct results in ipsilateral pharyngeal paralysis with contralateral paresis of the arm and leg (Wallenberg's syndrome).
4 Parkinson's disease. Akinesia impairs swallowing; up to 50% of PD patients have dysphagia. Levodopa and speech therapy may help.
5 Myasthenia gravis. Rare but important, because of good response to anticholinesterases, e.g. pyridostigmine.
6 Achalasia. More of a problem in younger patients but may be an aspect of presbyoesophagus.

NB: Nasogastric (NG) tube feeding is usually only justified short term when recovery is anticipated. Fine-bore tubes should be used, ideally when the patient can cooperate. Bridled loop NG tubes can be useful for patients with dementia who are likely to pull the tube out, but again use should be short term. If long-term treatment is contemplated, consider percutaneous endoscopic gastrostomy (PEG) feeding. See Chapter 7.

External pressure on the oesophagus

1 Pharyngeal pouches. All pouches become more common with increasing age. Zenker's diverticulum, through the posterior pharyngeal wall at the upper level of cricopharyngeus, may result from incoordinated contractions. When large and full, it may hinder passage of a food bolus. Symptomatic pouches can be removed surgically and endoscopic techniques permit operations on frailer patients. More rarely, pouches occur lower in the oesophagus.
2 Superior mediastinal obstruction – malignancy (usually carcinoma of the bronchus).
3 Dilated left atrium, in severe heart disease. A CXR, in conjunction with clinical signs, will usually be sufficient to make the diagnosis.
4 Aortic-arch dilatation.
5 Posterior pressure from spinal osteophytes (very rare).

Inflammatory lesions of the oesophageal epithelium

Oesophagitis

Inflammation in the lower oesophagus is associated with hiatus hernia and acid reflux. The patient often gives a long history of indigestion. Chronic inflammation can lead to strictures. Endoscopy is the best diagnostic modality as biopsies can be taken (essential if there is any suspicion of malignant change), and Barrett's oesophagus (see below) may be noted. Symptoms respond to antacids, but H2 antagonists (e.g. ranitidine) or proton-pump inhibitors (e.g. omeprazole) are necessary for healing. Strictures should be dilated.

Oesophageal candidiasis

Frail elderly people are at risk, especially if immunosuppressed, users of steroid inhalers or after antibiotics. The typical white patches of thrush are often (but not always) present in the mouth. Endoscopy confirms oesophageal involvement. Oral fluconazole is the treatment of choice.

Barrett's oesophagus

This is the development of intestinal metaplasia usually affecting the lower one-third of the oesophagus. Risk factors include being male, over 60, smoking and alcohol. It usually develops in combination with hiatus hernia, low oesophageal tone and duodenal reflux. It is premalignant and may progress to adenocarcinoma. Most elderly patients will die of other diseases, but fit elderly people without significant other pathologies should be offered regular surveillance.

Carcinoma of the oesophagus

- Commonly occurs in the sixth and seventh decades; 20 times more common in those aged over 65 compared with the younger population.
- UK incidence in men is 17.5 per 100,000; 8.8 per 100,000 women.
- Two main types: adenocarcinoma and squamous cell carcinoma.
  - o Adenocarcinoma is becoming more common in the West, is more common in men, affects slightly younger patients, and tends to affect the lower third of the oesophagus. The strongest risk factor is reflux and Barrett's oesophagus is a premalignant stage.
  - o Worldwide, squamous cell carcinoma is more common and is related to smoking, alcohol and vitamin deficiencies. The increased incidence in China is attributed to riboflavin deficiency.
- Symptoms: the patient complains of dysphagia, first for solids and then liquids. Weight loss is extremely common. Some patients experience retrosternal pain. Hoarseness indicates invasion of the left recurrent laryngeal nerve. Cough and breathlessness may be due to aspiration or direct invasion of the bronchial tree.
- Barium swallow is safest for initial evaluation and great care is needed during endoscopy because of risk of perforation.
- Endoscopy allows biopsy.
- CT scanning is useful for staging.

Management

Curative treatment is rare; tumours are discovered late and have often already spread, so palliation is the aim.

1 Patient should be discussed by a multidisciplinary upper GI team.
2 Oesophagectomy, for lesions at the lower end, is a massive undertaking unlikely to improve quality of life of frail older people.
3 Combinations of chemotherapy and radiotherapy may be an option for biologically fit patients with high performance status and localized disease.
4 Dysphagia can be reduced by debulking with endoluminal brachytherapy or photodynamic therapy.
5 Stent insertion: the treatment of choice for obstructive symptoms when other measures are not justified; pain and complications are common. If tumour blocks the stent, this can be debulked with a Yittrium Aluminium Garnet (YAG) laser or photodynamic therapy.
6 Patient support: patients and their families should be given the support of a specialist nurse and contact details for support networks (e.g. www.macmillan.org).
7 Nutrition: do not forget to optimize patient's oral intake by referring to the dietician for supplements where indicated and consider thickened fluids if there is risk of aspiration.
8 Palliative care: refer early for help with symptoms and further support (Chapter 17).

Intraluminal obstruction

Impacted objects may include food (especially if not properly chewed), missing dentures and other foreign bodies. Cognitively impaired patients are particularly at risk.

Complications of dysphagia

- Malnutrition.
- Aspiration pneumonia.
- Oesophageal rupture.

Dyspepsia

1 Indigestion is common at all ages (30% of the population); 2–3% of prescribed drugs are antacids.
2 In many elderly patients diagnosis is difficult as the symptoms are vague and non-specific.
3 As many drugs cause dyspepsia; a drug history is essential. Avoid NSAIDs, bisphosphonates and calcium channel blockers, and co-prescribe proton pump inhibitors (PPIs) with steroids.
4 *Helicobacter pylori* infection rises with age (up to 60% of elderly people are infected) and should be treated if demonstrated by biopsy, culture, breath test or serology.
5 The pathologies potentially responsible for indigestion become more common in old age. See box below.
6 Many patients will have more than one possible cause for their non-specific indigestion. A therapeutic trial may identify the responsible lesion as many of the conditions can be asymptomatic, e.g. 20% of hiatus hernia and up to 50% of gallstones.
7 Late-onset dyspepsia should be investigated. Endoscopy is the investigation of choice (except in the presence of dysphagia) and acceptable for most elderly patients; extra care is needed with pre-medication in those with poor respiratory reserve. Magnetic resonance cholangiopancreatography (MRCP) is useful in diagnosis in frail patients with biliary-tract disease. However, they may subsequently need ERCP for biopsies and treatment, e.g. to remove small biliary stones or insert stents.
8 Ultrasound examination is the best technique for suspected gallbladder and pancreatic disease.
9 Watch out for side-effects from medication, for example:

   o Metoclopramide may precipitate or worsen extra-pyramidal syndromes.
   o Cimetidine can cause delirium.
   o Avoid aluminium salts in constipated patients and magnesium in those with diarrhoea.
   o Bile salts have proved disappointing for dissolving gallstones and side-effects, especially diarrhoea, can be troublesome.
   o PPIs can cause hyponatraemia, diarrhoea, increase the risk of *Clostridium difficile* and long-term use has been linked to increased

risk of malignant change. There is uncertainty as to whether their interaction with clopidogrel is clinically relevant.
   o Patients with osteoporotic kyphosis are at increased risk of oesophageal perforation with bisphosphonates.

Lesions potentially responsible for 'indigestion'

- Hiatus hernia (affects 60% of over 70 year olds).
- Gastritis (especially drug-induced).
- Peptic ulceration (found in 20% of over 70 year olds).
- Carcinoma of the stomach.
- Gallstones (found in 38% of over 70 year olds).
- Pancreatic disease.
- Mesenteric ischaemia.
- Carcinoma of large bowel.

Gastro-oesophageal reflux disease (GORD)

This is return of gastric contents into the oesophagus.

- Heartburn is common, but GORD may cause respiratory symptoms such as chronic cough or asthma and non-cardiac chest pain.
- PPIs are the most successful treatment in conjunction with *H. pylori* eradication plus lifestyle changes (weight-loss, cessation of smoking, raise head of bed).
- Only endoscope if treatment fails to relieve symptoms.
- Oesophagitis, strictures, Barrett's oesophagus and adenocarcinoma are complications.

GI bleeding

Almost every cause of GI bleeding becomes more common with increasing age:

1 Hiatus hernia with oesophagitis.
2 Gastritis and gastric erosions: elderly patients on NSAIDs have a sevenfold increased risk of bleeding compared with the same age group not taking such drugs.
3 Gastric and duodenal ulcers.
4 Carcinoma of the oesophagus and the stomach.

5 Diverticular disease.

6 Ischaemic bowel disease, sometimes difficult to differentiate from chronic inflammatory disease, e.g. Crohn's disease.

7 Colonic polyps: 40% incidence in the over 65s in a post-mortem study.

8 Colon cancer.

9 Angiodysplasia.

10 Piles.

Acute blood loss

This is particularly dangerous in the elderly as the resulting hypotension may precipitate a stroke, MI, acute kidney injury or fracture. Timely treatment is required: initially blood transfusion but with ready access to surgical intervention if the bleeding persists.

Acute upper GI bleeding in the elderly often presents as melaena without haematemesis: endoscopy may therefore be helpful in locating the site of bleeding and mucosal injection may help to stop bleeding.

Acute, severe bowel ischaemia may present as rectal bleeding, and the ischaemia may be secondary to other pathology, e.g. a silent MI. A full assessment is therefore needed.

Chronic blood loss

Chronic GI bleeding is the most common cause of iron-deficiency anaemia in old age in the UK (see Chapter 14). The bleeding site is often asymptomatic. Examination of both the upper and lower tract is required in most cases. Discovery of a benign lesion should not prevent further exploration for more serious causes, providing the patient is sufficiently fit and willing to be investigated.

Suggested plan of investigation

1 Confirm the anaemia is due to iron-deficiency.

2 Is GI bleeding likely; faecal occult bloods now less commonly performed.

3 Endoscopy of upper GI tract. Barium swallow/ meal is indicated for dysphagia.

4 Flexible sigmoidoscopy followed by CT abdomen with oral and IV contrast to study the large bowel. Contrast CT of the abdomen is kinder than and almost as effective as barium enema in frail elderly patients and provides extra information about liver, pancreas and lymph nodes.

5 Colonoscopy, the gold standard, may require the patient to be hospitalized for bowel prep and like

barium enema may be poorly tolerated so the caecum may not be seen. It is often used after CT to confirm possible abnormality or reveal angiodysplasia. Biopsies can be taken and polyps can be removed.

6 Radioisotope-labelled red cells may be used to identify the site of GI bleeding in cases of brisk intermittent bleeding of unknown cause.

Treatment

1 Specific treatment for underlying cause.

2 Oral iron supplements: ferrous sulphate if tolerated.

3 Transfuse only if haemoglobin is very low, e.g. less than 8 g/dL, and causing symptoms; take care if risk of congestive heart failure is present.

The acute abdomen

This is a difficult diagnostic problem, but even more so in old age. The mortality rate in elderly patients may exceed 50%. There are four possible reasons for such depressing results:

1 Delay in presentation.

2 Atypical presentation ('silent').

3 Reluctance to operate on frail elderly patients.

4 Precipitation of other significant pathology during the acute episode, e.g. MI.

The NCEPOD report (2010) into the care received by elderly patients undergoing surgery made several recommendations (see box).

NCEPOD recommendations (2010)

- Review by senior surgeons/physicians, and more input from care-of-the-elderly physicians.
- Better fluid balance, pain relief and nutrition.
- Review of all medications including venous thromboprophylaxis.
- More awareness of prevention of acute kidney injury (see Chapter 13).
- Optimize time to theatre; investigate and stabilize the patient but avoid delaying surgery in life-threatening conditions.
- Plan high level post-operative care, e.g. high dependency or intensive care.

Common pathologies in patients aged over 75 undergoing emergency abdominal surgery are listed in Table 11.2.

Useful pointers in the elderly acute abdomen

1 Check hernial orifices.
2 X-ray for fluid levels, free air in peritoneal cavity and distended bowel (e.g. sigmoid volvulus).
3 Check serum amylase; about half the patients with acute pancreatitis are over 60.
4 Monitor presence of pulses and use ultrasound for detection of aortic aneurysm.
5 Do not forget ischaemic bowel (see below).

NB: Always consider the diagnosis of 'acute abdomen' in 'shocked' elderly patients. If supporting evidence is found on examination and emergency investigation, obtain an urgent surgical opinion.

Have a high index of suspicion before excluding an acute abdomen in the elderly

- Patients may down-play their symptoms.
- Symptoms may be vague.
- The abdomen may appear benign on examination.
- Late diagnosis in older people delays appropriate management.

Bowel ischaemia

1 Twenty percent of cardiac output is used to supply the GI tract, so any significant fall is likely to affect the perfusion of the bowel and precipitate ischaemia.
2 At least two major mesenteric arteries must be compromised for bowel ischaemia to occur.
3 Because of a poor anastomotic arrangement, the left side of the colon is the most vulnerable segment.
4 Mechanism:
  - Arterial occlusion: 50% of cases.
  - Non-occlusive mechanisms (low flow): 20–30%.
  - Venous occlusion: 5–10%.

Associated factors/conditions

1 Embolization, e.g. atrial fibrillation.
2 Reduced cardiac output, e.g. hypotension and biventricular cardiac failure.
3 Widespread atheroma.
4 Drugs, e.g. oestrogens, antihypertensives, psychotropic agents.
5 Vasculitis, e.g. rheumatoid arthritis and polymyalgia rheumatica.
6 Hypercoagulability.

Clinical course

Mild:

- Post-prandial abdominal pain, diarrhoea and weight loss.
- Mucosal swelling – 'thumb printing' on barium studies.
- Recovery, plus or minus scarring (stricture).

Severe:

- Sudden severe pain, but may be 'silent'.
- Movement of fluid into bowel lumen, vomiting, diarrhoea and shock.
- Rapid biochemical deterioration with hyperkalaemia and high lactate.
- Ischaemic bowel wall allows bacteria to cross from the lumen into the peritoneum, leading to peritonitis, plus or minus septicaemia.
- Death almost certain.

Treatment

Acute/mild:

- Support with fluids, broad-spectrum antibiotics, heparin and treat underlying cause to prevent recurrence.

Acute/severe:

- Consult surgeons regarding resection; supportive and symptomatic treatment.

Chronic:

- Small frequent meals; correct any nutritional deficiencies due to malabsorption.
- Consider warfarin and treat any underlying arrhythmia.
- Peritonism makes laparotomy or palliative care mandatory.

Acute diarrhoea

There is an arbitrary cutoff of < 2 weeks for 'acute' diarrhoea. The cause is usually obvious from the history.

Infective

Cultures must be taken and patient isolated while results are awaited:

- **Viral** most commonly *Norovirus* (also known as winter vomiting) which causes outbreaks, e.g. in hospitals, care homes and cruise ships. The incubation period is 12–48 h. Symptoms usually last for 24–60 h and include sudden onset projectile vomiting, abdominal discomfort and watery diarrhoea. Supportive measures are all that are usually required. Transmission is mainly faeco-oral, but also person-to-person, via fomites and airborne as the highly contagious virus is easily aerosolized in vomitus. Wash your hands – alcohol rubs are *not* effective as this RNA virus does not have a lipid envelope.
- **Bacterial** including *Salmonella* and *E. coli*; antibiotics are only justified in severe disease; in mild cases they may prolong symptoms and produce carrier states.

Clostridium difficile associated diarrhoea (CDAD)

This is the most serious cause of antibiotic-associated diarrhoea and occurs when competing bacteria in the gut flora have been wiped out by broad spectrum antibiotics. *Clostridium difficile* is a Gram-positive spore-forming bacillus. It produces two distinct exotoxins, A (enterotoxin) and B (cytotoxin). These bind to the intestinal epithelial brush border and trigger release of inflammatory mediators resulting in increased fluid secretion and inflammation. Biopsies reveal patchy necrosis with an exudate of fibrin and neutrophils. In severe disease, extensive necrosis and ulceration may result in development of a pseudomembrane, which can be seen at sigmoidoscopy/colonoscopy.

Symptoms

Usually a patient who has had a course of antibiotics develops malaise, abdominal pain, nausea, anorexia and very watery, foul-smelling diarrhoea. Worsening pain and diarrhoea may herald complications.

Examination

Low-grade fever, abdominal tenderness. High temperature and severe tenderness are signs of complications.

Investigations

Nurses have long claimed that they can recognize CDAD by its characteristic smell; this may be due to the volatile fatty acids produced. White cell count and CRP are raised. The most widely used diagnostic test is the enzyme-linked immunosorbent assay (ELISA) for toxins A and/or B. Abdominal X-ray (AXR)/CT of the abdomen are needed if complications are suspected and sigmoidoscopy will visualize the pseudomembrane.

Complications

Pseudomonas colitis, toxic megacolon and colonic perforation; all have high mortality rates in older people. Relapses are common and morbidity is high.

Treatment

Isolate any patient with suspicious diarrhoea immediately. Stop any culprit antibiotic and PPI whenever possible and replace fluid and electrolytes. First line therapy is usually oral metronidazole 500 mg t.d.s. Metronidazole is also effective when given IV because of hepatic metabolism. If this fails or the patient is allergic to metronidazole, use oral vancomycin 125 mg q.d.s. The dose can be increased to 250 mg q.d.s. in resistant cases. Consider using vancomycin instead of metronidazole for older people with poor oral intake because it is better tolerated.

Prevention

Prevention is extremely important; educate hospital staff and visitors about hand-washing with soap and water (alcohol gel is not effective). Hospitals invest in deep clean strategies with misting and proper disinfection of contaminated surfaces. Antibiotic policies reduce the use of antibiotics most likely to lead to CDAD. There is on-going research into whether probiotics, e.g. Actimel, reduce the risk of CDAD. Antiperistaltic agents, PPIs and opiates should be avoided.

Mandatory reporting

All acute Trusts have to report cases of CDAD to the Department of Health. There is a national drive to reduce the number of cases per Trust.

Chronic diarrhoea

This is incapacitating in old age, especially if the patient is already disabled and immobile due to other pathologies. It may result in faecal incontinence which patients and carers find very hard to manage.

A good history must be taken to exclude food poisoning, exposure to viruses or recurrence of *C. difficile*, especially if the patient lives in an institution or is a current or recent in-patient.

1 *Spurious*: i.e. obstruction with overflow, must be excluded first by rectal examination and then by sigmoidoscopy if necessary. The cause may be simple, e.g. faecal impaction, or serious, e.g. carcinoma of the rectum.
2 *Inflammatory:* Crohn's disease of the large bowel is the most common chronic inflammatory bowel disease in old age; diagnosis is made by barium studies and biopsy. Radioisotope white cell scans may be useful for determining extent of the disease. Microscopic colitis encompasses both collagenous and lymphocytic colitis. It is a cause of non-bloody diarrhoea that is increasingly common in old age. The mucosa looks normal at colonoscopy, but histology reveals an abnormal band of collagen above the basement membrane in collagenous colitis or lymphocytic infiltration in lymphocytic colitis. Treatment includes stopping drugs that may be exacerbating the diarrhoea, avoiding caffeine, looking for associated coeliac disease and a trial of steroids or mesalazine.
3 *Metabolic:* uncommon, but exclude thyrotoxicosis; some cases are secondary to diabetic neuropathy.
4 *Drugs:* antibiotic diarrhoea is common, especially after cephalosporins; consider purgative misuse; but also colchicine, PPIs, acetylcholinesterase inhibitors, e.g. donepezil, magnesium-containing antacids and iron.
5 *Iatrogenic:* gastrectomy/vagotomy.
6 Rule out *malabsorption*: see below.

Constipation

Fear of becoming constipated is an aspect of old age that is more common than the genuine symptom. Seventy percent of elderly people open their bowels once daily, 11% every other day and 14% twice daily. Difficulty passing motions is of greater importance than frequency of defecation.

Causes of constipation are listed below:

1 Faulty habits: low-residue diet, poor fluid intake, lack of exercise and ignoring the call to stool.
2 Poor appetite: leads to reduced gastro-colic reflex, but does not stop the bowels from working.
3 Immobility.
4 Drugs: check the drug chart for opiate analgesics, anticholinergics, diuretics, calcium channel blockers, etc.
5 Check for metabolic precipitants: diabetes mellitus, hypothyroidism, hypercalcaemia, hypokalaemia and hypomagnesaemia secondary to drugs, or bowel, endocrine or metabolic disease.
6 Psychiatric: depression, dementia.
7 Functional: irritable bowel, purgative abuse (cathartic colon).
8 Pain: from peri-anal disease such as piles and fissures.
9 Neurological causes include Parkinson's disease, spinal cord injury, multiple sclerosis and cerebrovascular disease.

Management

1 Identify the nature and duration (small, hard stools are often related to low-fibre diet or dehydration; soft stools in a dilated rectum suggest chronic laxative abuse).
2 Identify any precipitating causes from the list above.
3 Rectal examination must be performed and recorded in the notes before prescribing laxatives. Is there a rectal tumour?
4 If impaction is imminent, enemas are required.
5 If not impacted but a quick result is required prescribe a stimulant (senna); occasionally an osmotic laxative (magnesium sulphate) will be required.

6 For short-term treatment (associated with acute illness) ensure an adequate fluid intake and mobilize as soon as possible. Prescribe senna if stools are bulky and soft, co-danthrusate/co-danthramer if stools are small and hard in association with opiates. Macrogols (Laxido) or liquid paraffin and magnesium hydroxide emulsion (Milpar) may be acceptable alternatives.

7 Severe constipation in patients who are bed-bound: occasionally this can only be resolved by manual evacuation. Historically, this task is given to the most junior member of the team. Sensible precautions include a plastic apron, two pairs of gloves, lubricant such as KY jelly, plenty of wipes and a large clinical waste bag.

8 Review the need for laxatives once the patient is over the acute illness. Only prescribe laxatives on discharge from hospital if the need continues, e.g. prior usage or continuing precipitant.

9 For longer-term treatment, educating the patient and their family about a high-fibre diet, adequate fluid intake and exercise may be all that is required.

10 For longer-term treatment where non-drug treatment fails or is impractical, prescribe a macrogol or a bulking agent (ispaghula husk).

11 For intractable constipation try a combination of treatments or prucalopride in women.

12 For patients at the end of life on regular opiates titrate co-danthrusate/co-danthramer against response.

13 The high cost of lactulose can only be justified for hepatic encephalopathy.

14 Complications of constipation include: faecal impaction, overflow diarrhoea, obstruction and even perforation, megacolon predisposing to sigmoid volvulus and rectal prolapse, urinary retention and delirium.

Change in bowel habit

Alternating diarrhoea and constipation is always a worrying symptom. Carcinoma of the large bowel must be excluded, but diverticular disease, large-bowel ischaemia and irritable colon are more common.

As described for investigation of anaemia, abdominal CT with contrast and flexible sigmoidoscopy are often used in preference to barium enema or colonoscopy.

Faecal incontinence

- The incidence of faecal incontinence varies with age and where people live:
  o 7% of community-dwelling over 65s
  o 10–15% of those in residential homes
  o 55% of those living in nursing homes.
- This is not surprising, as faecal incontinence is a common reason for elderly people moving/being moved to institutional care.
- The true incidence is likely to be higher as faecal incontinence is under-reported: people are embarrassed or think it is a normal part of ageing.
- Women with faecal incontinence post-partum develop compensatory mechanisms, but co-morbidities affecting mobility or stool consistency cause the faecal incontinence to recur or become obvious in later life.
- The cost of managing faecal incontinence with pads is enormous.
- Most cases are multifactorial (see Table 11.3).
- Take a good history including food and fluid intake, history of gastrointestinal and neurological disease, medications and operations especially obstetric and rectal procedures.
- Examination includes the abdomen, rectal examination to assess anal tone and sensation, looking for fissures or fistulae and full neurological assessment.
- Initial management involves a trial of simple measures. In patients with disinhibition and lack of insight, e.g. those with dementia, try bulking preparations and regular toileting.
- Treat the underlying cause where possible, e.g. surgery for rectal prolapse.
- Some frail older people do well with codeine phosphate to cause constipation with enemas at regular intervals to empty the bowels.
- Other available devices include anal plugs which are placed in the rectum and swell up as they absorb fluid from the mucosa to block the rectum for several hours so that the patient can go out. Liaise with your local continence advisor.
- If the above fail and the patient is appropriate for surgical treatment, consider further investigations. Ano-rectal physiology is assessed using a pressure balloon to measure resting tone and active tone. An ultrasound probe can assess the integrity of the internal and external anal sphincters. This information can be used to determine whether the patient is best managed

Table 11.3 Causes, mechanisms, examples and management of faecal incontinence

Cause	Mechanism	Example	Management
Obstetric trauma	Third-degree tear Instrumental delivery	Large baby Forceps damage to pudendal nerve	Physiotherapy and biofeedback Anterior sphincter repair Overlying sphincteroplasty
Surgery	Trauma from anal stretch	Treatment of fistula, fissure, piles	As above
Colorectal disease	Weakness of internal anal sphincter	Rectal prolapse Haemorrhoids IBD Tumour	Delormes procedure Stoma as last resort
Neurological	Cerebral	PD Stroke	Sacral neuromodulation via implanted device
	Spinal Peripheral nerve	Spinal cord injury Diabetic autonomic neuropathy	
Overflow	Secondary to faecal impaction		Enemas, laxatives, good fluid intake, may need manual evacuation
Very loose stool	Infection Inflammatory bowel disease Irritable bowel syndrome	*C. difficile* Ulcerative colitis Crohn's disease	Appropriate antibiotics Steroids and mesalazine
Poor mobility	Unable to reach the toilet, unable to reach in time	OA Stroke PD	Reduce distance to toilet, use commode
Disinhibition	Dementia	See Chapter 4	Large signs over toilet doors Coloured toilet doors Red toilet seats

IBD, inflammatory bowel disease; OA, osteoarthritis; PD, Parkinson's disease.

with a surgical technique or neuromodulation; see Table 11.3.

Absorption

1 Small-bowel function declines with age, but nutritional deficiencies only occur when additional factors intervene, e.g. poor diet or ill health.
2 Causes usually considered in younger patients occur in old age, e.g. coeliac disease.
3 Maldigestion is more common than malabsorption, e.g. due to pancreatic disease.
4 Bacterial change in the small-bowel lumen due to stasis or diverticular disease is common (10%

of elderly people) and is frequently clinically significant.
5 Ischaemia is a special cause of malabsorption in old age.
6 Iatrogenic causes must always be considered, e.g. post-gastrectomy, alcohol and some drugs, e.g. biguanides.

Indicators of malabsorption

1 Weight loss (especially around the face) in spite of good dietary intake.
2 Low serum albumin.
3 Unexplained iron-deficiency anaemia (with negative faecal occult blood).
4 Macrocytic anaemia.
5 Osteomalacia, presenting as falls and weakness.

Table 11.4 **Common causes, evidence and treatment of malabsorption in older people**

Cause	Evidence	Treatment
Coeliac disease	Anti-tissue transglutaminase antibodies (tTGA), low total IgA	Gluten-free diet
Bacterial overgrowth	Positive hydrogen breath test, red cell folate very high	Course of antibiotics
Pancreatic insufficiency	Low faecal elastase	Creon capsules with every meal (including supplements)
Crohn's disease of the small bowel	Biopsy	Mesalazine, steroids
Atrophic gastritis, previous partial gastrectomy	Low B_{12}	Course of intramuscular hydroxocobalamin with 3-monthly top ups
Lymphoma	Biopsy results	Depending on type and grade of disease
Mesenteric ischaemia	Barium/CT appearance	Surgical in the fit patient, otherwise consider anticoagulation, palliation
Drugs, e.g. biguanides, cholestyramine	From drug history	Stop culprit drug wherever possible

6 Frank steatorrhoea is uncommon.
7 Abdominal distension secondary to gas.

Causes of malabsorption in old age

See Table 11.4.

Coeliac disease

- The incidence is around 1% of the population, most common in temperate European countries especially Ireland and Finland.
- Twenty-five percent of new cases are aged over 60.
- Cases are diagnosed ever later in life; even in the ninth decade.
- An autoimmune gluten-sensitive enteropathy. The gliadin component causes an immunologically mediated inflammation of the lining of the small intestine, causing subtotal villous atrophy.
- Gluten is found in wheat, rye and barley.
- Enteropathy leads to maldigestion and malabsorption.
- GI symptoms include chronic or intermittent diarrhoea, steatorrhoea, flatulence, borborygmi, weight loss, abdominal bloating and cramping.
- Features on examination might include evidence of weight loss, muscle wasting, oedema, cheilosis

and glossitis. Dermatitis herpetiformis is an exuberant, itchy erythematous rash often occurring in the axillae secondary to gluten intolerance.
- There are also non-gastrointestinal manifestations (see Table 11.5).
- Investigations: blood tests might show a mixed or macrocytic anaemia, low ferritin and folate levels, hypocalcaemia, hypokalaemia and low vitamin D. Coeliac disease is sometimes the underlying cause of persistently raised LFTs with no other explanation.
- NICE recommends using IgA anti-tissue transglutaminase IgA antibodies (tTGA) as the first line for diagnosis. If the result is equivocal, check IgA anti-endomysial antibodies (EMAs). The EMA is the most specific, but levels fall rapidly

Table 11.5 **Non-gastrointestinal manifestations of coeliac disease**

Non-gastrointestinal manifestations	Due to reduced absorption of:
Anaemia and fatigue	Iron and folate
Bleeding diathesis	Fat-soluble vitamin K
Osteomalacia and osteoporosis	Vitamin D
Neuropsychiatric	Calcium
Peripheral neuropathy	Folate
Dermatitis herpetiformis	

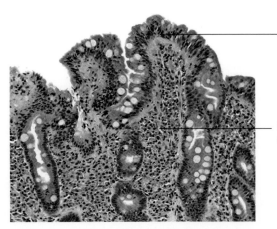

— partial villous atrophy

— lymphocytic infiltration of the lamina propria

Figure 11.1 Histology of coeliac disease. Source: Wikimedia.org. Released under the GNU Free Documentation License.

once gluten is removed from the diet. If both are negative, check total IgA levels.

- NICE recommends duodenal biopsy (Figure 11.1) to confirm the serological diagnosis.
- Ninety-five percent of people with coeliac disease are positive for HLA DQ2 and the remaining 5% are positive for HLA DQ8.
- Associated autoimmune conditions include thyroid disease, diabetes, primary biliary cirrhosis and Sjögren's syndrome. There is also an association with epilepsy, ataxia and dementia.
- Treatment: gluten-free diet. Patients are more likely to be compliant if they feel better when omitting gluten. Some gluten-free food is available on prescription.
- Correct vitamin deficiencies found at diagnosis.
- Patients and their families benefit from education at diagnosis from a dietician and a support group such as Coeliac UK (http://www.coeliac. org.uk/).
- Adherence to the gluten-free diet protects from malignant change including lymphoma and adenocarcinoma of the gut.

Diverticular disease

- Diverticula are small mucosal herniations through the bowel wall at the sites of weakness caused by nutrient vessels.
- The sigmoid bowel is the most common site as bowel contents are under the highest pressure.
- Diverticulosis describes the condition of non-inflamed diverticula.

- The prevalence of diverticulosis is over 50% of elderly people, and up to 70% of over 80s.
- Men and women are affected equally.
- A disease of the Western world thought to be due to low fibre diet, constipation and obesity. Interestingly, Westernization of the diet in Japan is leading to more cases there.
- Seventy-five percent of people with diverticulosis remain asymptomatic and require no treatment.
- Of the 25% with symptoms, 75% develop diverticulitis (and 25% of these develop complications which may include profuse haemorrhage).
- Diverticulitis occurs when faecal matter collects in a diverticulum and obstructs it. This leads to local inflammation with mucous secretions and bacterial overgrowth. This may compromise the vascular supply resulting in a microperforation.
- Mild diverticulitis may present with low-grade symptoms similar to those of irritable bowel syndrome (IBS) such as colic, bloating and flatulence. IBS co-exists in 30% of patients.
- Patients with severe disease and signs of peritonism must be admitted.
- Medical management includes:
  o Nil by mouth.
  o Nasogastric tube.
  o Intravenous fluids (watch fluid balance and renal function carefully).
  o Antibiotics: usually ciprofloxacin plus metronidazole, or piperacillin.
  o Good pain control, including opiates.
- Imaging: an erect CXR may show gas under the diaphragm if there has been a perforation.
- CT scanning of the abdomen may show colonic diverticula, pericolic fat stranding due to

inflammation, bowel wall thickening, inflammatory masses and abscesses.
- Small abscesses can be drained percutaneously with CT guidance.
- Serious complications requiring surgical intervention are:
  o Peritonitis following perforation and faecal leakage.
  o Uncontrolled sepsis.
  o Fistula: e.g. bowel/bladder in men and bowel/vagina in women.
  o Obstruction.
  o Uncontrollable bleeding, due to small vessels stretched over a large diverticular mass.
  o Concern about a masked carcinoma.
- The most common surgical procedure is a Hartmann's procedure to remove the affected bowel and to create an end-colostomy. The stoma can be reversed electively after a few months if the patient is sufficiently well.
- Remember the high mortality of surgery in very frail elderly patients and explain this to their relatives to ensure appropriate expectation management. See box p153 for NCEPOD recommendations.

Endoscopy in the elderly

Diagnostic and therapeutic techniques have been developing for almost 50 years and age alone should not exclude elderly patients from endoscopic procedures. However:

- Three percent of endoscopy patients die within 30 days of the procedure: the risks are highest in frail elderly patients.

The NCEPOD on therapeutic GI endoscopy (2004) noted the following:
- Nineteen percent of PEGs were considered futile.
- Sixty-eight percent of ERCPs were considered futile.
- Fourteen percent of patients developed respiratory complications secondary to sedation or local anaesthetics. Much lower doses of midazolam should be given to frail older people than fit younger people.
- 'Informed consent' was often questionable, i.e. in two-thirds of the patients with dementia or acute confusion.
- Procedures are not always performed by clinicians with documented competence.

- Common sense, compassion and practical skill are all needed if patients are to benefit and not suffer.

Percutaneous endoscopic gastrostomy (PEG)

- In patients over 50, 18% die within 1 month of the procedure, 44% die within 6 months, 54% within 1 year and 73% within 2 years.
- Only 9% of PEG-fed patients return to oral feeding, i.e. 90% have a PEG until death.
- Self-extubation occurs in 12% of patients.
- Many hospitals have a multidisciplinary feeding team to discuss the appropriateness of each individual patient.
- In patients with dementia there is no evidence that PEG feeding:

  o reduces aspiration pneumonia
  o promotes pressure sore healing
  o improves functional status
  o provides comfort
  o prolongs life.

Colonoscopy

- Indications are common in old age.
- The procedure is safe if care taken with selection, preparation and sedation, especially in those aged over 80.
- Complete examination rates (i.e. reaching the ileo-caecal valve) may be reduced to 50–60% in the very elderly.
- Abnormalities are common in the over-80s at about 80%. Diverticular disease is most common, but 11% reveal carcinoma, 25% polyps and 13% had multiple pathologies.
- It has both diagnostic and therapeutic potential, e.g. biopsy, polypectomy and stent insertion.

CT Abdomen

- The procedure is well tolerated by frail elderly patients. Modern machines take less than 15 min to produce the scan.
- CT has the advantage of demonstrating the bowel, other abdominal lesions causing extrinsic compression, plus disease in other solid organs, bones, the aorta and abnormal collections of fluid.

CT Colonography

- Computers are used to produce two- and three-dimensional views of the bowel and abdomen: the 'virtual colonoscopy'.

- The procedure is superior to CT at demonstrating the bowel lumen.
- It involves insufflation of the bowel with air or CO_2, and patients must be able to retain this.
- Intravenous contrast and antispasmodics are given. The usual care must be taken with patients with CKD.
- The patient must be able to turn over because views are taken supine and prone; they must also be able to follow commands about taking in deep breaths, etc.
- Radiation exposure from CT colonography is 8 mSv, compared with 5 mSv from an abdominal CT; annual background radiation is 1-3mSv.

Jaundice

- Surgical causes are common and must be identified rapidly before the condition becomes irremediable; ultrasound is the investigation of first choice.
- Medical causes of jaundice should be investigated and treated as in younger patients.
- Primary biliary cirrhosis and chronic hepatitis are more common in elderly patients than appreciated. Prognosis in late life is often better than in younger patients.

Chronic liver disease

All forms of chronic liver disease are becoming more common in older age, with an increased number of deaths from liver disease. Some cases are detected by chance with routine blood tests. Only 6% of liver biopsies are performed in over 80 year olds, but there is no evidence for increased risk. Diagnosis is important because of treatment options, e.g. anti-viral agents, immunosuppression, lifestyle advice. Ascites can be managed with spironolactone or paracentesis.

Ageing changes in the liver

- Size reduced by 20% in older age.
- Blood flow reduced by 30%.
- Reduced activity of enzymes such as cytochrome P450 and superoxide dismutase.

Alcoholic liver disease (ALD)

- Dubbed the 'invisible epidemic' of older people as there has been an increase in alcoholism in over 65 year olds and because of the increasing life expectancy.
- Twenty-eight percent of cases of ALD are over 65.
- More common in men than women, but the gap is narrowing.
- May present very non-specifically. Most have a prolonged course of 20–30 years leading to cirrhosis, 10 years with cirrhotic changes and an additional 5 years of severe symptoms in the period prior to death.
- Symptoms of jaundice and ascites develop late; 34% of older patients diagnosed with ALD are dead within 1 year.
- Watch for alcohol withdrawal when admitted to hospital.

Non-alcoholic fatty liver disease (NAFLD)

- The incidence of this is rising with increase of obesity and type 2 diabetes.
- Part of the metabolic syndrome.
- Twenty-six percent of cases are over 65.
- Diagnose early before irreversible fibrotic change occurs.
- Treat by lifestyle changes, i.e. weight reduction and more exercise.

Viral hepatitis

- Hepatitis C is the most significant cause, found in reformed drug users and recipients of blood and blood products prior to 1991. It is more common in people from Asia and sub-Saharan Africa.
- Treat with interferon and ribavirin, although side-effects are more common in older people.

Autoimmune hepatitis

- Check blood for raised IgG, and autoantibodies including antinuclear antibodies, smooth muscle antibodies and type 1 liver–kidney microsomal antibodies.
- Treat with prednisolone plus or minus azathioprine

Primary biliary cirrhosis (PBC)

- Fifty percent of cases of PBC are in over 65 year olds.
- More common in women than men.
- Antimitochondrial autoantibodies are present in 95% of cases.
- Some patients get symptomatic relief from urso-deoxycholic acid.

GI Malignancy

All parts of the GI tract can undergo malignant change – the commonest clinical problems in old age are described below.

Oesophagus

See above.

Gastric carcinoma

- Declining in incidence, but still quite common.
- The fall in incidence is variously attributed to reduced salt intake, refrigeration, increased intake of fresh fruit and vegetables and eradication of *H. pylori*.
- The rate for men is about twice that for women.
- Peak incidence is in the eighth decade and most (>80%) have advanced disease at diagnosis, underlining the importance of investigating late-onset dyspepsia. Five-year survival for all new cases over 70 is 5–12%.
- Most common site is the gastro-oesophageal junction.
- Risk factors include genetic predisposition and an association with blood group A, smoking, atrophic gastritis, pernicious anaemia, previous gastric resection and infection with *H. pylori*.
- There is considerable geographical variation in incidence and prognosis. It is particularly prevalent in Japan, but the outlook for the disease there is more favourable; earlier diagnosis, which 'improves' survival time, may account for some of this, but there are likely to be other factors involved.
- Prolonged use of PPIs may predispose to malignant change.
- Symptoms tend to reflect advanced disease, including weight loss, vomiting, haematemesis, melaena and abdominal pain.
- Diagnosis is usually made by endoscopic biopsy, followed by staging CT of the chest, abdomen and pelvis.

- Prognosis is poor and the treatment usually palliative. In early cases where the patient is biologically very fit, it may include gastrectomy, with adjuvant chemotherapy (e.g. etoposide and 5-fluorouracil) and radiotherapy or a bypass procedure.
- Once the cancer has metastasized, prognosis is likely to be only a matter of months, so the focus of care should move to good palliation (see Chapter 17).

Pancreatic carcinoma

- The incidence of pancreatic cancer is increasing in most developed countries although paradoxically not in Japan.
- Common in elderly men.
- Aetiological factors include cigarette smoking, high dietary fat and occupational exposure in chemical and metal industries.
- Eighty-five percent of cases have already metastasized by the time of diagnosis and the prognosis is grim (overall 20% 1-year survival).
- Weight loss is usually striking.
- There may or may not be abdominal pain, which characteristically radiates through to the back. Look for erythema *ab igne* on the epigastric skin from a hot water bottle used to ease pain.
- An ultrasound scan is a good initial investigation but CT is better able to define the extent.
- In most cases the head of the pancreas is involved, leading to obstructive jaundice.
- Radical surgery is usually not an option, but stenting procedures provide temporary relief from the symptoms of biliary obstruction.
- Chemotherapy prolongs life by a few months in trials, but does not improve quality of life.

Colo-rectal carcinoma (Figure 11.2)

- The most common malignancy of the GI tract and the second most common cause of death from cancer in the UK; it is rare in Africa and Asia.
- Lower grade of malignancy than gastric or pancreatic adenocarcinoma; the 5-year survival of all newly diagnosed cases has improved to around 50%. Survival is stage dependent and screening is being introduced to improve early diagnosis (see Table 11.6 below).
- Eighty percent of cases occur in people over the age of 60.
- Clinical presentation is often vague, but malaise, abdominal pain and change of bowel habit, rectal

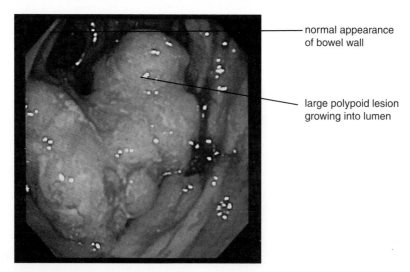

normal appearance of bowel wall

large polypoid lesion growing into lumen

Figure 11.2 Colonoscopic view of adenocarcinoma in the colon. Source: Wikimedia.org. Released under the GNU Free Documentation License.

bleeding, tenesmus or faecal incontinence, depending on the site of the lesion, are the usual pointers.
- Up to 30% of patients present with obstruction; they have a poor prognosis as 40% have secondaries at presentation and <20% survive 5 years.
- Diagnosis is confirmed by rectal examination and sigmoidoscopy, followed by abdominal CT and/or colonoscopy for biopsy and staging.
- The treatment plan will be discussed by a lower GI multidisciplinary team (MDT). The best option for cure is resection by a specialist colorectal surgeon, but chemotherapy is increasingly offered to older patients, depending on the staging, and monoclonal antibodies are promising. Stoma specialist nurses will be involved if a stoma is planned. Radiotherapy has a role in rectal cancers. Self-expanding intra-luminal stents offer some palliation for obstructive lesions.
- Patient education, support and good palliative care when appropriate are essential.

Screening programmes, based on occult-blood detection or sigmoidoscopy are currently being rolled out in the UK (see Table 11.6).

Clinical nutrition

The importance of food in the maintenance and recovery of health, which was obvious to past practitioners, is again being recognized amid the high tech of medicine.

Table 11.6 Screening for carcinoma of the colon

Investigation	Notes
Faecal occult blood (detects about 70% of cancers)	Bi-annual home testing kit, sent in post to those aged 60–75. Positives (2%) are offered colonoscopy, of whom 5 in 10 will be normal, 4 in 10 will have a polyp and 1 in 10 will have a cancer. False positives lead to anxiety and unnecessary investigation.
Flexible sigmoidoscopy (detects about 80% of cancers)	Once only between 55 and 64. Well tolerated.
Colonoscopy (detects almost 100% of cancers)	Expensive, requires full bowel preparation and has risk of complications. Only appropriate for screening very high risk groups.

Risk factors for carcinoma of the colon

- High red meat, processed meat and animal fat intake.
- Low fibre intake from fruit and vegetables.
- Low physical activity.
- Obesity.
- High alcohol intake.
- Genetic tendency to form polyps (but the major genetic conditions, familial adenomatous polyposis and hereditary non-polyposis colon cancer, present when young).
- Crohn's disease.
- Ulcerative colitis.

General nutritional standards in elderly people in the UK

Most older people in their own homes in the UK enjoy a reasonable diet. Their standards and practices are often higher than those of younger members of society. Elderly people (even old men) usually know how to cook and take a varied and balanced diet.

The 1997/98 National Survey of Elderly People in the UK (Finch et al. 1998) gave reassuring results. However, compared with the survey 30 years previously, the Medical Research Council (MRC) found that people were eating less (energy intake was down 15%) but were increasing in weight. In 1997/98, 66% were considered overweight and only 5% underweight. The fat content of the diet was only slightly over the recommended levels but sugar was 7% above recommendations at 18%. All but 8% appeared to take sufficient vitamins and minerals but blood levels for folate, iron and vitamin C were suboptimal in 10–15%. The adoption of a modified Mediterranean diet in a large cohort has demonstrated improved survival rates in participants of the EPIC study (Trichopoulou 2005).

Factors that impair dietary intake

- Illness – the most common and most serious.
- Poor dental state – restricts dietary choice.
- Poverty.
- Being male.
- Living in the north of Britain, especially Scotland.
- Being in an institution.

Percentage of elderly people regularly taking common foods

- Potatoes and bread: 70%.
- Cooked vegetables: 66%.
- Salads, raw vegetables and fruit: 50%.
- Nutritional supplements: 30%.

Subnutrition

In the UK, subnutrition is rarely due to poverty; it is more likely to be a consequence of eccentricity, loneliness or illness. Overnutrition, with excess carbohydrate, fat and calories, is more common than malnutrition and these excesses are often associated with inadequate dietary fibre. Alcohol abuse is another cause of poor diet.

Other important factors related to diet in old age are as follows:

- The incidence of subnutrition is difficult to determine as dietary assessment by recall (of foods eaten) or weighed surveys are unreliable in many elderly subjects, particularly the most vulnerable.
- There is doubt about the appropriateness of recommended intakes in older people.
- Surveys in the UK indicate levels of malnutrition of about 3–7%.
- Poor diets may be either the cause of or result of declining health.
- Other factors are social isolation and bereavement.
- Low blood levels of vitamins, etc. are common in old age, especially in the frail elderly, but their significance is uncertain (Table 11.7).
- Hyperhomocysteinaemia is associated with low folate and vitamin B_{12} levels and increased rates of vascular disease and thromboembolism.

Table 11.7 Prevalence of low blood levels of vitamins reported in elderly subjects

Subnutrition	Incidence
Haemoglobin < 12 g/dL	Up to 40% in institutions 6–9% of elderly at home
Serum iron	Approximately 20%
Red cell folate	Approximately 20%
Serum B_{12}	Approximately 20%
Vitamin C	Up to 50%

Note: Wide variation due to different groups studied and methods used – all incidences of low levels are more common than actual evidence of clinical deficiencies.

- In patients admitted to hospital levels of risk of malnutrition are high (32% in over 65s).

Causes of nutritional deficiency

1 Inability to shop or to prepare food, e.g. in cases of dementia, depression, poverty, loneliness, eccentricity, blindness or immobility due to arthritis or neurological disease; the 'tea and toast' diet.
2 Impaired appetite which may be part of general malaise, due to biochemical abnormalities, a consequence of drug side-effects or indicate underlying GI disease.
3 Malabsorption.

Assessment of nutritional status in old age

This is a very difficult task but the following criteria have been found to be of value in some instances (all have drawbacks):

- Dietary history.
- Weight change.
- Skinfold thickness.
- Muscle power.
- Blood levels of nutrients.
- Clinical evidence of nutritional disease.
- BMI under 15 (twice demispan may be substituted for height).
- Tools include the Malnutrition Universal Screening Tool (MUST) see Appendix and the Mini-Nutritional Assessment (MNA). Both include history and measurements.
- Taken in isolation most of these abnormalities have multiple causes. A diagnosis of malnutrition can only be made if several abnormalities are found – the cause of the malnutrition must then be explored and, if possible, corrected.

A simple recipe for a good diet

- Eat wholemeal bread not white bread.
- Have three portions of fresh vegetables daily.
- Eat two items of fresh fruit each day.
- Use 1/2 L (1 pint) of semi-skimmed milk daily, for drinking and in cooking.
- Have one portion of meat or fish per day (preferably oily fish).
- Drink at least 2 L of fluid a day.

Dietary deficiencies in old age

1 The most obvious are calories, protein and fluid.
2 Vitamin B group: refractory heart failure, macrocytic anaemia due to folate deficiency, also peripheral neuropathy, dementia, vascular disease and thromboembolism.
3 Vitamin C: scurvy.
4 Vitamin D: osteomalacia.
5 Zinc especially from animal protein. Deficiency is thought to be linked to macular degeneration.
6 Iron, calcium and selenium.
7 Fibre – diseases of 'Western civilization'.

NB: The routine use of vitamins and mineral supplements has not been proven to benefit 'free range' elderly subjects. Even in vulnerable groups (the ill and the institutionalized) there is no evidence for blanket supplementation, but if deficiencies are identified, they should be corrected.

Treatment of subnutrition in the community

1 Improve general health – treat underlying conditions.
2 Encourage supervised meals e.g. 'meals on wheels', luncheon clubs, meal preparation by home help, microwave meals.
3 Education of patients and carers.
4 A balanced diet is the best source of nutrition, vitamins and minerals. Supplements such as Fortisips and Forticreme should be used in addition to not instead of real food.

Treatment of subnutrition in institutions

According to Age UK, those admitted to hospital over the age of 80 are twice as likely to become malnourished as those under 50. The consequences are serious and lead to prolonged hospital stays due to:

1 Poor healing and recovery.
2 Increased risk of complications, e.g. infection, pressure sores and depression.

Attention needs to be paid at all times to:

- Suitable foods, e.g. familiar, easy to swallow, enjoyable and energy rich. Ask the patient or family what they like.

- Small, frequent meals and snacks.
- Protected mealtimes.
- Food and drink within reach.
- Provision of modified utensils.
- Assistance with feeding when necessary, from food being cut up to spoon feeding. A red tray system reminds staff who needs extra help and encouragement.
- Eating in selected groups at a table increases both pleasure and intake.
- Enriched food, supplements and artificial feeding when appropriate – see Chapter 16.

NB: These measures also apply to catering in care homes.

Overnutrition

- The epidemic of morbid obesity in the Western world includes older people.
- The cost to the NHS of managing obesity is estimated to rise to £9.7 billion by 2050.
- Obese people remain well whilst living within their limits. However, disaster may follow a significant change in health status.
- When obese patients become immobile secondary to an acute illness they rapidly lose strength. After just a few days it may become impossible for them to remobilize independently.
- Their weight will hinder attempts at assistance by care workers. Health and safety regulations will insist that hoists are used and this will undermine attempts at rehabilitation. These patients may (unkindly) be compared with beached whales: if not quickly refloated, they are doomed.
- The extra nutritional reserves they carry may be of benefit.
- However, their size will exaggerate the complications of immobility, especially hypostatic pneumonia and pressure sores. The latter are likely to develop in deep tissue between pressure points and only become obvious when an abscess suddenly discharges through the skin to reveal a necrotic cavity below.

Carrying excess weight into old age is detrimental to wellbeing through worsening of:

1 Angina.
2 Breathlessness.
3 Glycaemic control.
4 Blood pressure.
5 Arthritis in weight-bearing joints (hence pain and immobility).

6 Depression and low self-esteem.
7 Peri-operative complications.
8 Rehabilitation outcomes.

At retirement, all overweight patients should be encouraged to engage with improving their lifestyle.

In cases of sudden, unexplained weight gain, check the scales and look at the ankles. Heart failure with oedema is common; an endocrine cause (e.g. myxoedema) should not be missed but will rarely be the explanation.

REFERENCES

Finch S, Doyle W, Lowe C, et al. (1998) *People Aged 65 Years and Over, Volume 1. Report of the Diet and Nutrition Survey*. Stationery Office, London.

National Confidential Enquiry into Patient Outcome and Death (2004) *Scoping Our Practice*. http://www.ncepod.org.uk/pdf/2004/Full_Report_2004.pdf.

National Confidential Enquiry into Patient Outcome and Death (2010) *An Age Old Problem: A Review of the Care Received by Elderly Patients Undergoing Surgery*. http://www.ncepod.org.uk/2010eese.htm and http://www.ncepod.org.uk/2010report3/downloads/EESE_fullReport.pdf.

Trichopoulou A, Orfanos P, Norat T, et al. (2005) Modified Mediterranean diet and survival: EPIC – Elderly Prospective Cohort Study. *BMJ* 330: 991, doi: 10.1136/bmj.38415.644155.8F.

FURTHER INFORMATION

www.nice.org.uk/CG86Bouras EP, Tangalos EG (2009) Chronic constipation in the elderly. *Gastroenterology Clinics of North America* 38(3): 463–480.

Cancer Research: http://cancerhelp.cancerresearchuk.org/. For excellent statistics on cancers, patient information and up-to-date treatments see the relevant sections.

Coeliac UK Support Group: http://www.coeliac.org.uk/al.

Frith J, Jone D, Newton JL (2009) Review: chronic liver disease in an ageing population. *Age and Ageing* 38: 11–18.

Janes SEJ, Meagher A, Frizell FA (2006) Management of diverticulitis. *BMJ* 332: 271–275.

Lord DA, Bell GD, Gray A (2004) *Sedation for Gastrointestinal Endoscopic Procedures in the Elderly: Getting Safer but Still Not Nearly Safe Enough.* British Society of Gastroenterology. www.bsg.org.uk/pdf_word_docs/sedation_elderly.pdf.

McMinn J, Steel C, Bowman A (2011) Investigation and management of unintentional weight loss in older adults. *BMJ* 342: 754–759.

Medical Research Council: http://www.mrc.ac.uk/index.htm.

NICE Guidelines for Coeliac Disease: www.nice.org.uk/CG86.

Nutrition Screening Survey in the UK 2008: http://www.bapen.org.uk/pdfs/nsw/nsw_report2008-09.pdf.

Sassi F, Devaux M, Cecchini M, et al. (2009) *The Obesity Epidemic: Analysis of Past and Projected Future Trends in Selected OECD Countries.* OECD Health Working Papers, No. 45. http://www.oecd.org/officialdocuments/displaydocumentpdf/?cote=delsa/hea/wd/hwp(2009)3&doclanguage=en.

Surveillance of *Clostridium difficile* related diarrhoea: http://www.dh.gov.uk/en/PublicationsandstatisticsPublications/PublicationsPolicyAndGuidance/DH_4118344.

Talley NJ, Tangalos EG (2009) Gastroenterology in the elderly. *Gastroenterology Clinics of North America* 38(3): xi–xii.

12

Disorders of homeostasis and metabolism

Age changes

There is a reduction in lean body mass and body water and a relative increase in fat. When marked this is known as sarcopaenia and constitutes a marker of physical frailty. It is gaining acceptance as a geriatric syndrome.

Endocrine changes

Some elderly people have immeasurably low levels of growth hormone; in some, it fails to respond to an insulin tolerance test. Some male subjects have global muscle wasting, and the administration of human growth hormone has been shown to increase lean body mass and reduce adipose tissue but without clear benefit to quality of life.

Other hormonal changes

- Serum noradrenaline ↑ (but β-receptors ↓).
- Insulin ↑ (due to insulin resistance): carbohydrate tolerance diminishes.
- Arginine vasopressin (AVP) ↓ susceptibility to hyponatraemia ↑.
- Atrial natriuretic peptide ↑ and nocturia ↑.
- Oestrogen and progesterone in women ↓, follicle stimulating hormone (FSH) and luteinizing hormone (LH) ↑.
- Testosterone in men ↓, FSH and LH ↑.
- Renin and aldosterone ↓.

Adenomas are common in anterior pituitary, thyroid and adrenal glands and are usually of no clinical significance.

Fluid and electrolyte imbalance

Acutely unwell elderly patients are very often fluid-depleted or fluid-overloaded, and occasionally both.

Reasons for vulnerability to dehydration

1 Reduction in body water.
2 Inadequate intake due to:
  - Impaired thirst response.
  - Dementia or depression.
  - Immobility.
  - Reluctance through fear of being 'caught short'.
  - Swallowing difficulty.
  - Acute illness.
(Mainly affects intracellular compartment, with thirst, confusion and drowsiness.)
3 Increased loss:
  - Reduced concentrating ability by kidney.
  - Diuretics.
  - Diabetes, diarrhoea and vomiting.
Salt and water loss are often replaced by water, tea, etc. Mixed salt and water depletion presents

---

Lecture Notes Elderly Care Medicine, Eighth Edition. Claire G. Nicholl and K. Jane Wilson.
© 2012 John Wiley & Sons, Ltd. Published 2012 by John Wiley & Sons, Ltd.

with confusion, weakness, reduced turgor, tachycardia and postural hypotension, as the extracellular compartment is mainly affected.

Hyponatraemia

This is common and is due to too little sodium, too much water or both. Do not treat the sodium level in isolation. If the result is very odd was it taken from a drip arm? Depending on the assay, high lipids and high protein in myeloma can give false results. Decide whether the patient is dehydrated, euvolaemic or fluid overloaded. The most accurate clinical finding in dehydration is postural hypotension.

- If the patient is dry, salt and water have been lost either through the kidneys (diuretics especially thiazides, renal failure, osmotic diuresis), the gut (vomiting, diarrhoea, fistula, adenoma) or skin (burns).
- If the patient is oedematous, there is relative water excess due to fluid retention (in cardiac failure, liver failure or nephrotic syndrome) or excess water intake (usually overenthusiastic dextrose after surgery).
- If the patient appears euvolaemic, one of the preceding may be developing. However, if the urine is concentrated when it should not be (sodium > 20 mmol/L in the presence of hyponatraemia) and the plasma is dilute with a low plasma osmolality (< 260 mmol/kg), this is the syndrome of inappropriate antidiuretic hormone (SIADH). Accumulation of intracellular water in the brain causes confusion, headache, lethargy, coma and fits. The level of sodium and the rate at which it falls are important: if it happens slowly brain cells have time to adapt to extracellular hypotonicity. Similarly, rapid correction may lead to the irreversible osmotic demyelination syndrome: paresis, dysphagia, dysarthria, diplopia and loss of consciousness. In frail older people aim to correct by no more than 8 mmol/L/24 h.

The mechanism by which ADH affects water reabsorption in the renal collecting ducts is shown in Figure 12.1.

Hypernatraemia

This is usually due to water loss in excess of sodium loss and occurs where patients are unable to take in enough water to meet their needs.

Causes of SIADH

- Drugs, especially SSRIs, venlafaxine, opiates, antiepileptics, omeprazole.
- Malignancy especially small cell lung cancer.
- CNS, e.g. stroke.
- Chest disease, e.g. pneumonia.
- Post-operative pain.

Treatment

- Remove underlying cause.
- Water restriction/intravenous infusion of normal saline as appropriate. Correct abnormalities slowly.
- Demeclocycline (blocks action of ADH on tubule).
- Vaptans, e.g. tolvaptan (ADH-receptor antagonists produce dilute urine).

Oedema

If oedema is present to knee level in a patient in a chair, slip a hand under the thigh and, if oedema is present there too, lean the patient forward to check for a sacral pad. Not all leg swelling is oedema and not all oedema is due to heart failure.

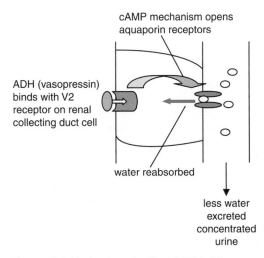

Figure 12.1 Mechanism of action of ADH at the collecting duct.

Causes of leg swelling

Raised venous pressure:

- Gravity (prolonged sitting).
- Cardiac failure.
- Pelvic mass.

The following causes are often unilateral:

- Venous insufficiency (side of hip surgery).
- DVT.
- Lack of muscle pump (side of hemiparesis).
- Over-active muscle pump in one leg (tremor in PD) makes bilateral oedema appear unilateral.

Fluid retention:

- Cardiac failure.
- Drugs (NSAIDs, steroids, calcium channel blockers, glitazones).
- Renal failure.

Hypoalbuminaemia:

- Nutritional, hepatic disease or protein loss via kidney (dip-stick urine for protein),
- Leak from bowels or extensive skin loss.

Lymphatic obstruction:

- Usually malignant.

Inflammatory:

- Cellulitis.

Hypokalaemia

Low potassium (K) is common in elderly patients, often due to diuretics or GI loss (remember the laxative abuser), exacerbated by inadequate dietary intake (deficient in fruit, vegetables and meat). Mild Conn's syndrome is probably under-recognized. It has been reported that sick elderly females, in particular, may develop 'acute transient hypokalaemia', probably due to a shift into the cells, which usually self-corrects within a few days. Hypokalaemia exacerbates digoxin toxicity. Replace orally or by slow intravenous infusion if severe. If the response is poor, check for low magnesium, as correcting this helps.

Hyperkalaemia

This occurs in renal failure and rhabdomyolysis (which may follow a collapse and long lie).

However, drugs are the common culprits. In old age, cardiac failure can often be managed with furosemide alone without needing the addition of potassium-retaining amiloride. A combination of an ACE inhibitor and spironolactone may be evidence-based treatment for cardiac failure, but, particularly if co-amilofruse is also prescribed, will usually result in dangerous hyperkalaemia with older kidneys!

If the ECG is abnormal give intravenous calcium gluconate first, then insulin and glucose. Low dose oral calcium resonium can be useful in the long term, e.g. if the patient is not suitable for dialysis, and is more palatable than a low K diet. Doses of ACE inhibitor, ARB and potassium-sparing diuretic that control heart failure when the patient is well, may in hyperkalaemia and renal failure in an intercurrent illness causing dehydration. On admission, hold the next dose of such drugs until you have confirmed that the creatinine and electrolytes are acceptable. Omit if BP is low or may drop, e.g. if surgery for hip fracture is planned or the patient develops diarrhoea. If the drugs are restarted teach 'sick-day' rules: omit the drug if vomiting or diarrhoea develops.

Diabetes mellitus

Definition

Diabetes mellitus (DM) is a metabolic disorder with heterogeneous aetiologies characterized by chronic hyperglycaemia and disturbances of carbohydrate, fat and protein metabolism resulting from defects in insulin secretion, insulin action or both.

The WHO Diabetes Programme (2011) recommends an HbA1c cut-off of 6.5% (48 mmol/mol) for diagnosis of diabetes.

- Advantages: reflects average glucose over 8–12 weeks, avoids day to day variability; test can be done at any time of day without fasting or a glucose load.
- Disadvantages: assays may lack standardization, affected by anaemia, haemoglobinopathies, red cell turnover, e.g. malaria and renal failure.
- Effect on incidence: this criterion alone will identify fewer 'diabetics' than the old criteria, but as it is more convenient more people may be tested.

The old WHO criteria (1999) remain valid and can be used in parallel; the ranges of blood glucose indicative of DM are:

- Random venous plasma glucose ≥ 11.1 mmol/L or
- Fasting plasma glucose ≥ 7.0 mmol/L or
- Plasma glucose ≥ 11.1 mmol/L at 2 h after a 75-g oral glucose load (oral glucose tolerance test).

Epidemiology

Prevalence rises with age up to the highest age band studied (84 years) and is higher in AfroCaribbean and South Asian people than white people in the UK. Since 1996 the number of people diagnosed with diabetes has increased from 1.4 million to 2.6 million. By 2025 it is estimated that over 4 million people will have diabetes because of our ageing population and increasing numbers of obese people; 90% of adults with DM have Type 2. Half the diabetic population and a quarter of insulin users are elderly. A common 'ballpark' figure is that over 10% of people aged 70 have known diabetes and the same number have unrecognized impaired glucose tolerance. In care homes around a quarter of residents have diabetes. Figure 12.2 shows the effect of age on the prevalence of diabetes in England.

Mechanism

The impairment of glucose tolerance in old age is mainly caused by reduced tissue sensitivity to insulin at post-receptor level. There is also beta-cell dysfunction; the pancreas is less able to secrete insulin in response to a glucose load and the rapid post-prandial spike of secretion is lost. The older diabetic usually has Type 2 diabetes, although the number of Type 1 graduates to old age will increase steadily. Occasionally, Type 1 diabetes occurs *de novo* in an older person.

Effects

Diabetics aged 65–75 have twice the cardiovascular and all-cause mortality – but thereafter it tends to revert towards normal for age. One-third have visual impairment, more often due to cataract than to retinopathy, and the amputation rate is enormously increased and cognitive and psychosocial function is generally impaired. A common end stage comprises poor cardiac function, renal failure and marked oedema.

Management

Management of the diabetes must be part of a holistic approach to cardiovascular risk and will depend greatly on the circumstances of the patient; a frail nursing home resident requires different care to an otherwise fit and independent 75 year old who should have access to the same resources as a younger person. Stopping smoking and treating high blood pressure and lipids have more effect on outcome than maintaining tight glycaemic control.

Aims include a feeling of well-being, avoidance of glycosuria at all ages (osmotic diuresis gives rise to symptoms but as the renal threshold increases with age tight control is not needed to achieve this) and tight enough control to reduce complications in younger elderly patients. Hypoglycaemia (which only occurs once the person is on hypoglycaemic drugs or insulin, NOT on diet alone) can cause brain damage or injury if the patient collapses and should be avoided.

- Education: about diabetes and how lifestyle changes will help.

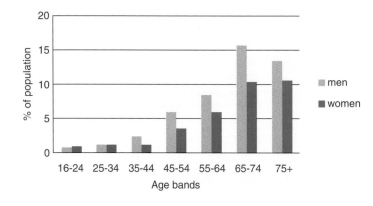

Figure 12.2 Prevalence of DM (percentage of population in England by age group) in 2006.

- Diet: weight reduction in the obese, reducing fat intake and ensuring that carbohydrates are of a high-fibre, unrefined, polysaccharide type. Because of the failure of the post-prandial insulin spike, the concept of the glycaemic index of food may be useful. Some carbohydrates are absorbed quickly and blood glucose levels increase very rapidly ('high GI' foods), while others release glucose slowly and have little effect ('low GI' foods). Carbohydrates are ranked on a scale of 1–100 with glucose being used as the reference point of 100.
- Exercise: highly beneficial (walking half an hour a day).
- Smoking: refer to the local quit service.
- Platelet stickiness: aspirin.
- Hypertension: treat vigorously if the patient can tolerate this. ACE inhibitors and ARBs have a particular role in reducing microscopic albuminuria.
- Hypercholesterolaemia: statins (at least up to 80 years).
- Drugs: if drugs are necessary, the best data come from the United Kingdom Prospective Diabetes Study (UKPDS).

Oral drugs:

- o Metformin, which decreases gluconeogenesis and increases peripheral utilization of glucose, is first-line. Patients usually lose weight. Care must be taken if there is renal impairment (contraindicated if eGFR < 30 ml/ min). Increase the dose gradually to minimize GI side-effects. Very unlikely to cause a hypo.
- o Sulphonylureas augment insulin secretion. Those with short half-lives (e.g. glipizide 3–6 h) are favoured (avoid chlorpropramide and glibenclamide). Weight gain may be a problem.
- o α-glucosidase inhibitor: acarbose, which delays starch absorption, is often not well tolerated because of flatulence but is safe and useful in those who can take it.
- o Meglitinides are, like sulphonylureas, insulin-secretagogues but bind to a different site on the ATP-sensitive potassium channel. Neither repaglinide nor nateglinide has been found to have much advantage over sulphonylureas.
- o Thiazolidinediones ('glitazones') activate the peroxisome-proliferator-activated receptor gamma (PPARγ) in the cell nucleus and increase glucose uptake and peripheral utilization. They were rarely used in the elderly as

they are contraindicated in heart failure. Unexpected osteoporotic fractures and cardiac side-effects lead to the withdrawal of rosiglitazone and reduction in pioglitazone use.
- o DPP-IV (dipeptidyl peptidase) inhibitors such as sitagliptin and vildagliptin are orally active inhibitors of the enzyme that inactivates endogenous GLP-1 (glucagon-like peptide 1). Saxagliptin can be used in moderate to severe renal disease. Physiologically, levels of GLP-1 rise in response to rising glucose after a meal and are responsible for the incretin effect, increasing pancreatic insulin secretion postprandially. The therapeutic effects of DPP-IV inhibitors are therefore analogous to the GLP-1 agonists; they are less potent but weight-neutral.

Injectable drugs:

- o GLP-1 agonists: these include exenatide and liraglutide. This new class of injectable therapy for Type 2 diabetes enhances post-prandial, glucose-dependent insulin secretion from the patient's own beta cells. This has physiological appeal, should make hypoglycaemia less likely and the drugs induce early satiety and thus weight loss. These are potential advantages over insulin but serious side-effects including pancreatitis have been reported.
- o Insulin: if control is poor, it is a mistake to be too reluctant to institute insulin, which makes the poorly controlled diabetic feel much better. A single daily injection of insulin glargine or detemir can achieve adequate control with minimal risk of hypoglycaemia. This is useful if the patient cannot inject their own insulin and must rely on a visiting district nurse as the exact timing is also not critical. A traditional twice-a-day mixed insulin regimen necessitates eating lunch at a relatively fixed time and having an evening snack to avoid nocturnal hypoglycaemia. Combinations of insulin and tablets are increasingly used. However, even where good control is not achieved, if the patient does not have the cognition, dexterity and vision to give their own insulin, intensifying the regimen can be impractical. Fit active elderly people will manage a basal bolus regimen just like younger people.

Further education is essential to make sure the patient understands how and when to take the drug, and how to manage hypoglycaemia. Simple glucose sweets should be carried for 'hypos' – blood sugar rises slowly after eating a Mars bar as the fat content delays gastric emptying! Check whether your patient drives and advise accordingly.

Foot care and regular chiropody are particularly important in the elderly diabetic and the usual checks including biochemistry and retinal photography are needed, usually in the context of an annual review. Once foot complications occur the patient's quality of life plunges and the costs of care increase dramatically. A long period in hospital usually culminates in an above-knee amputation.

Hyperosmolar crisis

Diabetic crises and complications do not present any special features in old people apart from hyperosmolar coma. This typically occurs in patients with Type 2 diabetes that has often hitherto caused very little problem. An osmotic diuresis leads to insidiously progressive dehydration and hypotension, culminating in stupor or coma. However, because there is still some endogenous insulin, the body does not switch to metabolic pathways resulting in ketone production. Extreme hyperglycaemia, hypernatraemia and uraemia are typical.

The aim here is steady correction of the metabolic derangement. Avoid doing things too rapidly and remember rehydration is more important than insulin. It is safest to give normal saline, as this will be relatively dilute in comparison with the plasma. Depending on the severity and the patient's cardiac status, give a litre over 1–2 h and **assess the effect**. Continue with a litre over 2, 4, 6 h, and so on. It may be necessary to give 10 L of fluid over and above output over the first 48 h, ideally monitored by the central venous pressure (CVP) line. Wait an hour before giving any insulin; the glucose often falls dramatically with rehydration, but if it is needed 1 unit per hour would be a typical dose. The risk of venous thrombosis is high so give a full preventative dose of heparin (e.g. 40 mg enoxaparin). Those who survive do not need insulin unless control remains poor.

Thyroid disease – function tests

Normal function is usually preserved until at least 80 years of age but in centenarians TSH and free T3 levels may decline. In the seriously ill patient, the TSH, T3 and T4 levels may all be misleadingly low ('sick euthyroid syndrome'). Amiodarone and anticonvulsants often interfere with thyroid-function tests (TFTs). Always check TFTs before starting amiodarone and remember that this will interfere with radioiodine treatment. Both hypo- and hyperthyroidism are difficult to diagnose clinically in old age and many geriatricians routinely check TSH in any significant illness.

Hyperthyroidism

Presentation is atypical – AF, heart failure, weight loss, proximal myopathy, functional decline. The thyroid may be nodular or impalpable – sometimes retrosternal. Treatment is carbimazole and a beta-blocker if the heart rate is high, prior to definitive therapy with ^{131}I (radioiodine). Carbimazole can be given in a dose aiming for normal thyroid hormone level, or a dose sufficient to block all production and giving levothyroxine replacement (see BNF), updated 6-monthly. Remember to give written advice about sore throat on carbimazole (neutropaenia). The management of amiodarone-induced thyrotoxicosis is controversial. Some advocate ignoring a raised free T_4 but treating raised T_3 with carbimazole and steroids.

Hypothyroidism

Hypothyroidism affects 5% of people aged over 60 and it may be due to Hashimoto's disease, I^{131} treatment, surgery, idiopathic or, occasionally, secondary to pituitary failure. Clinical pointers include impaired cognition and slow-relaxing reflexes. Treatment is with levothyroxine 25 µg, with similar increments every 3–4 weeks until, on a daily dose of around 100 µg, the patient feels well and the TSH confirms euthyroidism. If a profoundly hypothyroid woman is admitted and 100 µg levothyroxine tablets are brought in with her, do not just write them on the chart – it is very likely she has not been taking them. Get advice and if in doubt build up from a low dose to avoid precipitating an MI.

Adrenal disease

Cushing's syndrome

The commonest cause is iatrogenic: older people are often left on higher doses of steroid than they need, particularly for polymyalgia rheumatica, which usually burns itself out after a couple of years. Older people are particularly prone to fluid retention, heart failure, diabetes, proximal myopathy, skin thinning and bruising and osteoporosis (always give bone protection) and high doses may lead to acute confusion ('steroid psychosis').

Addison's disease

Adrenal insufficiency may occur acutely, usually when there is an acute severe illness in a patient with iatrogenic adrenal suppression due to long-term steroid treatment. Chronic adrenal insufficiency is due to idiopathic atrophy (likely autoimmune) or adrenal destruction, e.g. TB or metastases. You must consider the possibility to make the diagnosis because the presentation is insidious even in middle age. Postural symptoms are common. If the patient is ill and suspicion is high, send a cortisol sample urgently and treat straight away with 100 mg hydrocortisone IV 6-hourly and fluids. Otherwise do a short Synacthen test. Long-term treatment is hydrocortisone, ideally 10 mg in the morning, 5 mg at lunch and 5 mg early evening, with 100 mcg fludrocortisone daily, then tailored to the person's needs.

Autonomic nervous system

The autonomic nervous system (ANS) is most closely involved in homoeostatic mechanisms. There is some age-related decline in function and more obvious problems result from central or peripheral neurological damage, e.g. diabetes, alcoholism, PD (multi-system atrophy is less common but more severe), uraemia, drug-induced neuropathies, amyloidosis, autoimmune disorders and paraneoplastic syndromes. Common manifestations are orthostatic hypotension, erectile dysfunction, impaired bladder emptying, gastric paresis, diarrhoea or constipation. A battery of tests for autonomic function may be used.

Paraneoplastic endocrine syndromes

These arise from tumour secretion of hormones, peptides or cytokines. The four commonest syndromes are SIADH, hypercalcaemia, Cushing's syndrome and hypoglycaemia. Treatment of the

tumour produces the best results, but endocrine treatment may be needed.

SIADH

This was first described as a paraneoplastic condition and is due to tumour cell production of ADH and atrial natriuretic peptide which has natriuretic and antidiuretic properties see p. 170.

Hypercalcaemia

This occurs in up to 10% of all patients with advanced cancer and carries a poor prognosis see page 83. There are four principal mechanisms, though 3 and 4 are very rare:

1 Secretion of parathyroid hormone (PTH)-related protein (PTHrP) by tumour cells: 80% of cases, most commonly squamous cell tumours.
2 Osteolytic bone metastases: 20% of cases, especially breast cancer, multiple myeloma and lymphomas.
3 Tumour secretion of vitamin D.
4 Ectopic tumour secretion of PTH.

Paraneoplastic Cushing's syndrome

This arises from tumour secretion of adrenocorticotropic hormone or corticotropin-releasing factor. Patients often present with symptoms of Cushing's syndrome before a cancer diagnosis is made. Unlike a pituitary source, paraneoplastic Cushing's syndrome does not respond to high-dose dexamethasone suppression. Drugs are used to inhibit steroid production; ketoconazole is first-line treatment.

Hypoglycaemia

Tumour-associated hypoglycaemia is rare. It can be caused by insulin-producing islet-cell tumours or extrapancreatic production of IGF-2 or insulin.

Accidental hypothermia

Clinical features

Above 32 °C the features may be those of an underlying disease or of functional decline. Below 32 °C the features are as described for the aforementioned patient and, below 27 °C, 75% of the patients are comatose. Pancreatitis, hypoglycaemia

Accidental hypothermia: a salutary tale

One day, neighbours notice that the old lady who lives alone next door has not taken the milk in or opened the curtains and there is no sign of life. They have a key, so they let themselves in and, after shouting for her with no response, they eventually find her in her bedroom, on the floor, in a dazed condition, wearing only her nightdress. Hesitant to move her, they call the GP.

The GP notices that the room is cold; there is no heating and the window is open. The GP checks to exclude an obvious injury from the fall, such as a hip fracture, and that there is no obvious illness that may have caused her to fall, such as a hemiplegia. She hypothesizes that the old lady has a debilitating illness, e.g. pneumonia, that made her collapse as she tried to get out of bed to visit the toilet. She is drowsy, croaky, very slow of movement and response, and her limbs are strikingly rigid. Her abdomen feels unnaturally cool. Her pulse rate is 50 b.p.m., her BP 100/70 and the tympanic thermometer reveals a core temperature of 31 °C. **Why?**

- It has been a cold night.
- She has a serious illness – pneumonia (alcohol and drugs such as phenothiazines also predispose to hypothermia).
- She is only wearing a nightdress and has spent most of the night on the floor.
- Her ability to detect a falling ambient temperature is less than that of a young person. The previous evening, she forgot to put on her woolly nightcap, not realizing that up to 15% of the body's heat may be lost through the scalp. She also failed to close the window and to plug in the fan heater. She has never had central heating installed.
- As her body temperature started to fall, her ANS failed to cut down heat loss by cutaneous vasoconstriction and failed to increase heat production by shivering.

The three main factors that have combined to produce this typical clinical picture are: systemic illness, exposure to cold and ANS dysfunction; if sufficiently severe, only one of these factors need be present to cause accidental hypothermia (core temperature less than 35 °C).

and ventricular arrhythmias are among the complications. Everyone seems to remember the J waves (at the R-ST junction or 'J point' – Google for multiple examples), but you diagnose hypothermia with a low reading thermometer, not an ECG. Over 30 °C the mortality is about 33%, but below 30 °C it approaches 70%.

Management

At a core temperature just below 35 °C, it is reasonable to re-warm the patient at home and counsel to prevent recurrence. More serious cases (30–34 °C) have traditionally received gradual passive re-warming in hospital at 0.5–1.0 °C per hour to avoid sudden profound hypotension. Avoid instrumentation, which may precipitate serious arrhythmia. Below 30 °C some would argue that admission to the ITU is required. However, most elderly patients have to take their chance on an open ward with active re-warming using a 'Bair hugger' or forced-air warming system.

Other dangers of extreme weather

Cold kills in other ways, and in an average winter there are 40,000 deaths in England and Wales above the expected number, mainly due to vascular causes. Platelets, haematocrit, blood viscosity, plasma cholesterol and, in old men at least, systolic BP tends to rise on exposure to the cold. Blood fibrinogen levels may rise during the winter months. Slipping on icy pavements is a further hazard.

The incidence of strokes and the mortality rate also tend to rise among elderly people in the UK during heat waves (see also Chapter 1). Food poisoning is another hazard of hot weather.

 REFERENCES

UK Prospective Diabetes Study – overview of multiple publications (1977–97). Turner R and colleagues. http://www.dtu.ox.ac.uk/ukpds_trial/index.php.

WHO (2011) *Consultation paper 2011. WHO/NMH/CHP/CPM/11.1 Use of Glycated Haemoglobin (HbA1c) in the Diagnosis of Diabetes Mellitus.* http://www.who.int/diabetes/publications/report-hba1c_2011.pdf.

→ FURTHER INFORMATION

Allan LM, Ballard CG, Allen J, et al. (2006) Autonomic dysfunction in dementia. http://jnnp.bmj.com/cgi/rapidpdf/jnnp. 2006.102343v1.

Biswas M, Davies JS (2007) Hyponatraemia in clinical practice. *Postgraduate Medicine Journal* 83(980): 373–378, doi: 10.1136/pgmj.2006.056515.

Cruz-Jentoft AJ, Baeyens JP, Bauer JM et al. (2010) Sarcopenia: European consensus on definition and diagnosis. Report of the European Working Group on Sarcopenia in Older People. *Age Ageing* 39: 412–423, doi: 10.1093/ageing/afq034.

Diabetes UK: www.diabetes.org.uk. Has lots of information for patients, carers and professionals: check diagnostic criteria, the latest on the NSF, etc.

Diabetes in the UK 2010. Key statistics on diabetes: http://www.diabetes.org.uk/Documents/Reports/Diabetes_in_the_UK_2010.pdf.

Diabetic foot problems: inpatient management of diabetic foot problems. NICE Clinical Guideline 119 (2011; NHS evidence accredited): www.nice.org.uk/CG119/.

Laurberg P, Andersen S, Carlé A, Karmisholt J, Knudsen N, Bülow Pedersen I (2011) The TSH upper reference limit: where are we at? *Nature Reviews Endocrinology* 7: 232–239, doi: 10.1038/nrendo.2011.13.

NICE (2009) Type 2 diabetes: the management of type 2 diabetes. NICE Clinical Guideline 87 (2009; NHS evidence accredited): www.nice.org.uk/CG87/.

NICE Quality Standards for Diabetes 2011: http://www.nice.org.uk/guidance/qualitystandards/diabetesinadults/diabetesinadultsqualitystandard.jsp.

Practical guidance on diabetes diagnosis and management: www.diabetesbible.com/.

Practical guidance on endocrine diagnosis and management: www.endobible.com/.

Pelosof LC, Gerber DE (2010) Paraneoplastic syndromes: an approach to diagnosis and treatment. *Mayo Clinic Proceedings* 85: 838–854, doi: 10.4065/mcp.2010.0099.

SIGN Guidelines for Management of Diabetes (2010): http://www.sign.ac.uk/guidelines/fulltext/116/index.html. A super website with a wide range of material.

SIGN Guidelines for PD (2010): http://www.sign.ac.uk/guidelines/fulltext/113/index.html.

Pimenta E, Calhoun DA (2006) Primary aldosteronism: diagnosis and treatment. *Journal of Clinical Hypertension* 8: 887–893.

Prabhakar VKB, Shalet SM (2006) Aetiology, diagnosis and management of hypopituitarism in adult life. *Postgraduate Medicine Journal* 82: 259–266, doi: 10.1136/pgmj.2005.039768.

UK Department of Health: www.doh.gov.uk/. With press releases explaining latest policies. Relevant examples here include 'Keep warm, keep well' and 'Supporting vulnerable people during a heatwave'.

13

Genitourinary disease

Age changes

1 In old age, renal function is reduced to about 50% of the peak at 30 years.
2 Serum urea may remain in the normal range despite deteriorating renal function.
3 Creatinine reflects muscle bulk; so beware the frail elderly patient with a 'normal' level of creatinine.
4 The estimated glomerular filtration rate (eGFR) can be calculated using the creatinine, gender and age. This only applies in steady states, not in acute deterioration.
5 Ability both to concentrate urine and to process an extra water load quickly is impaired. This is one explanation for nocturia in old age. Maximum urine concentration falls from 1300 to 850 mOsm/L.
6 There is loss of renal mass, affecting the cortex more than the medulla, in half of 'normal' elderly kidneys.
7 Reduced renal function is due to:
   - Loss and sclerosis of glomeruli leading to fewer functioning nephrons.
   - Reduced renal blood flow, particularly to the cortex.
   - Diminished response to antidiuretic hormone (ADH).

These effects are exaggerated in hypertension, diabetes and after pyelonephritis.

8 The combination of ageing changes and systemic or renal disease may lead to rapid, dramatic deterioration in renal function.
9 Atrophic changes occur in the urogenital tract of post-menopausal women as oestrogen levels fall.
10 Prostate size increases and cancerous foci become common.
11 The incidence of unstable bladder increases due to sudden uncontrollable surges in bladder pressure secondary to contractions whilst filling (detrusor instability).

Acute kidney injury (AKI) in old age

AKI is now the preferred term for acute renal failure. AKI is defined as an abrupt rise in serum creatinine, usually accompanied by a decrease in urine output. AKI is common in older people admitted to hospital, but is also a frequent complication during admission (in up to 20% of cases). The ageing kidney does not have sufficient reserve to tolerate insults such as dehydration and sepsis; AKI is usually multifactorial and iatrogenic factors such as drugs and inadequate fluid management often contribute. Pre-existing renal damage from hypertension and diabetes, cardiovascular comorbidity and poor nutrition increase the vulnerability of old kidneys to common acute insults. As the outcome of AKI is poor in old age, identify at-risk patients and manage them carefully to prevent AKI.

Causes

See Table 13.1.

History

- Evaluate for all causes of volume depletion and hypotension (e.g. poor oral intake, vomiting,

Lecture Notes Elderly Care Medicine, Eighth Edition. Claire G. Nicholl and K. Jane Wilson.
© 2012 John Wiley & Sons, Ltd. Published 2012 by John Wiley & Sons, Ltd.

Table 13.1 **Causes of acute kidney injury in older people**

Pre-renal	Renal	Post-renal
Dehydration	Acute tubular necrosis results from ischaemia (usually from a pre-renal cause)	Prostatic hypertrophy
Blood loss	Nephrotoxins, e.g. drugs, contrast agents	Ureteric stones
Pump failure	Myoglobinuria secondary to rhabdomyolysis (falls)	Prostate cancer
Over-treatment of hypertension	Allergic interstitial nephritis	Gynaecological cancer
Sepsis (vasodilation)	Systemic diseases – myeloma, gout, etc.	Bladder cancer
Renovascular disease	Glomerulonephritidies	Retroperitoneal fibrosis

diarrhoea, GI bleed, sepsis, over-diuresis, ACS and antihypertensives).

- New onset postural dizziness suggests volume depletion.
- Ask about all drugs including over-the-counter (OTC) herbal preparations as some cause allergic interstitial nephritis.
- Confused, elderly inpatients may not drink enough, and may be given medications (including diuretics, ACEi) that they had stopped taking at home long ago.
- Lower urinary tract symptoms (LUTS).
- Past medical history: prostate, bladder and ovarian, cervical or uterine cancer.
- Review previous blood results to check baseline function.

Examination

- Assess fluid status (patients with oedema can still be intravascularly depleted).
- Check lying and standing blood pressures and heart rate. A postural drop and tachycardia indicate hypovolaemia.
- Check the jugular venous pressure (JVP) carefully.
- Palpable bladder?
- Rectal examination; size and character of the prostate.

Investigations

1 Urgent electrolytes: hyperkalaemia is the most immediately life-threatening abnormality.
2 Hypernatraemia is common in severe dehydration with drowsiness leading to poor oral intake; prognosis is very poor.

3 ECG to check for effects of hyperkalaemia (see Figure 13.1).
4 FBC, CRP and ESR to check for sepsis or inflammation. Normocytic anaemia may indicate CKD.
5 Urea and creatinine.
6 Glucose/HbA1c.
7 Bone profile – high phosphate suggests CKD.
8 ABG and lactate – ?acidotic.
9 CXR: cardiomegaly, pneumonia, pulmonary oedema and infiltrates (vasculitis).
10 Ultrasound: assess for bladder outflow obstruction, hydronephrosis and also kidney size (if small, suggestive of chronic renal disease).

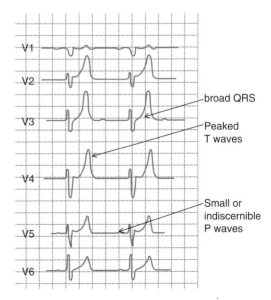

Figure 13.1 ECG in hyperkalaemia. *Source:* Wikimedia Commons (public domain).

11 Urinalysis: leucocytes and nitrites suggest infection; blood and protein suggest renal disease.

12 Midstream urine (MSU): microscopy for casts and culture.

13 Further tests, guided by the results of the above, might include creatine kinase, protein electrophoresis and Bence–Jones protein, uric acid, autoantibodies, CT scan.

Management

1 Treat hyperkalaemia: intravenous calcium gluconate first (10% in 10 mL aliquots by slow push) and then 50 mL 50% dextrose with 10 units of insulin over 20 min.

2 Fluid resuscitate: if in doubt, give 250 ml 0.9% saline stat, review and repeat as needed.

3 Catheter to relieve urinary obstruction and to monitor urine output.

4 Antibiotics for sepsis.

5 Stop nephrotoxins, especially NSAIDs and diuretics, ACEi, ARBs plus other antihypertensives if the patient is dry or hypotensive. Check ALL drugs on the chart in the BNF – do not rely on your memory.

6 Reduce the dose of drugs metabolized by the kidneys, e.g. enoxaparin.

7 Daily weight helps guide fluid balance.

8 A nephrostomy tube inserted under ultrasound guidance reduces unilateral hydronephrosis. If this is secondary to a stone blocking the ureter, the patient is referred to urology for insertion of a J-J stent. If the hydronephrosis is secondary to tumour, it may be more appropriate to leave the nephrostomy in situ for symptomatic relief.

9 Refer to nephrology for advice, consideration of temporary haemofiltration (to allow acute tubular necrosis to resolve) and longterm renal replacement therapy. Age alone is not a contraindication to dialysis. However, co-morbidities such as low output heart failure make haemodialysis challenging.

Complications

- Acidosis.
- Hyperkalaemia.
- Oedema.
- Sepsis.
- Respiratory failure.
- Encephalopathy.
- Haemorrhage.

Chronic kidney disease (CKD) in the elderly

- Observe caution when interpreting creatinine because older people tend to have a lower muscle mass and therefore a lower creatinine level whatever the renal function.
- CKD is diagnosed using eGFR which is based on the MDRD (Modification of Diet in Renal Disease) calculation.
- CKD is common – 70% of > 70 year olds have CKD 3 – this reflects vascular disease and renal ageing; these patients are more likely to die from vascular disease than kidney failure.

Causes

> **Common causes of CKD in older people**
>
> 1 Diabetes mellitus
> 2 Hypertension
> 3 Obstructive uropathy
> 4 Chronic pyelonephritis
> 5 Cardiac insufficiency
> 6 Renovascular disease
> 7 Myeloma
> 8 Systemic vasculitis
>
> Biopsy is rarely helpful if the kidneys are small.

Symptoms

Table 13.2 shows the stages of CKD. Symptoms appear usually only in CKD 4/5 – poor appetite,

Table 13.2 Stages of CKD

Stage	Description	eGFR (mL/min/1.73 m^2)
1	Normal or increased eGFR	≥ 90
2	Mildly decreased eGFR	60–89
3	Moderately decreased eGFR	30–59
4	Severely decreased eGFR	15–29
5	Kidney failure	< 15

nausea and vomiting, tiredness, breathlessness, peripheral oedema, itch and cramps.

Signs

Assess fluid balance to exclude hypovolaemia due to infection, dehydration or overload; palpable bladder, enlarged prostate or uraemic frost (anaemia plus uraemia).

Investigations

As for AKI. Look for anaemia (decreased epo production from renal fibroblasts) and renal bone disease (increased PTH due to deficient 1α hydroxylation of vitamin D in proximal tubule mitochondria and phosphate retention).

Management

- The objectives are to prevent progression, reduce complications, treat cardiovascular risk factors and control symptoms. If there are no contraindications use aspirin or simvastatin; target BP < 138/80 if possible without inducing symptomatic postural hypotension.
- The best drugs to reduce blood pressure and proteinuria are ACEi and ARBs, but they reduce renal blood flow and may worsen renal function if the patient is hypovolaemic. Start with a small dose and monitor!
- Fluid retention may need high dose loop diuretics with cautious use of metolazone watching the potassium.
- Review medications, reducing doses and monitoring levels where appropriate. See 'Drugs and the kidney' below.
- Erythropoietin injections/iron infusions for symptomatic anaemia.
- 1α calcidol/phosphate binders (Calcichew, sevelamer).
- Renal diet (low sodium, potassium and phosphate) is often unpalatable, and not necessary for end-of-life patients.
- Education regarding diet, regulating fluid intake and concordance with medications.
- Renal replacement therapy: in the UK 46% of dialysis patients are aged over 65 and 33% are aged over 70 years.
- Many elderly patients adopt a philosophical approach, which makes them suitable for continuous ambulatory peritoneal dialysis (CAPD).
- Palliative care when needed.

Complications of CKD

Renal osteodystrophy

- Hypocalcaemia
- Hyperphosphataemia
- Secondary hyperparathyroidism (increased PTH)

Cardiovascular: increased risk of stroke, amputation, MI

- Hypertension
- Atherosclerosis

Anaemia
Metabolic acidosis
Malnutrition: secondary to anorexia, renal diet, increased protein catabolism

---

Intrinsic renal disease

Specific kidney diseases are less common than pre- and post-renal causes of renal failure in elderly patients.

- **Nephrotic syndrome**. In a series of patients aged over 50 (diabetics were excluded), the underlying cause in order of incidence was:
  - Membranous glomerulonephritis.
  - Proliferative glomerulonephritis.
  - Amyloid: usually secondary to long-standing inflammatory disease, e.g. bronchiectasis, osteomyelitis or rheumatoid arthritis.
  - Minimal-change glomerulonephritis.
- **Diabetic nephropathy** – common, no special features in old age.
- **Hypertensive damage** – common.
- **Myeloma**: see Chapter 14.
- **Nephrocalcinosis/stones**. Exclude excess vitamin D, gout and hyperparathyroidism, all more common in old age.

Urinary-tract infection (UTI)

- Very common in old age: 20% of people over the age of 65.

- This increases to 50% of women in institutional care.
- Female-to-male ratio: 3:1.
- *Escherichia coli* is the most common pathogen. Others include *Proteus mirabilis*, *Pseudomonas* and *Klebsiella*.
- Catheter-related infections are hard to eliminate unless the catheter is changed.
- Asymptomatic bacteriuria with no pyuria does not require treatment.
- Pyelonephritis is responsible for 20% of cases of renal failure.

Precipitating factors for UTI in old age are:

1 Urinary stasis:
  - Incomplete voiding.
  - Outflow obstruction, including constipation.
  - Increased bladder diverticula, e.g. secondary to BPH.
2 Loss of acidity of the female urethra, atrophic vaginitis and urethritis due to reduced oestrogen.
3 Associated disorders:
  - Diabetes.
  - Immobility.
  - Indwelling catheter.
  - Poor fluid intake.
4 Urinary-tract stones.

Presentations of urosepsis in old age

1 Increased frequency and dysuria are common, but there may be other vague symptoms such as nausea, vomiting and lethargy.
2 Delirium: catheterization may be required to obtain specimen; alternatively organisms may be isolated from a blood culture. NB: UTI is rarely the sole cause of the delirium!
3 New urinary incontinence; infected urine irritates the bladder mucosa.
4 Increasing drowsiness due to worsening renal impairment.

Management

1 Culture organism from urine or blood.
2 Appropriate antibiotics (as per local guidelines).
3 Maintain good fluid input (greater than 2 L/day).
4 Reverse precipitating causes, if possible.

Obstructive nephropathy

Obstructive nephropathy is secondary to a blockage anywhere along the urinary tract. See Figure 13.2.

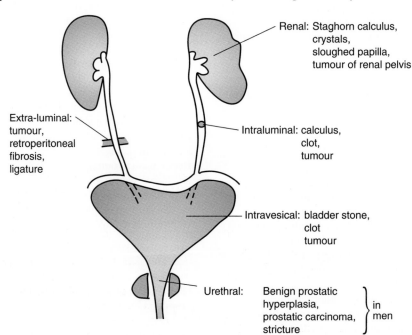

Figure 13.2 Causes of obstructive uropathy.

Bladder outflow obstruction

Benign prostatic hyperplasia

1 By the age of 60, 50% of prostates contain areas of hyperplasia of the glands and connective tissue. By 85 years, 90% of prostates are affected, i.e. this is part of normal ageing (sometimes, incorrectly, referred to as hypertrophy).
2 Within the prostate, 5α reductase converts circulating testosterone to dihydrotestosterone (DHT), which acts locally to cause cellular proliferation.
3 Lower urinary tract symptoms (LUTS) are classified as filling or irritative (frequency, urgency, dysuria, nocturia) and voiding or obstructive (poor stream, hesitancy, terminal dribbling, incomplete voiding, overflow incontinence).
4 Fewer than half of all men with benign prostatic hyperplasia develop symptoms.
5 Mild cases or patients who are a poor surgical risk can be effectively treated with selective α-adrenoceptor antagonists. There are receptors in the smooth muscle, capsule of the bladder and bladder neck, and α-blockers relax the muscle. Tamsulosin has more α_1 specificity and causes less orthostatic hypotension than doxazosin or terazosin.
6 5α reductase inhibitors such as finasteride work by blocking conversion of testosterone to DHT and inhibit prostate growth. Warn the patient it will take 6 months for the finasteride to reach optimum efficacy.
7 Rectal examination is the first essential step in diagnosis, although prostatic enlargement may need to be confirmed by rectal ultrasound.
8 If suspicious nodules are detected on rectal examination, it may be appropriate to measure the prostate-specific antigen (PSA). See 'Cancer of the prostate' below.
9 Transurethral prostatectomy (TURP) has been the mainstay of treatment for very symptomatic benign prostatic hyperplasia, but complications include perioperative haemorrhage and absorption of irrigation fluids, urethral strictures and incontinence. Repeat surgery may be needed.
10 If malignant cells are found in a TURP specimen, the management remains problematic as many patients will live trouble-free.
11 Minimally invasive procedures are being developed which can be performed with local anaesthetic. Heat is used to cause cell death and reduce outflow obstruction. Examples include:

- Transurethral incision of the prostate (TUIP): useful for small prostates in men unable to tolerate TURP.
- Transurethral microwave therapy (TUMT): heat is delivered to the prostate via a catheter or per rectum.
- Transurethral needle ablation (TUNA): high frequency radiowaves are used as above.

Cancer of the prostate

Prostatic cancer is the third most common cause of death in men aged over 55 years. It is very common in the over 70s, when it is usually indolent, i.e. 'many men die with it rather than from it'. However, invasive disease has a mean survival time of 4 years. The unpredictability of the clinical course makes management a challenge. Thus the patient's preferences must be taken into account. Screening continues to be highly controversial because, despite much anecdotal evidence of improved outcome in individuals, there is no large body of evidence to demonstrate increased survival rates.

Clinical features

- Often asymptomatic.
- There may be LUTS such as poor stream, post-micturition dribbling and nocturia, but usually only late in the disease.
- If the cancer has spread, there may be bony pain, lower limb lymphoedema and cachexia.
- Rectal examination reveals a hard, craggy prostate.

Investigations

- Measurement of PSA is readily available but still lacks sensitivity and specificity. The ratio of free to total PSA may give extra specificity. A low ratio implies a greater chance of discovering cancer if the prostate is biopsied. A very high PSA suggests metastatic disease.
- Multiple prostatic biopsies are taken under transrectal ultrasound guidance.
- Histology of prostate chippings following TURP.
- Bone scintigraphy is a sensitive way of detecting bone metastases.
- MRI scans may demonstrate local and widespread disease.

Treatment

- Treatment can relieve symptoms but does little to prolong survival.
- Transurethral resection may be necessary to relieve bladder-neck obstruction.
- If there is evidence of spread beyond the gland, hormone therapy is generally indicated, but not all would agree with treatment in the absence of symptoms, even at this stage. Hormonal 'control' fails eventually, possibly due to 'clonal selection' of hormone-independent malignant cells.
- Radical prostatectomy gives no better results in over 65s and morbidity is far greater than with hormonal manipulation.
- External beam radiotherapy or brachytherapy (radioactive implants placed in the prostate) are also used, especially for anaplastic tumours (even when confined to the prostate) and for localized metastases.
- Blood transfusions are helpful for the patient with slowly progressive metastatic disease and severe anaemia.

In advanced disease, the aim is to reduce androgen stimulation of the tumour to levels found in castrated men, with minimal adverse effects. Loss of libido, erectile dysfunction, breast tenderness, hot flushes and mood swings are common. All current approaches are palliative and include:

- Bilateral subcapsular orchidectomy is simple, cheap and effective but can have adverse psychological effects.
- Antiandrogens, e.g. cyproterone acetate 200–300 mg daily in divided doses, are first-line drugs despite the extra cost and risk of severe depression. More recently, flutamide has been used, with less risk of depression but with adverse cardiovascular effects similar to stilboestrol.
- LH releasing-hormone agonists, e.g. goserelin (monthly or 3 monthly subcutaneous injections). More expensive than anti-androgens and must be covered by anti-androgen (cyproterone or flutamide) during the first 1–2 weeks of treatment to reduce risk of 'disease flare'.

Drugs and the kidneys

In view of the changes to renal function that accompany old age, and the increased risk of AKI and CKD, it is essential to scrutinize every older patient's list of medications to review ongoing indication and dosage.

1 Nephrotoxic drugs:
  - Antibiotics, e.g. gentamicin, vancomycin and tetracycline.
  - Analgesics, e.g. NSAIDs and COX 2 inhibitors, disrupt the regulation of renal medullary blood flow and salt and water balance. This effect is exacerbated by diuretics and ACEi.
  - Disease-modifying anti-rheumatic drugs (DMARDs), e.g. penicillamine and gold.
2 Too high a dosage of drugs acting on kidneys, i.e. diuretics leading to dehydration, hypotension and electrolyte imbalance, to the extent of causing marked renal failure. Remember to reduce/omit diuretics when patients are admitted with hypotension and dehydration.
3 Drug toxicity due to accumulation secondary to reduced renal excretion, the best example is digoxin.
4 ACE inhibitors may precipitate renal failure if used in patients with silent renovascular disease.
5 Remember to check the BNF whenever prescribing for patients with AKI or CKD: it may be necessary to omit or reduce the dose of many medications including metformin, allopurinol, enoxaparin, ciprofloxacin, lithium and digoxin.

Blood pressure and the kidneys

1 Renal disease may cause hypertension, e.g. chronic interstitial nephritis.
2 The overtreatment of high blood pressure will impair renal function. Yet, untreated hypertension may result in renal failure!
3 About one-third of elderly patients with hypertension have impaired renal function.
4 Hypotension, e.g. after bleeding, myocardial infarction or pulmonary embolus, may result in renal shutdown and acute renal failure especially where renal function is already compromised by extreme old age or pathological changes.
5 Renal artery stenosis (RAS) may first present as a marked deterioration in renal function after treatment with an ACE inhibitor. However, ACEi are useful in other causes, but should be commenced at a low dose. Renal function and electrolytes should be checked regularly.

6 Bilateral renal artery stenosis can also present as 'flash' pulmonary oedema, which is thought to be due to the combination of the RAS and fluid overload plus diastolic ventricular dysfunction.

Haematuria

See Table 13.3.

Renal cell carcinoma

Risk factors

- Smoking, obesity (especially in women) and hypertension.
- Median age at diagnosis is 64 years.
- Up to 30% of cases are asymptomatic and discovered incidentally on scans done for other reasons.

Symptoms

- Haematuria (45%).
- Flank pain (40%).
- Weight loss.

Signs

- Flank mass, evidence of secondaries, e.g. lung, liver or bone metastases.
- Renal cell carcinoma is associated with a high incidence of paraneoplastic syndromes secondary to the release of cytokines such as IL6, erythropoietin and nitric oxide.

Investigations

- Calcium levels.
- Urine cytology.
- Ultrasound.
- CT scanning.
- Bone scintigraphy.

Treatment

- For fit older people with non-metastatic disease, nephrectomy may be curative. Some patients have very indolent disease and die with the renal cell carcinoma rather than of it. Bevacizumab and pazopanib have been appraised by NICE (2010) and may be used as first-line therapy for metastatic renal cell carcinoma, with sorafenib or sunitinib as potential second-line therapies.
- Other treatment options are radiotherapy for cord compression or bone metastases. Renal artery embolization can reduce severe haematuria.

Table 13.3 Causes, investigations and management of haematuria

Cause	Investigations	Management
Bleeding diathesis	Abnormal clotting, low platelet count, abnormal platelet function	Review need for anticoagulants, check liver function, clotting screen
Urosepsis, pyelonephritis	MSU, blood cultures, ultrasound	Antibiotics guided by MSU result, treat predisposing factors
Transitional cell carcinoma of the bladder	Cystoscopy	Transurethral resection of bladder tumour with regular review
Ureteric stones	Intravenous urogram (IVU), ultrasound	Extracorporeal shockwave lithotripsy, endoscopic removal, preventative measures
BPH	Rectal examination, bladder ultrasound	Alpha blockers, 5 alpha reductase inhibitors, TURP
Carcinoma of the prostate	Biopsy, PSA	Treat as appropriate
Intrinsic renal disease	Consider renal biopsy if appropriate	Treat as appropriate
Renal cell carcinoma	Ultrasound or CT abdomen, urine cytology	Nephrectomy for early disease, embolization for continuous haematuria
Contamination with vaginal blood	Obtain clean catch specimen, with catheter if necessary	See vaginal bleeding
Immune complex disease, e.g. bacterial endocarditis	Blood cultures, echocardiography (see Chapter 9)	Treat underlying condition

Bladder carcinoma

- Bladder cancer is the fourth most common cancer in the UK.
- Median age at diagnosis is 68 years.
- Transitional cell carcinoma (TCC) accounts for 90%, squamous cell 5% and adenocarcinoma only 2% of cases in the West. However, 75% of cases in the developing world are squamous cell carcinomas; this is thought to be due to infection with *Schistosoma haematobium*.
- TCC is four times more common in men than women. It may occur anywhere along the renal tract – renal pelvis, ureter, bladder or urethra.

Symptoms

Painless haematuria.

Signs

Often nothing abnormal to find on examination.

Investigations

- Urine cytology, cystoscopy for diagnosis, histology.

Treatment

- Transurethral bladder tumour resection (TURBT)
- Once tumour has breached muscle layer, cystectomy is the only cure.

Urinary incontinence

Urinary incontinence is defined as 'the complaint of any involuntary urinary leakage'.

- Incontinence affects 50% of older people in hospital and nursing homes and 35% of those living in the community.
- It is often concealed by the patient because of embarrassment.
- Only 25% of affected women consult a doctor, possibly because it is assumed that incontinence is normal with increasing age or that little can be done about it.
- It is twice as common in women as in men. This is because of the anatomy of the female urethra, and because low oestrogen levels lead to reduced mucosal cohesion of the urethra, making it patulous.

Complications

- Embarrassment leads to fear of going out, which leads to social isolation.
- Depression.
- Embarrassment may lead to avoiding sex.
- Huge burden on older people and their carers: both financial (pads and new mattresses are expensive) and increased workload (extra washing).
- The cost of incontinence in the USA in 1995 was £7 billion. It is estimated that the current annual cost to the NHS is £536 million with a further £207 million paid by affected individuals.
- Increased risk of institutionalization (second only to dementia).
- Skin irritation and maceration may lead to pressure sores (see Chapter 14).

Reversible causes

The mnemonic 'diappers' is helpful! See Table 13.4.

Table 13.4 Reversible causes, examination, investigations and management of urinary incontinence

Cause	Examination and investigations	Management
Delirium	MSU, CXR, FBC, U&Es, CRP	Treat underlying cause
Infection	MSU, CRP	Treat infection
Atrophic urethritis	Pelvic examination	Topical oestrogen in females
Pharmaceuticals: sedatives, caffeine, diuretics, doxasosin, antidepressants, alcohol	Drug and alcohol history	Use alternatives if possible, or try lower doses. Reduce intake of caffeine and alcohol
Psychiatric: secondary to dementia, behavioural problems	Assess mental state and cognition	Exclude treatable causes, toilet regularly, ensure toilets are well-signposted and consider red toilet seats
Excess urine production	Serum glucose, calcium	Treat diabetes, hypercalcaemia
Restricted mobility	Joint and neurological examination	Physiotherapy, walking aids, commode, disabled toilets
Stool impaction	Rectal examination	Adequate fluid intake, regular laxatives, may need suppositories or manual evacuation

Assessing urinary incontinence

1 Best practice is to ask the patient to keep a bladder diary for at least 3 days. This should record whether they are continent or incontinent throughout the day and night including the volumes of urine passed, document fluid intake, and any symptoms that might help to diagnose the type of incontinence, e.g. leaking urine whilst sneezing.

2 Take a full history to determine the likely type of urinary incontinence. If the patient is wet all the time, consider a urogenital fistula. The aim is to determine the likely type of incontinence. Don't forget to ask about haematuria, recurrent bladder pain, recurrent UTIs and faecal incontinence.

3 Examine the abdomen for a palpable bladder secondary to urinary retention. If the patient is obese, consider a bladder ultrasound or an 'in and out' catheter to exclude retention.

4 Rectal examination to assess prostate size in men, exclude faecal impaction and check integrity of anal sphincter.

5 Vaginal examination to exclude atrophic vaginitis and urethritis and to look for prolapse.

6 Neurological examination to exclude spinal cord problems.

7 MMSE to assess cognitive function especially where there is double incontinence.

8 Assess medications: are there alternatives to diuretics that would not produce large volumes of urine?

9 Current advice is that all women with stress or mixed incontinence should have a trial of 3 months of pelvic floor exercises. Ideally the first 6 weeks are supervised by a specialist physiotherapist.

10 Patient education; suggest the following:
   • Trial of reducing caffeine intake.
   • If the patient is obese, aim to lose $^1/_2$ stone.
   • Regular toileting.
   • Regulate fluid intake to around 1.5 L/day (greater volumes increase the risk of incontinence but concentrated urine is more irritant to the bladder lining, provoking incontinence).
   • Ensure patient is aware of self-help groups where appropriate.
   • Radar key (disabled toilet facilities).

11 All patients with incontinence should have urinalysis, and if this is positive, an MSU should be sent. UTIs should be treated according to sensitivity.

12 Referral to continence advisor if no improvement with simple measures.

13 Further investigations such as urodynamics, cystometry and cystoscopy are not indicated prior to conservative management but can be useful if surgery is planned and there are concerns regarding overactive bladder or bladder dysfunction.

Types of incontinence

1 **Stress incontinence:** involuntary leaking of urine associated with increased intra-abdominal pressure, e.g. when sneezing, coughing and exercising. Most common in multiparous women and those who have had pelvic surgery. In men the most common cause is sphincter damage after radical prostatectomy.
   • *Non-surgical treatments:* pelvic floor exercises remain the gold standard. They should be prescribed for the individual woman and supported by a therapist for the 6 weeks. The patient must be encouraged to continue with the exercises long term, or the benefit is lost. Some patients benefit from biofeedback techniques, so that they understand which muscles they should be contracting.
     o Ring pessaries are useful for women with significant vaginal prolapse who are not fit for or do not wish to have surgery.
     o Duloxetine is a serotonin-noradrenalin reuptake inhibitor, which works at the level of the spinal cord increasing urethral sphincter tone. It improves continence in 50% of women who take it, but nausea is a very common side-effect.
   • *Surgical procedures:* there are now two minimally invasive procedures available.
     o Collagen implant improves continence. Collagen is injected into the urethral sphincter via a cystoscope under local anaesthetic; the procedure needs to be repeated every 6–18 months.
     o Tension-free vaginal tape (TVT) can be used to raise the middle portion of the urethra and improve continence. This is done as a day case under local anaesthetic so it is cheap and recovery is fast.
       If this fails and the patient is fit enough, she can go on to have an open colpo-suspension to elevate the bladder neck, or an anterior repair for prolapse.

2 **Urge incontinence:** frequent and urgent passing of small amounts of urine, sometimes with so

little warning that the patient does not reach the toilet in time. This is due to detrusor instability. It increases with age and is associated with hyper-reflexia in neurological conditions such as stroke, multiple sclerosis and Parkinson's disease.

- *Drug treatments:* antimuscarinic anticholinergic agents such as oxybutynin and tolterodine. As oxybutynin is the cheapest, NICE (2006) suggests it should be used first line treatment. Solifenacin is said to be more specific to the bladder muscarinic receptors and therefore causes less dry mouth and confusion. Trospium does not cross the blood–brain barrier and is therefore even less likely to cause confusion. Patients should be warned about these side-effects and urinary retention.
- *Surgical devices:* the overactive bladder can be managed using sacral stimulation where other treatments have failed. A lightweight (50 g) device, e.g. InterStim, is implanted above the buttock and stimulates the third sacral nerve. It has achieved 1-year success rates approaching 85% for controlling urgency, urge incontinence and nocturia.
- *Botulism A:* can be injected into the detrusor muscle of those suffering from hyper-reflexic bladder, with good results.

3 **Mixed incontinence:** a combination of the symptoms of stress and urge incontinence, and probably the most common presentation in older people.

4 **Overflow incontinence:** most common in men with benign prostatic hypertrophy (BPH), but may also be secondary to prostatic carcinoma, constipation or urethral stricture. It is also associated with neurological deficits, e.g. diabetes. If the cause is BPH, treatments include α-blockers such as tamsulosin, or TURP.

5 **Nocturia and nocturnal enuresis:** there are usually multiple causes. Sensible solutions to start with are fluid restriction in the evenings and avoiding caffeine. BPH may respond to tamsulosin. Nocturia associated with urge incontinence may respond to solifenacin. Nocturia due to diabetes insipidus and PD can be treated with desmopressin if there is no heart failure. Patients with marked peripheral oedema are advised to lie on the bed for an hour in the afternoon to cause a diuresis prior to going to bed. Failing this, try a small dose of furosemide in the afternoon.

Management

> **Management strategies for irreversible incontinence**
>
> - Pad and pants.
> - Condom-type (Conveen) catheters for men, especially at night, but often fall off!
> - Intermittent self-catheterization.
> - Suprapubic or urethral catheter.
> - Catheter with valve.
> - Support groups for incontinence such as the National Association for Continence: www.nafc.org.

Catheters

Indications

- Acute urinary retention, or chronic retention with hydronephrosis causing impaired renal function.
- Bladder irrigation post surgery or clot retention.
- Preoperative abdominal or pelvic surgery.
- Monitoring urine output.
- Allowing healing of macerated sacral sores.
- Some patients with severe urinary incontinence prefer catheters.

Complications

- UTIs: catheters account for 86% of hospital acquired UTIs; more common in women, multiple catheterizations, longer duration of catheter, poor hygiene; reduce the risk by giving prophylactic antibiotics on insertion and using silver-coated catheters.
- Encrustation and blockage of the catheter tip, especially in presence of *Proteus mirabilis* infection; can lead to formation of bladder stones.
- Trauma to epithelium during insertion and removal especially if the catheter is pulled out with the balloon inflated by a confused patient.
- Development of urethral stricture, which might lead to obstructive uropathy.
- Urine bypassing catheter: try catheter with finer bore and an oral antispasmodic.
- Incontinence once the catheter has been removed: risk can be reduced by using a valve that maintains bladder tone and gives the patient control of emptying the bladder.

- Use of a female (short) catheter in a man in error causes severe trauma if the balloon is inflated.

Vaginal bleeding

Bleeding from the genital tract long after the menopause must always be taken seriously, because there are pre-malignant or malignant as well as benign causes. The patient may present with stained underwear or bed sheets. If she is also incontinent of urine or has an anal lesion, the source of the loss may be unclear. Physical examination should locate the site. The heavier the bleeding, the more likely the cause is to be malignant.

Ask especially about hormone treatment for cancer or hormone-replacement therapy, also trauma (including abuse). Even very old women can be subject to this, either from coitus or a foreign body in the vagina. Once sure that you are not dealing with haematuria or rectal bleeding refer to gynaecology for further investigation.

Causes of post-menopausal bleeding are:

- Atrophic vaginitis, which will respond to topical oestrogen cream.
- Hormone replacement therapy: assess risk versus benefit for the individual.
- Ulceration from prolapse or foreign body, e.g. ring pessary.
- Endometrial hyperplasia, which may be premalignant.
- Benign tumours, such as cervical or endometrial polyps.
- Cancer of the genital tract, involving vulva, vagina, cervix or endometrium. Endometrial cancer is managed aggressively with total abdominal hysterectomy and bilateral salpingo-oophorectomy in fit patients.

Vaginal prolapse

- Risk factors include trauma secondary to childbirth, striated muscle weakness and neuromuscular disease.
- Cystocoele: the bladder bulges through the anterior vaginal wall. This can be associated with stress incontinence, but a large cystocole can impair bladder emptying.

- Rectocoele: bulging of the posterior vaginal wall by the rectum, which can impair defecation. Some women use a finger to push against the posterior vaginal wall to aid emptying.
- Conservative management consists of topical oestrogen, pelvic floor exercises and pessaries. Ring or shelf pessaries placed high within the vagina hold the uterus in place. They need to be changed 3–6 monthly and may cause vaginal discharge (especially if forgotten!).
- Surgery, e.g. anterior or posterior repair for selected fit elderly women.

Disease of the vulva

Scrupulous hygiene continues to be important in older age; avoiding soap and perfumed products and wearing cotton underwear reduce the risk of many common conditions and infections of the vulva. The most common symptoms are pruritus, discharge and pain, or a lump may have been noted by the patient or their carer.

Ask about co-morbidities including diabetes, atopy, skin conditions including psoriasis, urinary and faecal incontinence.

- The most common cause of vulval itch and discharge in older women is *Candidiasis*, which responds to topical 1% clotrimazole ointment or a single dose 500 mg pessary.
- For cases of itch with no discharge, rule out diabetes, jaundice and uraemia.
- Allergic dermatitis responds well to topical steroids. Don't forget to avoid precipitants such as detergents or highly perfumed soaps.
- Lichen sclerosus et atrophicus is an autoimmune condition which affects older women. Initially the vulval skin is red, but with time the skin appears thin and wrinkled and white shiny plaques may develop. A biopsy is required to confirm the diagnosis, as it may be premalignant in 4% of cases. Treatment is with topical 2% testosterone.
- Carcinoma of the vulva in older age is usually squamous cell. Early disease can be managed surgically with radiotherapy to the inguinal nodes. Invasive disease confers a very poor prognosis.
- If the vulva looks beefy red, this may be Paget's disease; as in the breast, this is adenocarcinoma in situ.

Sex in old age

Many people continue to enjoy a sexual relationship until the end of life. However, others stop having sex for a variety of reasons:

- Decline in sex drive.
- Erectile dysfunction affects 15–25% of men by the age of 65. It is more common in men suffering from diabetes, hypertension and renal disease, but stress, anxiety and depression play an important part. Drugs such as β-blockers, alcohol and luteinizing hormone-releasing hormone (LHRH) agonists are also culprits. Premature ejaculation is less common.
- Longer time to arousal.
- Longer time to orgasm.
- Reduced genital sensitivity.
- Loss of lubrication in women secondary to reduced oestrogen.
- Reduced satisfaction.
- Reduced mobility, e.g. from arthritic hips, previous stroke.
- Anxiety about provoking myocardial or cerebrovascular events. However, the evidence suggests that sex with a familiar partner is unlikely to precipitate a fatal event.
- Low mood.
- Disinhibition in one partner secondary to dementia may be off-putting to the other partner.
- Loss of partner.
- Moving to a residential home with reduced privacy.

Advice for maintaining a healthy sex life in later life

- 'Use it or lose it.'
- Plenty of exercise to keep physically fit.
- Try different positions to find the most comfortable to allow for arthritic joints.
- Stop smoking.
- Avoid excess alcohol.
- Use artificial lubricants.
- Consider phosphodiesterase type 5 (PDE5) inhibitors, e.g. sildenafil or tadalafil, to achieve erection. (Use is contraindicated in patients taking nitrates or who have a history of recent myocardial infarction or stroke.)

- Consider intermittent self-catheterization or a suprapubic rather than urethral catheter for incontinence.
- Sex does not have to be penetrative; other physical contact can also be pleasurable and satisfying.
- Seek help early for difficulties.

 REFERENCES

NICE (2006) *CG40. Urinary Incontinence: The Management of Urinary Incontinence in Women.* http://www.nice.org.uk/nicemedia/pdf/word/CG40quickrefguide1006.pdf.

NICE (2010) *TA219. Everolimus for the Second-line Treatment of Advanced Renal Cell Carcinoma.* http://www.nice.org.uk/guidance/TA219.

→ FURTHER INFORMATION

Dawson C, Whitfield H (2006) *ABC of Urology.* BMJ Books, London.

Department of Health (2005) *The National Service Framework for Renal Services – Part Two: Chronic Kidney Disease, Acute Renal Failure and End of Life Care.* DH, London.

Dwinnell BG, Anderson RJ (undated) *Diagnostic Evaluation of the Patient with Acute Renal Failure,* Chapter 12. http://www.kidneyatlas.org/book1/adk1_12.pdf.

Kessel B (2001) Sexuality in the older person. *Age and Ageing* 30: 121–124.

Kidney Alliance Patient Association: www.kidneyalliance.org/docs/twoone.htm.

Naikar SS, Liu KD, Chertow GM (2007) The incidence and prognostic significance of acute kidney injury. *Current Opinion in Nephrology and Hypertension* 16: 227–236.

National Association for Continence: www.nafc.org.

National Confidential Enquiry into Patient Outcome and Death: Adding Insult to Injury? http://www.ncepod.org.uk/2009aki.htm.

Royal Association for Disability and Rehabilitation: www.radar.org.uk.

SIGN Guidelines for the Diagnosis and Management of CKD: http://www.sign.ac.uk/guidelines/fulltext/103/index.html.

The UK eCKD Guide: www.renal.org/whatwedo/InformationResources/CKDeGUIDE.aspx.

Wilt TJ, Thompson IM (2006) Clinically localised prostate cancer. *BMJ* 333: 1102–1106.

14

Blood and bone marrow

Normal elderly people have normal peripheral blood films. However, abnormalities increase with increasing age. Presentations such as anaemia or polycythaemia need to be explored and corrected if possible. Haematological diseases in old age are important because they:

1 are common;
2 aggravate other pathologies/symptoms, e.g. breathlessness, dizziness, confusion;
3 are often treatable.

Age changes

The following facts are given because they are interesting, but they are of more theoretical than practical importance.

Red blood cells

There is evidence of reduced deformability in health and this is even more marked in those with cerebrovascular disease.

White blood cells

1 More marked granulation (probably due to lysosymes) and lobulation of granulocytes.
2 Tendency towards leucopenia, with a normal leucocyte count in the range of 3.0–8.5×10^9/L in old age.
3 The lymph nodes and the lymphoid tissue of the GI tract and spleen are much reduced. The thymus is atrophied by middle age, but thymic remnants are thought to remain active into extreme old age.

4 The B-cell population is well maintained, but there is a reduction in T-cell numbers and function.
5 Some impairment of phagocytosis by neutrophils and macrophages has been reported.

Plasma proteins

Conflicting reports on age changes relate to the difficulty in distinguishing those changes solely to age from those due to other factors, such as malnutrition or disease. The main points to emerge are as follows:

1 Low levels of total protein and of the individual fractions are pathological.
2 Increased globulin fractions indicate disease; however, asymptomatic individuals with very high levels of gamma globulins may have monoclonal gammopathy of unknown significance (MGUS) rather than myeloma.
3 Abnormal immunoglobulins are increasingly common with age; present in about 3% of those aged > 70 years and 20% aged over 90.
4 Auto-antibodies are more prevalent with ageing and the female preponderance is lost.

Anaemia

- Estimates of the prevalence of anaemia vary dramatically.
- Prevalence in over 70s in the community is 15%; 24% in nursing homes.
- People with anaemia have a higher mortality, greater risk of hospitalization, poorer mobility

Lecture Notes Elderly Care Medicine, Eighth Edition. Claire G. Nicholl and K. Jane Wilson.
© 2012 John Wiley & Sons, Ltd. Published 2012 by John Wiley & Sons, Ltd.

and functional abilities and a higher risk of falls compared with those who do not.

Haemopoiesis and ageing

1 There is a gradual loss of active haemopoietic tissue initially in the long bones and later in the flat bones; vertebral marrow persists.
2 In health, the cellular composition of the residual haemopoietic tissue is normal. However, the response to stress such as haemorrhage and hypoxia is reduced.

Basic investigations

Anaemia is the most common abnormality and the red cell size (mean corpuscular volume, MCV) and morphology often suggest the aetiology (Figure 14.1). Always request a peripheral blood film; it is inexpensive and easy and will often lead you directly to the cause. White cell morphology will also be helpful, especially in myeloproliferative disorders.

Measurement of the acute-phase response is also useful. ESR is the cheapest investigation but it reflects changes slowly (i.e. days). CRP is better for monitoring more rapid changes (i.e. hours). A protein electrophoretic strip is needed to diagnose myeloma.

Clinical history and examination

The symptoms of anaemia, i.e. tiredness, breathlessness and general malaise, are too common and non-specific to be of great value. Anaemia may exacerbate symptoms due to other pathologies, e.g. angina, heart failure, intermittent claudication, increased confusion in dementia, and falls may occur more frequently. The patient's symptoms may therefore be greater than expected from the haematological abnormality.

The history may suggest the cause. Ask about previous surgery and transfusions, family history (pernicious anaemia), medication and dietary change, weight loss, GI symptoms and blood loss. Physical examination may not be helpful, but look for pallor, jaundice, lymphadenopathy, abdominal organomegaly, rectal masses and neurological abnormalities, as these may direct you to the correct diagnosis.

Two important final points: remember that anaemia is a sign of disease and is not a diagnosis and that there are often multiple causes in each patient.

Types and causes of anaemia

The WHO definition of anaemia is haemoglobin of less than 13 g/dL in males or less than 12 g/dL in

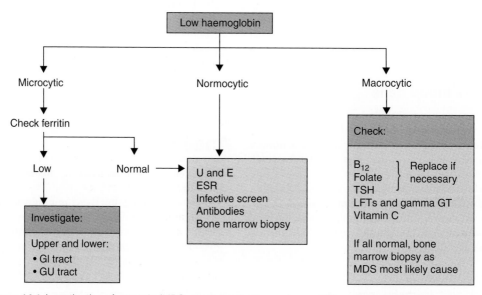

Figure 14.1 Investigation of anaemia (MDS, myelodysplastic syndrome; GU, genitourinary tract).

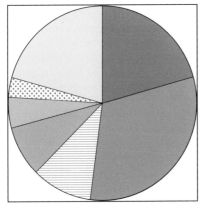

Iron deficiency
Chronic disease
B₁₂/folate deficiency
CKD
Myelodysplasias
Hypothyroidism
Unknown

Figure 14.2 Causes of anaemia in older people.

females. The validity of this definition in older people is often disputed, but it improves the pick-up rate of disease.

The main categories (see Figure 14.2) are:

1 Red cell/haemoglobin loss:
  • Due to bleeding.
  • Due to cell destruction (haemolysis).
2 Impaired red cell/haemoglobin production:
  • Deficiency states.
  • Marrow dysfunction.
  • Anaemia of chronic disease.

Iron-deficiency anaemia (microcytic)

Iron-deficiency anaemia, the most common cause of microcytic (low MCV) anaemia, affects 2–5% of the older population.

Aetiology

1 Iron-deficiency anaemia is usually due to chronic blood loss, especially from the GI tract and, less often, from the genitourinary tract or elsewhere.
2 Defective absorption may be a contributory (but rarely the sole) factor. Causes include achlorhydria secondary to chronic gastritis, previous gastrectomy or small-bowel disease. Look for clinical or biochemical evidence of malabsorption, such as steatorrhoea, osteomalacia, folate and vitamin B deficiencies.

3 Inadequate intake may stem from inability to shop or prepare meals as a result of physical or mental disorder or from poverty.

History

1 Symptoms may be non-specific.
2 Ask specifically about weight loss, problems swallowing, indigestion, change in bowel habit, black tarry stool, blood in the urine, haemoptysis and postmenopausal bleeding. Do not forget to ask about alcohol intake.
3 Restless legs syndrome is sometimes secondary to iron deficiency.
4 Past medical history: peptic ulcer disease, gastrectomy, diverticular disease, bowel resection for carcinoma.
5 Document all drugs including OTC medications especially aspirin, ibuprofen and Rennies.

Examination

See also Chapter 11 for full gastrointestinal examination.

• General: pallor, lymphadenopathy or jaundice.
• Tachycardia, hypotension, murmurs if there is volume loss from bleeding.
• Mouth: stomatitis, telangiectasia around the mouth and palate.
• Hands: koilonychia (spoon-shaped nails associated with iron deficiency).
• Abdomen: epigastric tenderness, masses, scars from previous surgery, hepatomegaly or splenomegaly.

- Examine the rectum for masses and exclude melaena.

Investigations

- Peripheral blood film: the red cells are small, hypochromic and vary in size (anisocytosis) and shape (poikilocytosis). There may also be pencil cells and target cells.
- Red cell distribution width (RDW) may increase reflecting greater variability in the size of red blood cells. Remember that if there is also B_{12} or folate deficiency, the red cells may not be microcytic.
- A low serum ferritin is good evidence of iron deficiency. However, it is an acute-phase protein and may be falsely elevated in the context of inflammation, in which case CRP will also be high.
- A raised reticulocyte count implies bleeding or haemolysis with appropriate increased bone marrow activity.
- As 10–15% of patients have both upper and lower GI causes of anaemia, most patients need both an oesophago gastro duodenoscopy (OGD) with duodenal biopsies and at least a CT abdomen with contrast (see Chapter 11).

Treatment

- Oral iron should be continued for 3 months to replenish the iron stores; it is sufficient to prescribe ferrous sulphate 200 mg twice daily, as more than this may not be absorbed and increases side-effects such as constipation or diarrhoea. Warn the patient that their stools will become black and gritty. Encourage the patient not to chew the tablets or their teeth or dentures may become stained.
- If the response to oral iron treatment is not satisfactory (i.e. 2 g/dL after 2 months), check the patient is taking the tablets and that any bleeding has stopped. Also consider additional diagnoses that may explain the problem, such as co-existent anaemia of chronic disease. Consider giving ascorbic acid to increase absorption.

Blood transfusion
- Blood transfusion is needed after acute haemorrhage, commonly a GI bleed. If there has been volume loss, there is no need to give furosemide to prevent overload.
- Injuries such as scalp lacerations, large haematomas and hip and pelvic fractures may cause substantial blood loss (especially in those taking warfarin) which may not be obvious. Watch for a drop in haemoglobin and transfuse if symptomatic or the Hb drops below 8.
- Patients with acute anaemia who are not shocked need full investigation but emergency transfusion is not needed – transfuse in the day which is less disruptive and safer.
- Patients with chronic anaemia may benefit from transfusion. The usual cutoff is below 8 g/dL, but the threshold may be higher if the patient has symptoms such as angina. Usually, 2 units are sufficient; oral or IV furosemide is usually needed.
- In conditions like myelodysplastic syndrome, regular transfusions can be done in day care facilities.

Haemolytic anaemia

- Haemolysis is the premature destruction of red blood cells. When the bone marrow can no longer match the rate of haemolysis, the patient becomes anaemic.
- Haemolytic anaemias are rare in old age and therefore in danger of being overlooked, especially as the peripheral blood film may not show any specific features.
- Autoimmune haemolytic anaemias are more common in older age as part of an autoimmune illness (e.g. SLE), due to antibody production secondary to infection (hot and cold antibodies following a viral infection) or as an iatrogenic disease (e.g. methyldopa treatment).
- Patients with hypersplenism may also have a haemolytic element to their anaemia.
- Most patients with metal heart valves have minor haemolysis.
- Relevant investigations are those indicating increased red cell destruction, i.e. raised bilirubin level, lactate dehydrogenase, raised reticulocyte count (raising the MCV), haptoglobins and direct antibody test (Coombs' test).
- Supportive management includes stopping culprit drugs, replacing folate and transfusions only for severe cases.

Deficiency states causing macrocytosis

The macrocytic (high MCV) anaemias are usually secondary to deficiency of folic acid, vitamin B_{12} or, more rarely, thyroxine. They are much less common than anaemia due to iron deficiency or chronic disease. The bone marrow precursors are

Table 14.1 **Causes of macrocytosis**

Folate deficiency
B_{12} deficiency
Alcohol excess
Hypothyroidism
Myelodysplastic syndromes
Liver disease
All causes of reticulocytosis
Drugs:
- Folic acid antagonists (methotrexate, phenytoin)
- Purine synthesis antagonists (6-mercaptopurine)
- Pyrimidine antagonists (cytosine arabinoside)

Spuriously raised MCV – cold agglutinins, paraproteins

megaloblastic in B_{12} and folate deficiency and drug toxicity (as DNA replication is affected). In other macrocytic anaemias the marrow is normoblastic. See Table 14.1 showing causes of macrocytosis.

Vitamin B_{12} deficiency

- Pernicious anaemia (PA) is the cause of B_{12} deficiency in 80% of cases in the UK.
- Other causes are gastrectomy, bacterial colonization of intestinal strictures or diverticula and disorders of the terminal ileum, especially Crohn's disease.
- Only strict vegans are likely to suffer from dietary vitamin B_{12} deficiency.
- B_{12} stores last for several years, hence the lag between a pathology affecting B_{12} absorption and clinical manifestations.

Pernicious anaemia

- PA develops insidiously due to autoimmune gastric atrophy and failure of intrinsic factor secretion.
- The incidence is said to be 1:10,000 with a female preponderance.
- Cancer of the stomach occurs in about 10% of cases.
- Other complications are peripheral neuropathy, subacute combined (corticospinal and dorsal column) degeneration of the spinal cord so with the neuropathy there are UMN and LMN signs. There may be cognitive impairment.
- These features may predate the haematological changes and continue if folate is given when B_{12} is low.
- There may be a family history of other autoimmune conditions such as Hashimoto's thyroiditis, vitiligo and Addison's disease.

Clinical features

- Symptoms and signs of anaemia, with lemon tinge to skin (jaundice secondary to mild haemolysis).
- Glossitis, anorexia and weight loss.
- In severe cases, hepatosplenomegaly and heart failure.
- Neurological signs.

Diagnosis

1 The blood film contains large oval red cells and occasionally hypersegmented neutrophils. The reticulocyte count is reduced (they are abnormally fragile). Platelets may be low.
2 The bone marrow is megaloblastic.
3 Serum B_{12} is low.
4 Serum autoantibodies are positive to gastric parietal cells in 90% of cases, to intrinsic factor in 60% and to thyroid in 40%.
5 The Schilling test would confirm that vitamin B_{12} can only be absorbed when given with intrinsic factor but is rarely done (involves 24 h collection of radioactive urine and the outcome does not affect treatment).

Treatment of vitamin B_{12} deficiency

1 Hydroxocobalamin 1 mg intramuscularly three times a week for 2 weeks, to replenish body stores and thereafter 1 mg every 3 months for life.
2 There is often associated iron deficiency, necessitating a course of oral iron.
3 Blood transfusion is generally not indicated.

Folate deficiency

Folate deficiency is much more common than vitamin B_{12} deficiency and is usually due to poor diet, with or without malabsorption, e.g. due to coeliac disease. Other factors are increased demand, e.g. in lymphoma, infection and haemolysis. Anticonvulsant drugs and chronic alcoholism cause low levels by increasing the hepatic metabolism of folate. The body only stores sufficient folate for 6 months or so.

Clinical features

The clinical features include:

1 Irritability, depression, confusion and occasionally dementia.
2 Peripheral neuropathy and subacute combined degeneration of the cord (as with PA) in more severe cases.

Diagnosis

- The peripheral blood and marrow picture is identical to that of vitamin B_{12} deficiency.
- Red cell folate is low. Folic acid absorption tests are not used routinely.

Treatment

1 Lifestyle advice to improve diet, reduce alcohol abuse; stop offending drugs, when practicable.
2 Oral folic acid tablets for a few months to replenish stores, and then stop; long-term use may mask a developing PA.
3 Do not give folic acid until vitamin B_{12} deficiency excluded; otherwise there is a risk of precipitating subacute combined degeneration of the cord. If in doubt, give both vitamins concurrently; the patient may need iron also.
4 Prophylactic use in malabsorption states and in epileptics on anticonvulsants may be justified.

Hypothyroidism

The macrocytic normoblastic anaemia, which occurs in over 50% of cases in myxoedema, is usually mild, never megaloblastic and responds slowly to levothyroxine replacement. It is thought to be caused by reduced renal erythropoietin production in response to the lower oxygen demand of the lower basal metabolic rate. Co-existing iron deficiency will require replacement. About 10% of patients also have autoimmune PA.

Scurvy

The macrocytic normoblastic anaemia of scurvy is commonly associated with other nutritional deficiencies. Ascorbic acid is necessary for the reduction of folate into its active metabolite. Clinical signs include bleeding gums (if the patient has teeth), vascular purpura secondary to fragile blood vessels, and occasionally blood loss can be severe. Vitamin C replacement, followed by a balanced diet, is curative.

Marrow dysfunction

The peripheral red cells are normally normochromic and normocytic but may on occasion be macrocytic. The underlying fault may be inherent in the marrow itself, and examination of the marrow is needed for diagnosis as either an aspirate or a trephine.

Myelodysplastic syndromes (MDS)

This is a group of clonal haemopoietic disorders (now considered as blood cancers). Often a single mutant stem cell will multiply suppressing the production of other cell lines. Any of the three cell lines can be affected.

- Incidence of MDS increases with age; most common in males over 80.
- Most are spontaneous, a few occur after chemotherapy or radiotherapy.
- Twenty-five percent are discovered incidentally on blood film requested for another reason.
- Fifty-five percent of cases present as a refractory macrocytic anaemia (MCV > 100).
- Twenty percent present with neutropenia (sepsis) or thrombocytopenia (bruising, epistaxis, bleeding gums).
- Ten percent have splenomegaly.
- The blood film may show a single cytopenia or, as the disease progresses, a pancytopenia. There may also be giant platelets and juvenile neutrophils.
- The marrow is hypercellular due to stem-cell hyperplasia but poor haemopoiesis.
- The clinical course is very variable. Mean survival from diagnosis is 2 years; some cases are indolent, others are aggressive with early transformation into acute myelocytic leukaemia (AML) or the patient may succumb to infection secondary to poor white cell function.
- Most cases are managed with repeated blood transfusions (consider desferioxamine to prevent iron overload).
- In view of toxicity, only fit older people are considered for chemotherapy. NICE has approved azacitidine which slows progression to AML in high grade MDS.

Aplastic anaemia

Aplastic anaemia is a rare, potentially life-threatening failure of haemopoiesis characterized by pancytopenia and hypocellular bone marrow. At least two of the following are needed for diagnosis:

Haemoglobin $< 10\,g/dL$
Platelet count $< 50 \times 10^9/L$
Neutrophil count $<1.5 \times 10^9/L$

- Most cases are idiopathic.
- Known causes are drugs (NSAIDs, antibiotics, thiazides and cytotoxic drugs), radiotherapy, toxins (benzene) and viral infections.

- Treatment is supportive with blood and platelet transfusions, and antibiotics for infection. More aggressive therapies include cyclosporin A, antithymocyte globulin, high-dose methyl prednisolone and bone marrow transplantation, but these are often not appropriate in older people if there is frailty or co-morbidity.

Leucoerythroblastic anaemia

This is an anaemia with immature red and white cells in the peripheral blood. The marrow examination may reveal the malignant cells that have infiltrated and impaired function.

Anaemia of chronic disease

This is usually a normochromic normocytic anaemia and does not respond to haematinics. It may be improved by treatment of the underlying condition.

- Seventy-five percent of cases are associated with malignancy; the remaining cases are associated with infection or inflammation such as rheumatoid arthritis.
- Ferritin is normal or high.
- There are increased levels of iron in the reticulo-endothelial system.
- The underlying problem seems to be defective iron transfer to red cell precursors.
- Anaemia of chronic disease can be differentiated from iron deficiency anaemia by measuring the number of transferrin receptors. They are upregulated in anaemia of chronic disease, but normal in iron-deficiency anaemia. This assay is expensive and not yet widely used.

Mixed picture anaemias

In clinical practice, many anaemias have several causes with features of deficiencies, blood loss, haemolysis and marrow dysfunction. The blood picture will only improve if the underlying conditions can be alleviated. The most common examples are discussed below.

Rheumatoid arthritis

In addition to 'anaemia of chronic disease', look for blood loss (NSAIDs), low folate due to poor nutrition and increased utilization and B_{12} deficiency (autoimmune). Complications of rheumatoid disease, such as vasculitis or amyloidosis, increase the severity and complexity of the anaemia.

Malignant disease

Usually there are a number of causes: anorexia, blood loss, anaemia of chronic disease, malabsorption and/or haemolysis. Additionally, there may be marrow infiltration, with development of leuco-erythroblastic anaemia.

Chronic kidney disease

The anaemia in renal disease may be related to the underlying cause, e.g. myeloma or SLE. It is also associated with reduced production of erythropoietin. Biologically fit elderly patients with chronic kidney disease and anaemia are offered subcutaneous recombinant erythropoietin or darbepoetin once any iron deficiency is corrected.

Alcohol abuse

This can contribute to anaemia via several mechanisms:

- Bleeding from oesophagitis, gastric or duodenal ulceration, or varices.
- Anorexia.
- Dietary deficiency of folate.
- Direct effect of alcohol on the bowel, reducing absorption.
- Suppressed marrow function.
- Hypersplenism from chronic liver disease.
- Malabsorption from chronic pancreatitis.

Myeloproliferative disorders

These heterogeneous malignant conditions are due to uncontrolled proliferation of marrow cells. The predominant cells produced and speed of progression define the disease and diagnosis is made on the appearance of the blood film and bone marrow. A cytoplasmic enzyme of the tyrosine kinase group, Janus Kinase 2 (JAK2), plays a central role in initiating signal transduction from the erythropoietin receptor. In most patients with polycythaemia vera (PV) the receptor is activated all the time due to lack of auto-inhibition caused by an abnormal JAK2 enzyme (the V617F mutation which results in valine being substituted by phenylalanine). This is also found in half of cases of essential thrombocytosis and myelofibrosis.

The leukaemias are considered separately.

Polycythaemia (rubra) vera

Abnormal clonal red cells suppress normal stem cell growth and maturation.

- Peak incidence is 50–70 years old.
- Symptoms include:
  - Hyperviscosity leading to headache, dizziness, vertigo, tinnitus, visual disturbance, angina and claudication.
  - Pruritus secondary to release of histamine, especially after a hot bath.
  - Gout from increased cell turnover.
- On examination: facial plethora, 70% have splenomegaly and 50% have hepatomegaly.
- Treatment: venesection to reduce hyperviscosity, or hydroxycarbamide which is well tolerated.

Essential thrombocytosis

This results in uncontrolled production of platelets, splenomegaly and episodes of thrombosis and haemorrhage.

Myelofibrosis

This is a cause of massive splenomegaly. The patient may complain of abdominal pain or shoulder tip pain. Other symptoms include weight loss, fatigue secondary to anaemia and frequent infections secondary to white cell dysfunction.

Leukaemias

Leukaemias are a group of cancers of the blood-forming cells in the bone marrow. There are four broad categories: myeloid or lymphocytic, and acute or chronic. Overall 5-year survivals are:

- CML (chronic myeloid leukaemia) 55%,
- CLL (chronic lymphocytic leukaemia) 80%,
- AML (acute myeloid leukaemia) 10%,
- ALL (acute lymphoblastic leukaemia) 66% (better in children).

Diagnosis and active treatment require specialist haematology.

Acute myeloid leukaemia (AML)

- This is a disease of the elderly with the maximum incidence at 80–84 years.
- The development of the haemopoietic precursors is arrested at an immature stage. In AML, the bone marrow contains at least 20% blasts.
- Normal maturation of all cell lines is affected, leading to anaemia, thrombocytopenia and neutropenia.
- The patient may present with symptoms and signs of any of the above.
- More common in the Western world.
- More common in men as the most common risk factor is transformation of MDS.
- Also evolves from other blood disorders including aplastic anaemia and PV.
- AML is aggressive and most elderly patients are best managed with good supportive care including blood and platelet transfusions and antibiotics as necessary.
- A small minority of patients have a good response to daunorubicin and cytarabine, and newer agents such as azacitidine.

Acute lymphoblastic leukaemia (ALL)

ALL is thought of as a disease of childhood, but it has a bimodal age distribution and the highest incidence in adults is in the over 75s.

- Prognosis is usually very poor.
- B-cell and, more rarely, T-cell types.
- The Philadelphia chromosome (see below) occurs in about 20% of adult cases.
- Treatment of ALL combines prolonged chemotherapy (remission induction, consolidation and maintenance) and supportive measures.

Chronic lymphatic leukaemia (CLL)

- Caused by clonal expansion of immature B cells which resemble normal lymphocytes but are functionally incompetent with an abnormally long survival because of suppression of apoptosis.
- Unknown aetiology but evidence of a genetic element; it arises at a younger age in successive generations of some families.
- Accounts for 25% of all haematological malignancies.
- Affects older people; the incidence is 50/100,000 per year in the population aged over 70, and this increases with increasing age.
- Thirty percent of cases are detected incidentally on a blood film, e.g. pre-operative assessment.
- It does not require treatment if asymptomatic.
- May convert to an acute disorder; any intervention should be in conjunction with a haematologist.

Clinical features

- Superficial symmetrical cervical lymphadeno-pathy.
- Anaemia.
- Splenomegaly in 40% of cases.
- Hepatomegaly in 15%.
- Purpura and bruising secondary to low platelet count.
- Often presents as pruritus.
- Occasionally presents with florid herpes zoster.

Diagnosis

- The blood film contains multiple small lympho-cytes, sometimes $\geq 300 \times 10^9$ lymphocytes/L and occasional smear cells.
- There may be a normocytic normochromic or autoimmune haemolytic anaemia.
- Bone marrow aspirate shows replacement of the normal marrow with lymphocytes.

Treatment

Many elderly people have a benign form of the disease, which requires no treatment, and survive for up to 10 years. The mainstay of treatment of those with more aggressive disease is steroids plus alkylating agents such as chlorambucil. Rituximab is also used. Survival in these cases is usually 3–5 years.

Chronic myeloid leukaemia (CML)

CML is less common than CLL. It is of interest because it is the best worked out genetically: the translocation of genes from the long arm of chromosome 9 to chromosome 22 creates the Philadelphia chromosome and this produces the BCR-ABL fusion gene. This in turn produces an abnormal tyrosine kinase which triggers uncontrolled cell growth.

- Incidence is 1–1.5/100,000 per year.
- Affects people of all ages, mean range 40–50 years, but increasingly common with increasing age.
- Slightly more common in men than women.

Clinical features

- Bone marrow failure.
- Hypermetabolism (weight loss, anorexia and night sweats).
- Splenomegaly may be massive.

- More rarely, leucostasis causing priapism, visual impairment and hyperuricaemia.

Investigations

- Leucocytosis, 50–200 × 10^9/L, with the full spectrum of myeloid cells seen in the peripheral blood film.
- Bone marrow is hypercellular with granulocytes.
- Philadelphia chromosome may be detected in the peripheral blood or bone marrow.
- Normochromic normocytic anaemia.
- Platelet count often elevated, but may be normal or low.
- Raised uric acid.

Progression and treatment

Usually the disease remains in the chronic phase for 3–5 years. If it is not treated, it will progress to the acute blast phase. When the disease enters its acute phase, deterioration may be rapid, with median survival being 3–6 months.

Philadelphia positive CML can be treated in the chronic phase with imatinib which is a BCR-ABL inhibitor.

Myeloma

Myeloma is the abnormal monoclonal proliferation of plasma cells (the specialist B cells that make antibodies). Usually a large amount of just one antibody is made; this is known as a paraprotein. Usually more light chains than heavy chains are produced. Free light chains in the urine are known as Bence–Jones protein. Myeloma accounts for 10% of haematological malignancies. It is more common in men than women and in black populations more than white. It is a disease of older age, the mean age of onset being over 70 years.

The aetiology is unknown, but possibilities include toxins and the human herpes virus HH8. There may be a genetic component as it occurs in family clusters.

Clinical syndromes

Common
- Malaise secondary to anaemia.
- Bone pain and pathological fractures in 70% of cases in some series.

- Recurrent infections secondary to immuno-paresis and neutropenia.
- Renal failure due to deposition of immune complexes, or the development of amyloid (the building block of the amyloid in myeloma is over-produced light chain). Renal function can also deteriorate secondary to hyperuricaemia.
- Bleeding secondary to abnormal platelet function.

Less common
- Confusion secondary to hypercalcaemia.
- Rarely, hyperviscosity syndromes, amyloidosis or cord compression.

Investigations

- Normochromic normocytic anaemia.
- Red cell rouleaux.
- Thrombocytopenia.
- Raised ESR greater than 100.
- Increased plasma viscosity.
- The bone marrow contains greater than 10% plasma cells.
- Hypercalcaemia.
- Abnormal monoclonal plasma-protein band, usually IgG seen on plasma electrophoresis.
- Bence–Jones proteins in the urine.
- Lytic bone lesions on skeletal survey are caused by overexpression of receptor activator of nuclear factor kappa-B ligand (RANKL) leading to increased osteoclast activity.

Treatment

This depends on how the patient presents:

- Careful fluid balance for renal failure, and dialysis in selected cases.
- Fluids and bisphosphonates for hypercalcaemia. Some studies show that patients treated with bisphosphonates do better in the long term.
- Radiotherapy for bone pain and cord compression.
- Analgesics, opioids often needed.
- Treat infections, usually bacterial respiratory infections.
- It is important to assess the patient carefully before commencing chemotherapy: consider aggressive treatment with a view to bone marrow transplant in younger and fitter patients.
- If chemotherapy is deemed appropriate, the mainstay is melphalan, usually given with prednisolone. Myeloma usually responds to this but then relapses again. Thalidomide is being used with some success. Lenalidomide, which is structurally similar, is giving encouraging results. However, even with treatment the mean survival is still only 4 years.

Monoclonal gammopathy of unknown significance (MGUS)

Sometimes a paraprotein is found in the serum but there is no definite evidence of myeloma; no bone lesions and no Bence–Jones proteins in the urine.

Some of these patients, but not all, will eventually develop full myeloma.

Lymphoma

There are two main types of lymphoma:

1 **Hodgkin's disease.** This mainly affects adolescents and people in their 30s (mean 25 years), but there is a second peak in 80 year olds. Reed–Sternberg cells are pathognomonic of Hodgkin's disease; they are multinucleated giant cells found in the peripheral blood. The clinical features include lymphadenopathy which is typically localized and above the diaphragm. It may be accompanied by constitutional symptoms such as fever and weight loss.
2 **Non-Hodgkin's lymphoma.** The incidence increases with increasing age from 50, peaking at 80 years. Any lymphoid tissue may be affected (up to 20% of cases arise in the GI tract, bone, liver or CNS). Symptoms include general malaise, pyrexia of unknown origin, night sweats, pruritus and weight loss. Hepatosplenomegaly is more common in NHL. general malaise, pyrexia of unknown origin, night sweats, pruritus and weight loss. Compression of neighbouring structures may also lead to symptoms e.g. superior vena caval obstruciton. Cerebral lymphoma presents with subacute progression of confusion or other neurological symptoms such as dizziness. It is more common in immunosuppressed patients.

Investigations

- Lymph node biopsy.
- Blood film: leucocytosis.

- Normochromic normocytic anaemia.
- Bone marrow.
- Raised ESR and LDH.
- Very high CRP with no evidence of infection.
- CT abdomen, pelvis and chest.

Treatment

Treatment depends on histology and staging. The agents used most frequently are cyclophosphamide and chlorambucil, often given with steroids. This is obviously a problem when patients have co-morbidities including diabetes, osteoporosis, heart failure, etc. Thus, each patient must be assessed individually to determine whether or not they would benefit from chemotherapy.

Coagulation disorders

Clotting disorders

- DVT is the most common clotting problem in geriatric practice.
- Age alone is a risk factor, but most patients also have other precipitants, such as immobility, trauma (accidental and surgical), underlying malignancy, inflammatory disorders and dehydration.
- Other conditions in which the blood has increased viscosity, e.g. myeloma, polycythaemia, hyperosmolar non-ketotic diabetic coma and hypothermia, also increase risk of venous thrombosis.
- All older people in hospital are at increased risk of venous thromboembolism and should be offered prophylactic low molecular weight heparin unless there is a contraindication. Thromboembolic device stockings (TEDS) are useful in reducing post-phlebitic syndrome. See Chapter 9 for more information about venous thromboembolism.

Bleeding disorders

The most common cause of prolonged bleeding is medical treatment or overtreatment with anticoagulants such as warfarin. As the indications for anticoagulation of elderly patients increase, so will the episodes of overtreatment. Elderly patients are particularly at risk because of the problem of compliance (with both drug regime and regular monitoring), plus the changing pharmacodynamics and complication of drug interactions, for example with analgesics and NSAIDs. Patients with usually stable INRs treated for infection with antibiotics especially ciprofloxacin can present with very deranged INRs and severe haemorrhage, or haematoma if they have fallen.

High INRs not complicated by haemorrhage or shock can be managed by giving a small dose of vitamin K orally (assuming the warfarin is to be continued). If there is severe haemorrhage with hypovolaemic shock bleeding into a confined space, then the warfarin should be reversed with IV vitamin K and IV Beriplex.

Other elderly patients at risk are those with thrombocytopenia. This may be due to their underlying pathology, as in aplastic anaemia or autoimmune idiopathic thrombocytopenia, or as a consequence of powerful chemotherapeutic regimes for myeloproliferative and other neoplastic diseases. The risk of serious haemorrhage, e.g. stroke, is much higher in elderly subjects.

The increasing use of thrombolysis (see Chapter 9) is another example of elderly patients experiencing both greater benefits and greater risks. Careful selection is needed to avoid the increased risk of bleeding, especially into the brain.

Disseminated intravascular coagulation (DIC)

In DIC there is both thrombosis and haemorrhage. The initial thrombotic element is usually silent but the consumption of coagulation factors in the process leads to uncontrolled bleeding. Likely precipitants in old age are sepsis, disseminated malignant disease, trauma and fulminant liver failure. Only sepsis is likely to respond to active treatment. Supportive treatments are blood transfusion for bleeding, Beriplex and fresh platelet transfusions. In general, 50% of patients die, and a higher percentage of very frail elderly patients succumb.

⊙ FURTHER INFORMATION

Green AR, Hoffbrand V, Catovsky D, et al. (2010) *Postgraduate Haematology*, 6th edn. Wiley–Blackwell, Oxford.

Hoffbrand V, Moss P (2011) *Essential Haematology*, 6th edn. Wiley-Blackwell, Oxford.

Leukemia and Lymphoma Society Facts 2010–11: http://www.lls.org/content/nationalcontent/

resourcecenter/freeeducationmaterials/general cancer/pdf/facts.pdf.

Liu D (2011) Chronic lymphocytic leukaemia. eMedicine: *emedicine.medscape.com*/article/199313-overview.

Macmillan Cancer Support: http://www.macmillan.org.uk/Cancerinformation/Causesriskfactors/Pre-cancerous/Chronicidiopathicmyelofibrosis.aspx. Also has comprehensive patient information.

Patient information about leukaemia: http://beat-bloodcancers.org/home.

Patient information plus articles written for non-specialist doctors dealing with common leukaemias: http://www.patient.co.uk/patientplus.asp.

Uprichard J, Bain BJ (2009) Practice: rational testing: investigating suspected anaemia. *BMJ* 338: b1644. http://www.bmj.com/content/338/bmj.b1644.full.

15

Eyes, ears, mouth and skin

Eyes

Age-related changes

1 Eyes appear sunken due to loss of periorbital fat.
2 Arcus senilis (deposition of calcium and cholesterol salts in a ring at the edge of the cornea) is common but not clinically significant.
3 The muscles in the iris weaken so the pupil becomes small (miosis) and less light reaches the retina. The pupil is slow to react to light and accommodation becomes impaired.
4 Dark adaptation slows because of the reduced rate of regeneration of rhodopsin.
5 The sclera appears more yellow due to dehydration and lipid deposition.
6 The conjunctiva contains fewer mucus-secreting cells so becomes drier. Conjunctival vessels are more fragile leading to conjunctival haemorrhages.
7 The vitreous contains more floaters and cholesterol deposits. It may become more liquid, increasing the risk of retinal detachment.
8 Presbyopia, the deterioration of vision with age, occurs because the lens becomes inelastic, so that focusing on near objects becomes difficult.
9 Entropion (in-turned lashes) is common and causes irritation of the cornea. It must be corrected surgically to avoid corneal damage.
10 Ectropion (out-turned lashes) is very common and the most frequent cause of epiphora (watery eye). Again, this can be surgically corrected. The everted eyelid can be mistaken for 'red eye'.

Examination of the fundus in old age

Age-related miosis can make it difficult to examine the fundi of older people. Short-acting eye drops are recommended, usually tropicamide 0.5% (rapid onset and effects last 4–6 h). Reversal with pilocarpine is usually unnecessary and can be painful. The risk of acute closed-angle glaucoma is minimal, but beware the small eyeball with a shallow anterior chamber and small-diameter cornea.

Loss of vision

Approximately 70,000 persons over the age of 65 years in the UK are registered as partially sighted, i.e. about 1% of the elderly population. Figure 15.1 lists the causes of blindness in older people. Many more are visually disabled but remain unregistered. Registration of disability is essential for special benefits and visual aids.

Criteria for being registered blind/partially sighted

• Severely sight impaired/blind:
  o Visual acuity (VA) of less than 3/60 with a full visual field.
  o VA between 3/60 and 6/60 with severe field reduction, such as tunnel vision.
  o VA of 6/60 or above, but with a much reduced field of vision, especially in the lower part of the field.
• Sight impaired/partially sighted:

  o VA of 3/60 to 6/60 with a full field of vision.
  o VA of up to 6/24 with a moderate reduction of field of vision or central vision that is blurry.

Lecture Notes Elderly Care Medicine, Eighth Edition. Claire G. Nicholl and K. Jane Wilson.
© 2012 John Wiley & Sons, Ltd. Published 2012 by John Wiley & Sons, Ltd.

Causes of visual impairment

Slow loss:
- Age-related macular degeneration, 45%: central vision is lost but peripheral vision is maintained.
- Cataracts, 33%.
- Retinopathy (diabetes mellitus), 17%.
- Open-angle glaucoma (chronic), 15%: central vision is maintained until late in the disease.

Sudden loss:
- Acute glaucoma.
- Vitreous haemorrhage, more common in diabetics.
- Central retinal artery occlusion, secondary to embolus from carotid bifurcation or mitral valve.
- Venous occlusion: more common in patients with hypertension or hyperviscosity.
- Retinal detachment.
- Ischaemic optic atrophy, secondary to giant-cell arteritis or atherosclerosis.

NB: If one eye is affected, the other is at risk.

- o VA of up to 6/18 if a large part of the field, for example a whole half field or a lot of peripheral vision, is missing.

Advantages of being registered blind

- Fifty percent reduction in television licence fee; free for over 75s anyway!
- Blue badge scheme for the driver.
- Free eye tests; free for over 60 year olds anyway.
- Free loan of equipment from Low Visual Aid clinics.

The painful eye

1 Closed-angle glaucoma (acute).
2 Infection:
   - o Conjunctivitis.
   - o Uveitis.
   - o Herpes zoster: when the ophthalmic branch of the facial nerve is affected, there may be involvement of the forehead, eyelids and conjunctiva. The patient must see an ophthalmologist urgently.
3 Trauma, e.g. corneal abrasion or a foreign body.

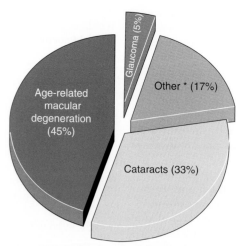

* Including diabetic complications

Figure 15.1 Causes of blindness in old age. *Source:* ABPI (1991) *The Challenges of Ageing.* ABPI, London.

Primary open angle/chronic glaucoma

- A silent and progressive disease which may result in blindness if not treated.
- Accounts for 15% of blindness fulfilling criteria for registration in the UK.
- Risk factors include increasing age, family history, African or Caribbean descent, diabetes, myopia and hypertension.
- There may be cupping and atrophy of the optic disc.
- Early cases are best detected by regular eye tests, with ocular-pressure measurement.
- Affects peripheral vision first, only affecting central vision late in the disease.
- May affect one eye more than the other.
- Treatment is aimed at reducing the intraocular pressure:
  o Once daily prostaglandin agonists give excellent results, e.g. latanaprost. Intraocular pressure is reduced by increased drainage of aqueous humour via the trabecular meshwork.
  o Beta-blockers, e.g. timolol eye drops and alpha$_2$ adrenergic agonists, e.g. brimonidine eye drops, reduce the production of aqueous humour by the ciliary body.
  o Carbonic anhydrase inhibitors act on the carbonic anhydrase in the ciliary body, e.g. dorzolamide. They are less effective than other treatments so are often used as adjuncts.
  o Educate the patient about the efficacy of treatment and the high risk of blindness without it, to engage them in persevering with eye drops for life.

- If treatment with eye drops fails, trabeculoplasty with an argon laser or surgical trabeculectomy will improve aqueous flow.

Acute glaucoma

- Less common than chronic glaucoma.
- More common in females because the anterior chamber is more shallow.
- Most common in 6th and 7th decades.
- Easier to detect because it presents with sudden painful loss of vision in a red eye.
- Often associated with ipsilateral headache and vomiting.
- The patient may describe haloes around lights secondary to corneal oedema.
- The patient may report a precipitating event such as exposure to very dim light or mydriatic treatments such as anticholinergics and sympathomimetics.
- The pupil is mid-dilated and non-reactive.
- Visual acuity is reduced.
- Slit lamp examination may show corneal oedema and an irregular pupil.
- The intraocular pressure will be increased.
- Emergency treatment is IV and oral acetazolamide or IV mannitol plus topical beta-blocker eye drops. Steroid drops reduce inflammation.
- Analgesia and anti-emetics reduce the distress of the patient which also helps reduce the pressure.
- Laser iridotomy reduces the pressure acutely.

Table 15.1 summarizes the differences between acute and chronic glaucoma.

Table 15.1 Summary of differences between acute and chronic glaucoma

	Acute – closed-angle	Chronic – open-angle
Symptoms	Sudden pain in eye, blurred vision, vomiting and prostration	Insidious loss of vision, leading to tunnel vision; family history common
Signs	Painful red eye with reduced vision. Eye tense, irregular fixed pupil, cornea and conjunctiva congested	Painless normal looking eye. Raised pressure on tonometry, scotoma on field testing; cupped disc
Pathology	Sudden impairment of anterior-chamber drainage – may be precipitated by anticholinergics and mydriatics	Gradual increase in intraocular pressure – idiopathic
Treatment	Constrict pupil, analgesia, carbonic anhydrase inhibitor – urgent action needed	Prostaglandin, beta-blocker and/or pilocarpine drops, drainage operation

Age-related macular degeneration (AMD)

- Affects people aged 50 and over, and becomes more common with advancing age.
- The most common cause of visual impairment in the industrialized world.
- Affects 1.5 million people in the UK currently, and predicted to rise to 1.9 million by 2020 because of the ageing population.
- As the macula is the area damaged, central vision is affected more, with peripheral vision being preserved.
- Loss of central vision means loss of face recognition and difficulty reading.
- AMD is usually bilateral, but may affect one eye earlier or more than the other.
- Age-related maculopathy: mild or moderate non-exudative changes in the macula.

Risk factors for AMD

Increasing age
Female preponderance
Positive family history
Smoking (inhibits complement factor H)
Hypertension
White ancestry, especially with light-coloured eyes
Obesity
Cataract surgery
Sun exposure
Diet low in vitamins A, C and E, and zinc

AMD is divided into two broad types:

1 'Dry' or non-exudative AMD, characterized by atrophic and hypertrophic changes and drusen (yellow extracellular deposits of proteins, lipids and debris) in the retinal pigment epithelium (RPE) underlying the macula.
- Develops slowly over months or years.
- No treatment, but encourage to stop smoking; some evidence that antioxidant supplements (vitamins A, C and E with zinc and copper) may be protective.
- Geographic atrophy (patchy loss of RPE cells) may signal development of wet AMD.
- Ten to twenty percent of patients progress to the wet type.

2 Wet AMD or exudative AMD, characterized by choroidal neovascularization. Tissue hypoxia stimulates the release of vascular endothelial growth factor (VEGF). This in turn stimulates the production of new vessels growing into the choroid which are fragile and 'leaky'.

- More rapidly progressive and causes more visual impairment.
- New treatments have been developed to inhibit VEGF: pegaptanib sodium (a direct antagonist) and ranibizumab (a monoclonal antibody). Both are given as monthly intraocular injections and need to be continued for at least 2 years to preserve vision. 'Rationing' of these expensive treatments by imposing strict eligibility criteria (likely to increase in the current economic climate) creates controversy,
- NICE (2011) only recommended ranibizumab. Criteria for treatment include best corrected vision 6/12 and 6/96, no permanent structural damage of fovea (central macula), lesion less than 12 disc areas, evidence of disease progression and response to initial treatment.
- Side-effects: conjunctival haemorrhage, eye pain, vitreous floaters, vitreous haemorrhage, retinal detachment and increased intraocular pressure.
- Ranibizumab improves vision in 40% of cases and prevents further deterioration of sight in most patients.
- NICE supports photodynamic therapy for wet AMD with definite choroidal neovascularization. Verteporfin (a light-sensitive drug given intravenously) sticks to the new vessels and is activated using a cold laser to seal the vessels.
- Exciting developments in the genetics of AMD point to a single nucleotide polymorphism in complement factor H (CFH) gene on chromosomes 1 and 10. CFH is an inhibitor of the complement pathway and abnormal CFH leads to inflammation.
- If vision is severely impaired, refer to the Low Vision Service.

Table 15.2 summarizes the differences between dry and wet AMD.

Driving

- Legally, the patient must be able to read a car registration plate at 20 m, in good light with glasses if appropriate.

Table 15.2 Differences between dry and wet AMD

	Dry AMD	Wet AMD
Frequency	80–85%	10–15%
Symptoms	Asymptomatic until late stage	Rapid loss of central vision over days to weeks
	May notice loss of central acuity	Metamorphopsia
	Peripheral vision preserved	Decreased colour and contrast sensitivity
	Sudden deterioration of vision suggests	Slow dark adaptation
	progression to wet AMD	
Appearance	Focal hyperpigmentation, drusen,	Larger more confluent drusen, more
	geographic atrophy	pigmentation and new vessels, scarring
Management	Stop smoking	Intravitreal ranibizumab
	Increase dietary antioxidants	Photodynamic therapy

- A patient with visual field defects, regardless of cause (e.g. glaucoma, stroke or pituitary disease), should not drive unless allowed by the ophthalmologist.

Cataracts

- So called because the world appears blurred as if seen behind a waterfall.
- Arise because of protein breakdown and dehydration of the lens.
- Are very common and easily detected and corrected, resulting in marked improvement of quality of life.
- In the USA 300,000–400,000 cases occur annually.
- Responsible for around 36% of cases of blindness in Africa.
- Short-sighted patients may report an improvement in near vision ('second sight') because progression temporarily increases the power of the lens. As the cataract progresses further, near vision is lost again.
- Other visual problems include reduced contrast sensitivity and increased glare from daylight or car headlights at night.

Types

1 Central – early visual loss.
2 Peripheral – late visual loss and vision impaired by scattering of bright light.

Multifactorial pathogenesis.

Causes

- Ageing.
- Hereditary.
- Diabetes mellitus.
- Hypertension.

- Iatrogenic, e.g. steroids.
- Alcohol.
- Environmental – bright sunshine (increased incidence in the tropics).
- Nuclear cataracts seem to be related to smoking.

Examination

Thorough assessment of both eyes is essential to exclude problems, e.g. AMD which will not be resolved by cataract extraction, to ensure a good outcome from surgery. This includes acuity, fields, assessment of pupillary reflexes, indirect and direct ophthalmoscopy and slit lamp examination.

Treatment

Surgery
Timing depends on individual need, e.g. earlier in those who read a lot, but may be delayed in those whom the distortion, change in magnification and reduced visual fields caused by wearing glasses post-operatively would be a hindrance.

Contraindications
1 Early stages.
2 Where vision is compromised by other ocular co-morbidities such as AMD or severe retinopathy.
3 In the presence of severe mental impairment.
4 Avoid oral alpha-blockers such as tamsulosin in the month prior to cataract surgery to avoid 'floppy iris' syndrome.

Surgical procedure
- Usually done as a day case under local anaesthetic.
- The anterior chamber of the eye is incised. Phacoemulsification is the process of fragmenting

the opacified lens by ultrasound. This debris is removed, leaving the lens capsule intact. An artificial lens is inserted into the capsule.

- The power of the new lens is selected to optimize vision so that the patient does not have to wear thick aphakic spectacles.

Complications of treatment

1 Dilatation of the pupil may precipitate glaucoma.
2 Lens implant: possible failure and risk of infection.
3 Posterior capsular opacification: may occur several months after the cataract extraction and is treated by Yittrium Aluminium Garnet (YAG) laser capsulotomy.

Giant-cell arteritis (GCA)

See also Chapter 9.

Clinical features

1 This is a vision-threatening disease: a systemic vasculitis of large and medium sized arteries. Arteritis affecting the posterior ciliary arteries can cause ischaemic optic neuropathy leading to blindness.
2 May present with loss of vision which is sometimes transient (amaurosis fugax), or with abnormal purple vision (photopsia).
3 Associated with headache, usually localized to the temples, plus scalp tenderness when combing the hair. Jaw ache when chewing secondary to ischaemia of the masseter muscles, occipital headache secondary to occipital artery claudication, or more rarely tongue claudication also occur.
4 The patient is often systemically unwell and febrile.
5 Often overlaps with polymyalgia rheumatica: proximal limb girdle ache, early morning stiffness.
6 Fundus examination is usually normal, but if there is visual loss, it may reveal a pale swollen optic nerve head.
7 Diagnosis is supported by a raised ESR and CRP and confirmed by temporal artery biopsy (ultrasound of the temporal artery improves the diagnostic yield).
8 Alkaline phosphatase is often elevated.
9 The histology remains characteristic of GCA for up to 4 weeks after commencing steroids, so do not wait for biopsy result before treating.
10 The treatment is high-dose oral steroids: 1 mg/kg.

11 Evidence suggests that co-prescribing aspirin 75 mg for the first month reduces the increased risk of stroke associated with inflammation.
12 The disease often lasts for up to 2 years. The steroids should be weaned down slowly according to the clinical picture and fall in ESR and CRP.
13 Don't forget gut and bone protection.

Simple measures to assist patients with visual impairment

1 Check visual acuity – provision or change of lenses may help. Reflective coatings reduce glare.
2 Keep patient and spectacles together, especially in hospital!
3 Keep spectacles clean.
4 Consider a magnifying glass for reading. Some have a marker to aid patients with AMD keep their place when reading.
5 Appropriate lighting is the best visual aid: the bulb should be shielded from the eye-line and glare should be reduced.
6 Encourage the patient to be registered as partially sighted or blind. In the UK this is done by a consultant ophthalmologist.
7 Seek advice about the availability and use of low-visual aids. Examples include telephones and computers with large buttons labelled in large print or Braille, talking clocks and watches. A Kindle is good for reading.
8 Optimize hearing ability.
9 Recommend a support charity, e.g. the Royal National Institute of Blind People website: www. rnib.org.uk.
10 Subscribe to talking newspaper, talking-book library, etc.
11 Aids to staying in your own home: entry phone, community alarm, contrasting colours around doorways and steps; good lighting as above.

Treatable precipitating/aggravating factors in vascular causes of visual loss

1 Diabetes.
2 Hypertension/hypotension.
3 Arteritis.
4 Polycythaemia.
5 Paraproteinaemia.

Ears

Ageing changes

1 Wax becomes more viscous and needs to be removed in one-quarter of elderly people.
2 Age-related hearing loss (presbycusis) is insidious, progressive loss of hearing, most affecting higher pitched sounds. Consonants and word endings are missed, impairing word discrimination in speech. High frequency sounds are lost because the outer hair cells of the organ of Corti (located in the basal cochlear) are more vulnerable to free radical damage. Recruitment may be problematic. Soft sounds, e.g. <50 dB, may be inaudible, but slightly louder sounds, e.g. >80 dB, are uncomfortable or distorted. This occurs as more neurones are switched on or 'recruited' to try to compensate for the loss of hair cells.
3 The brain is slower at processing auditory information.
4 Seventy percent of the over 70s have hearing loss and should be considered for a hearing aid.
5 Impaired hearing leads to impaired health.
6 The WHO predicts that by 2030, age-related hearing loss will be in the top 10 health burdens (above cataracts and diabetes) in the UK and other Western countries.
7 Progressive loss of hair cells in the semicircular canals impairs balance.
8 Degeneration of otoliths in the saccule makes benign paroxysmal positional vertigo (BPPV) more common. See Chapter 5.
9 Reduction in the number of vestibular nerve cells contributes to increased risk of dizziness with age.

Causes of hearing impairment

1 Nerve deafness:
 • Presbycusis.
 • Ototoxic drugs, e.g. gentamicin and furosemide in high dosage.
 • Nerve compression, e.g. acoustic neuroma and Paget's disease of the bone.
2 Conduction deafness:
 • Impacted wax.
 • Otosclerosis is hereditary so early onset is likely.
 • Post-infective, e.g. chronic suppurative otitis media.
 • Paget's disease.
At present only conductive forms of deafness in old age are treated surgically; although cochlear implants may be useful in profound presbycusis they are deemed too expensive.

> 70% of over 70 year olds have hearing impairment (range of quietest sound heard given in brackets):
>
> • Mild – 27%; difficulty following conversations in a noisy room (25–39 dB).
> • Moderate – 36%; have difficulty following speech without a hearing aid (40–69 dB).
> • Severe – 6%; may have to lip-read/sign even with hearing aids (70–94 dB).
> • Profound – 1%; likely to rely on lip-reading/signing (>94 dB).

Management of hearing impairment

1 Check for wax. Administer softening drops, e.g. sodium bicarbonate or olive oil, and then microsuction if necessary.
2 If deafness persists after wax removal, refer for audiometry.
3 If appropriate, a hearing aid should be offered (see the following box).
4 Ask if the patient thinks they are deaf. If they do not, they are unlikely to use a hearing aid.
5 Educate the patient and their family about equipment:
 • Environmental aids, e.g. flashing telephones and doorbells, vibrating-pillow alarm clocks and smoke alarms.
 • Advise about use of 'T' switch, used in conjunction with induction loop systems to amplify television, telephones, at cinemas, etc.
6 Inform the patient about national charities and local support groups:
 • www.actiononhearingloss.org.uk/.
 • www.deafcouncil.org.uk/CAMTAD.htm.
 • www.yourlocalcinema.com – gives information about whether a loop system or subtitles are available.

Advantages of digital hearing aids

• Sound is digitally processed so the quality is better.
• The aid is programmed for the individual's pattern of frequency loss; these frequencies are amplified more than others.

Getting the most from hearing aids

- Warn the patient that even the best hearing aids can only amplify sound and cannot restore normal hearing. Otherwise, people are so put-off by the general increase in noise that they do not persevere.
- People do better the more they practise with the aid early on (brain plasticity).
- Bilateral aids give the best result in bilateral hearing impairment if tolerated.
- The characteristic whistling is caused by feedback; check the aid is sitting properly in the ear, that the canal is not blocked by wax and that the volume is not turned up too high.
- Teach maintenance of aid, i.e. cleaning of tubing and battery replacement (see Figure 15.2).
- Follow-up to encourage use of the aid is essential; volunteers can help.
- Behind-the-ear analogue aids are still most frequently used. See Figure 15.3 for correct insertion.
- Body-worn hearing aids are the most powerful and used in profound hearing loss.
- In-the-ear aids have the advantage of being discrete but are easily plugged with wax, are awkward if manual dexterity is reduced and are readily lost, especially in hospital. They are unsuitable for patients with otitis externa (inflammation of the pinna and ear canal).

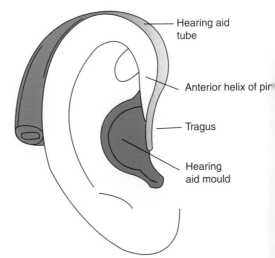

Figure 15.3 Correct insertion of behind-the-ear hearing aid.

- Feedback, which occurs when sound from the speaker travels back into the microphone and is amplified again, is reduced because the aid is programmed to filter it out.
- The aid may have several programmes, e.g. to compensate for background noise, concerts, meetings. Top-of-the-range models switch programme automatically.
- Open ear fitting: soft ear pieces sit in the ear comfortably and allow more air to circulate; only appropriate for mild to moderate hearing impairment.

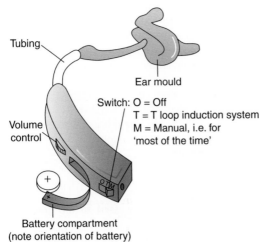

Switch: O = Off
T = T loop induction system
M = Manual, i.e. for 'most of the time'

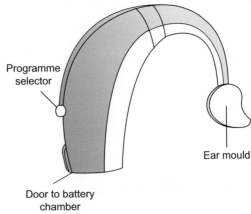

Figure 15.2 Behind-the-ear analogue and digital hearing aids.

- Technology is improving all the time: there are aids that have Bluetooth connectivity for use with Bluetooth mobile phones.
- Automatic volume control.
- Directional microphones.
- People used to analogue aids may find it difficult to switch to digital.

How to communicate with people who have hearing impairment

1 Do not shout, as this just increases the distortion of your voice (recruitment) and lips (making it more difficult for lip-readers).
2 Speak clearly and slowly but not in an exaggerated way.
3 Face the patient and make sure your face is well lit in order to assist lip-reading.
4 Do not obscure your mouth.
5 Ask the patient if they can hear you, adjust tone of voice or try rephrasing your question.
6 Check that, if patient has an aid, it is properly worn and functioning.
7 All clinical areas should have available a simple portable microphone and headphones, or 'communicator'.
8 If all else fails, write down your questions.

Complications of deafness

1 Social isolation, withdrawal from friends and family, especially at large gatherings.
2 Sense of loss.
3 Depression and anxiety.
4 Increased risk of accidents because of reduced auditory warnings.
5 Associated tinnitus.
6 Associated dizziness and unsteadiness.

Tinnitus

1 Noises in the ears which may be continuous or intermittent. Often described as a rushing, buzzing or roaring in the ears. If full sentences are heard, a psychiatric cause should be excluded.
2 Most commonly associated with presbycusis: one theory is that the noise is generated by the brain to replace the sound that is 'missing'.
3 Can be noise induced.
4 Affects over 20% of over 65 year olds.
 - Severe symptoms in 5%.
 - Incapacitating in 0.5%.

5 Pulsatile tinnitus: the noises beat in time with the pulse; suggests a vascular lesion such as an arteriovenous malformation, or a glomus tumour.
6 When tinnitus is unilateral, request an MRI of the internal auditory meatus to exclude an acoustic neuroma (benign Schwanoma). These tumours are very slowly progressive; the dilemma is choosing when to operate, as surgery always causes hearing loss.
7 Discontinue implicated drugs: aspirin, NSAIDs, loop diuretics, aminoglycosides.
8 Treatment:
 - Research suggests that patients should be told that tinnitus is often self-limiting; health care professionals should avoid negative suggestions such as 'nothing can be done'.
 - Hearing aids may help if the tinnitus is associated with hearing loss.
 - Advise the patient to minimize stress and tiredness as these tend to aggravate the symptoms.
 - Sometimes a masker, which produces 'white noise', is beneficial.
 - Fill quietness with music or predictable noises such as a fan just above the volume of the tinnitus.
 - If the tinnitus causes depression, antidepressants are helpful.
 - In severe cases, consider cognitive behavioural therapy.
 - Seek support from self-help organization, e.g. British Tinnitus Association (www.tinnitus.org.uk/).
 - The NMDA receptor blocker neramexane is a possible treatment, but has not yet been licensed.

Dizziness

See Chapter 5.

The mouth and its contents

The lips

1 Herpes simplex, as in younger patients may indicate systemic disease.
2 Angular stomatitis is usually due to the escape of saliva due to poor lip closure. The corners of the mouth become red and sore, especially if

complicated by fungal (*Candida*) infection; most common in the edentulous.

Oral mucosa

1 Pemphigoid and pemphigus produce blisters in the mouth; see below.
2 Lichen planus presents as white patches/ulceration (see Table 15.3).
3 *Candida* infections are white patches on the tongue or oral mucosa, especially in patients taking oral or inhaled steroids and antibiotics, or with diabetes or dentures.
4 Aphthous ulcers are round, shallow and well-circumscribed and are usually self-limiting.
5 Oral cancers: are usually squamous cell in origin and are strongly linked with smoking.

Tongue abnormalities

1 Smooth and shiny – iron deficiency.
2 Red and sore – glossitis, e.g. vitamin B group deficiency.
3 Geographical/furred tongue – usually not significant.
4 Injury to the lateral borders – think of epilepsy.
5 Ulceration – consider malignancy, but trauma from teeth most common.
6 Fasciculation – motor neuron disease (LMN).
7 Asymmetrical protrusion – points to side of weakness, e.g. base of skull tumour.
8 Small spastic tongue: pseudobulbar palsy (UMN lesion).

The teeth

1 In the UK 65% of people aged 65–74 have no natural teeth and this rises to 82% in those over 75.
2 In the past, every effort was made to rescue surviving teeth. Modern dentists work more to preserve periodontal health as tooth implants are so effective. Regular dental review is important; with age the dental pulp atrophies so caries cause less toothache.
3 Sixty percent of patients are unhappy with their dentures, usually complaining of looseness.
4 Twelve percent of those with dentures never wear them.
5 The edentulous need to continue to consult dentists: gum ridges recede with age and new dentures will be needed.
6 Dentures should only be supplied to those who are prepared to wear them.
7 Dentures should be left in situ in a cardiac arrest, unless they are obstructing the airway.
8 Dignity and nutrition are best maintained if well-fitting dentures are worn; the presence of surviving teeth helps to secure dental plates and improves the fit.
9 Dentures should be labelled to avoid loss if owner is admitted to an institution.

NB: In wild animals, non-accidental death (i.e. due to 'old age') is most commonly due to starvation secondary to dental loss.

Skin

Age changes

- Most age changes in the skin are proportional to the extent of environmental damage from sun and wind or heat, as in erythema ab igne.
- Thinning of epidermis and dermis, which become more transparent, increasingly fragile and less elastic.
- Skin becomes drier, due to reduction in sebum secretion.
- Reduced subcutaneous fat and vascularity, which both reduce the ability of the body to maintain its temperature.
- Increased capillary fragility (lax connective tissue).
- Reduced epidermal turnover and repair of damage to the skin.
- Reduced sweating due to both reduced numbers and function of sweat glands.
- Reduction in the production of vitamin D_3 from 7-dehydrocholesterol.
- Age-related blemishes of cosmetic significance only include senile purpura (on hands and forearms), lentigo (brown macules on back of hands), Campbell de Morgan spots (trunk), sebaceous warts (face and back) and telangiectasia (face).

Damage to skin

Leg ulcers and pressure sores are common, serious and expensive conditions in geriatric practice.

Leg ulcers

These are usually situated in the distal third of the lower leg. When associated with varicose veins, eczema and swollen ankles, they are usually

Table 15.3 Causes, clinical features, examples and treatment of itch in older people

Cause	Clinical features	Examples	Treatment
Xerosis	Abnormal maturation of keratocytes causes dryness and roughness of skin with fine scale	Associated with PVD and neurological disease	Avoid soap, use emollients
Eczema	Exacerbations in winter/dry conditions Exposure to allergen	Atopic	Emollients, topical steroids
		Contact Seborrhoeic	Remove allergen Nizorel shampoo to scalp
Psoriasis	Erythematous plaques with silver scale, commonly on extensor surfaces.	Exacerbated by stress, alcohol and drugs such as beta-blockers	Treat with topical calcipotriol, Psoralen + UVA treatment (PUVA), methotrexate in severe disease
	Tear-drop lesions on trunk	Guttate psoriasis, triggered by streptococcal infection	
	Lesions on palms and soles	Pustular psoriasis	
Lichen simplex chronicus	Localized raised plaque caused by habitual scratching		Consider covering the lesion with dressing, e.g. Duoderm + emollients
Drugs	Ask about new medications	Opiates, phenothiazines, aspirin, quinine	Stop suspect medications where possible
Urticaria	Type I hypersensitivity reactions to drugs, food, cold, sunlight	Sensitivity to penicillin, sulphonamides, nuts, chocolate	Avoid cause, short course of prednislone
Lichen planus	Itchy purple papules on flexures of wrist	May be triggered by gold and photochemicals	Topical steroids; systemic in severe disease
Dermatitis herpetiformis	Itchy vesicles on extensor sites, buttocks	All patients have gluten enteropathy, but may be subclinical	Avoid gluten in diet
Pityriasis rosacea	Itching red rash on trunk in 'Christmas tree' distribution		Usually self-limiting, if necessary try sedative antihistamine or topical steroids
Bullous pemphigoid	Irritating deep bullae	See text	Oral steroids
Infestations	Straight or 's'-shaped burrows in webs of fingers and anterior surface of wrist. More often a generalized allergic rash is seen. Other members of the household will be affected	Scabies	Shower/bathe in antibacterial soap. Topical permethrin solution. Wash clothes and bedclothes. Treat household and close contacts
Infection	Dermatophytes	*Candida* in intertriginous areas; Tinea corporis, pedis and cruris	Treat with topical antifungal, e.g. clotrimazole
Neoplasia	Fever, weight loss, itch	Mycosis fungoides Lymphoma	Treat as appropriate
Metabolic	Hypothyroid facies Uraemic frost	Hypothyroidism Renal impairment	Levothyroxine Relieve cause where possible

(continued)

Table 15.3 (*Continued*)

Cause	Clinical features	Examples	Treatment
	Jaundice/raised alkaline phosphatase	Hepatic impairment, e.g. Primary biliary cirrhosis	Relieve cause where possible, ursodeoxycholate, menthol cream
	Iron deficiency	Gastrointestinal disease	Look for and treat cause

secondary to venous insufficiency. When well demarcated and painful, arterial insufficiency is most likely to be responsible. In many cases there will be a contribution from both venous and arterial disease (Table 15.4).

Treatment

1 Keep clean, warm and hydrated. Cleanse with saline, water or chlorhexidine.
2 Debride wound either surgically or with preparations as per local policy.
3 Cover or pack if large, with paraffin gauze if healing. Use hydrogel, hydrocolloid or alginate dressings if exudate present.
4 Bandage from toes to knee.
   • Crepe bandage in presence of ischaemia or cellulitis.
   • Where there is a lot of oedema, four-layer bandaging can help heal ulcers. However, peripheral vascular disease must be excluded first (by Doppler measurement if necessary).
5 Encourage mobility, but at rest elevate the feet.
6 Use antibiotics if there is evidence of sepsis, but avoid topical preparations because of risk of contact dermatitis.
7 Dressings should rarely be changed more frequently than once daily. When healing has started, increase intervals between dressing changes. Hydrocolloid and similar dressings may be left in place for a week.

Cellulitis

This usually presents as painful, red, hot, swelling of the lower limb, and it is often bilateral. If the cellulitis is extensive, the patient may be systemically unwell and have a fever. Care must be taken to exclude a co-existing DVT (see Chapter 9). The most common pathogens are *Streptococcus pyogenes* and *Staphylococcus aureus,* but do not forget MRSA in cases of hospital acquired infection.

Risk factors include chronic leg oedema, trauma causing a pretibial laceration (check if tetanus toxoid is needed if the injury was sustained in the garden) and maceration between the toes secondary to *Tinea pedis* (athlete's foot).

Treatment depends on the severity of the infection. If the patient is unwell, then the best management is admission for intravenous antibiotics, usually benzyl penicillin, adding in flucloxacillin if *Staphylococcus* is suspected. Use erythromycin if the patient is allergic to penicillin. In the case of MRSA, treat with intravenous vancomycin. Oral antibiotics may be used for less severe cases. Treat any co-existing DVT or athlete's foot as appropriate (e.g. terbinafine).

Table 15.4 Differences between arterial and venous leg ulcers

	Arterial	Venous
History	Usually recent	Often years
Pain	Present	Often absent
Site	Medial or lateral leg or dorsum of foot	Gaiter area of leg
Appearance	Small, clean, punched out	Large, weepy, infected, surrounding pigmentation or eczema
Pulses	Absent or bruits in proximal vessels (not invariable in diabetes)	Present unless obscured by oedema
Proportion	15%	70%

Pressure sores

- Prevalence in the UK is quoted as 7–18%.
- Seventy percent of all pressure sores occur in the over-70-year-old population.
- Pressure sores are areas of necrosis due to persistent and unrelieved pressure that exceeds the perfusion pressure of the tissues.
- It only takes a pressure of 32 mmHg for 2 h to cause skin necrosis in fit younger patients.
- Affected areas are usually between bony prominences and an unyielding surface upon which the patient is lying. See box below for common sites.
- Shearing forces (e.g. between the patient's skin held stationary by friction on the sheets and gravity pulling the body down the bed) aggravate the problem.
- Persistent moisture (e.g. from incontinence) causes maceration of the skin which worsens the damage.
- Pressure sores are very expensive: in terms of dressings and increased nursing time. The NHS spends £4 billion per year on ulcer treatment. The cost per individual can be £11–40,000 for severe ulcers.
- Sores are painful and demoralizing and are therefore distressing to the patient and their family.
- Pressure sores are associated with increased morbidity and mortality, mainly due to infection.
- Nursing home residents who develop new sores have a mortality of 60–80% in the next 3 months.
- In debilitated patients, pressure sores may occur within hours, but may take months to heal or even prove to be fatal.
- Prevention is cheaper and more humane than expensive and prolonged treatment.
- However, the damage may have occurred before presentation, e.g. during a 'long lie' after a fall at home.
- If prevention fails, the extent of the damage must be minimized and healing promoted.
- With modern medicine keeping many frail, elderly patients alive and in hospital, the incidence of pressure sores is bound to rise.
- The prevention and management of pressure sores should be multidisciplinary.

Preventive measures

1 Pressure sores are now deemed 'never happen' complications: sores that are grade 2 or above (see box below) must be documented as clinical incidents.

Common sites of pressure sores (estimated incidence)

Ischial tuberosity (28%)
Sacrum (25%)
Greater trochanter (17%)
Heels (15%)
Occiput
Malleoli

Intrinsic risk factors for pressure sores

- Increasing age: ageing changes to the skin.
- Reduced mobility: spinal injury, stroke, fractures, plaster of Paris casts (POPs).
- Impaired level of consciousness.
- Sensory neuropathy; diabetes, alcohol.
- Acute, chronic, terminal illness.
- Urinary and faecal incontinence.
- Low BMI.
- Catabolic state secondary to surgery or infection.
- Poor nutrition/hydration: impairs healing.
- Co-morbidities: poor blood supply, e.g. peripheral vascular disease, infection, pain, medications.
- Poor cognition secondary to delirium or dementia.
- Previous pressure damage.

Extrinsic factors
- Skin hygiene.
- Medications, e.g. sedatives, opiates, which would further reduce mobility, steroids impair healing.
- Inadequate pressure relieving system.

---

2 Identify at-risk patients using a score such as the Waterlow Risk Assessment which has a 99% sensitivity. The score factors in age, gender, build, skin condition, mobility, continence, nutrition and special factors, e.g. diabetes, heart failure (see Appendix 9).

3 Reduce immobility. Avoid long lies on hard trolleys in the emergency department, radiology, etc. Patients going to theatre should be placed on adequate pressure mattresses. Ensure patients are not left sitting in one position in a chair for more than 2 h.

4 Minimize sedation.

5 Position patients carefully; a pillow between the knees prevents pressure on the medial aspects.

6 Relieve pressure when immobility is unavoidable, e.g. by regular turning, mechanical devices (low air loss mattresses which support the patient on multiple air-filled cells, air-fluidized mattresses, waterbeds, suspension techniques), or protect vulnerable areas, e.g. heel protectors, inflatable troughs, wheelchair cushions.

7 Monitor nutrition, and refer to dietician if necessary.

8 Maintain perfusion pressure, i.e. support BP and maintain good hydration.

9 Optimize general health: treat heart failure and maximize haemoglobin level, transfusing if necessary.

10 Keep the skin dry, consider catheterization.

Encourage healing

1 Measure the wound's length, width and depth accurately, and describe the edges: look for exudate, black eschar, necrotic tissue and granulation tissue. This allows effective monitoring of progress. A photograph may be useful.

2 Clean the sore, e.g. surgically, by debridement, or chemically, with preparations as directed by local policy. Choices include povidone iodine or normal saline.

3 Use appropriate systemic antibiotics for cellulitis, septicaemia or osteomyelitis of underlying bone; include cover for anaerobic organisms.

4 Consider nutritional supplements, including vitamin C and zinc, and correct anaemia.

5 Dressings depend on the nature of the ulcer.
   - Early, superficial ulcers can be managed with transparent adhesive films which are semipermeable but occlusive. They prevent secondary infection and maintain healthy margins.
   - For wounds with more exudate, hydrocolloid dressings combine with moisture in the wound to form a gel; they keep the skin moist, reduce odour, and can often be left in situ for several days.
   - Gel dressings keep the wound moist and reduce bacterial infection.
   - Calcium alginate dressings are very absorptive and are used for wounds with high levels of exudate. Do not allow deep sores to become sealed off: packing the cavity with colloid or alginate encourages healing from the base of the ulcer.
   - Charcoal dressings (to absorb smell) are useful in malignant ulcers, e.g. breast cancers. Metronidazole gel also helps reduce exudate and associated odour.

6 If the sore is large, enlisting the help of the plastic surgery team for split skin grafting may be the quickest form of healing.

7 Do not forget to treat pain.

European Pressure Ulcer Advisory Panel classification system of pressure ulcer grades

Grade 1: non-blanchable erythema of intact skin. Other warning signs include skin discoloration, warmth, oedema and induration which might be helpful in patients with darker skin.

Grade 2: partial thickness skin loss involving epidermis or dermis, or both. The ulcer is superficial and presents clinically as an abrasion or blister.

Grade 3: full thickness skin loss involving damage to or necrosis of subcutaneous tissue that may extend down to, but not through, underlying fascia.

Grade 4: extensive destruction, tissue necrosis, or damage to muscle, bone or supporting structures with or without full thickness skin loss.

Pruritus

This is common in older people, who are predisposed by dry skin (see Table 15.3).

- Significantly reduces quality of life.
- Can prevent patient and their partner/carers from sleeping.
- Can cause depression and agitation.
- Sometimes surprisingly intractable especially if patients unable to apply creams themselves because of arthritis, or compliance is limited because of dementia.
- The itch–scratch cycle occurs because scratching causes inflammation of the skin which releases mediators including histamine, serotonin, prostaglandins and cytokines which trigger

unmyelinated C nerve fibres which fire off to the thalamus via the spinothalamic tract. Motor fibres from the cortex lead to more scratching and the cycle continues. Eventually the skin is damaged and its barrier function is breeched, allowing superadded infections to occur.

An approach to management

- Take a good history to make diagnosis where possible.
- New onset itch might suggest a reaction to a new drug or infestation.
- Heat often worsens itch.
- Careful examination to exclude infestation/infection or other cause as in Table 15.3.
- Routine blood tests to exclude a metabolic or systemic cause: FBC, ferritin, urea, bilirubin, alkaline phosphatase, TSH.
- Encourage patient to drink plenty (at least eight glasses of water per day).
- Avoid hot baths. Use aqueous cream as soap/shower gel substitute.
- Pat skin dry, avoid rubbing.
- Moisturize within 5 min of leaving the bath, preferably with a ceramide lipid-based emollient which traps the absorbed water and reduces evaporation.
- Educate the patient to avoid scratching: trim fingernails!
- Use steroid creams or ointments for short periods only for true inflammatory eczema.
- Consider antihistamines for sedative effect.
- Cooling preparations, e.g. menthol, may help by masking the itch.

Other important skin conditions in geriatric medicine

1 **Shingles**: suspect wherever you see crops of vesicles and scabs in a dermatomal distribution. The subsequent pain and debility and risk of chicken pox to others present the most serious aspects of this condition (see Chapter 8).
2 **Pemphigus vulgaris** is an autoimmune condition where autoantibodies to desmoglein 1 and desmoglein 3 molecules on the keratinocyte surface cause loss of cell-to-cell adhesion, leading to severe superficial blistering and erosions of the skin. The lesions tend to start in the mouth and spread to other areas of the skin. It is a life-threatening condition because of the high risk of secondary infection and massive loss of protein. It requires treatment with high doses of steroids. There is much ongoing research into the use of immunomodulating agents such as tacrolimus and mycophenolate.
3 **Bullous pemphigoid** is a similar but more common and much less severe condition. It is more common in women. The blisters may be large and tense because the immunological lesion is deeper, targeting the basement membrane. IgG autoantibodies are directed to hemidesmosomal bullous pemphigoid antigens. Mouth ulceration is less common. The skin changes may be more localized and in practice the blisters often burst. Again, oral steroids are used, at high dose initially until the lesions are under control and then a lower maintenance dose.
4 **Intertrigo** is moist seborrhoeic eczema, which is often secondarily infected with fungi, e.g. *Candida*. It is especially common in obese individuals and where there is close skin-to-skin contact under pendulous breasts, abdominal aprons and between the buttocks. Better personal hygiene and treatment with antifungal preparations is required.
5 **Solar (or actinic) keratosis**: occurs on sun-exposed areas such as the face, ears, bald scalp, forearms and hands. It starts as a small rough area of skin but may develop into larger (3–10 mm) hyperkeratotic plaques. It is more common in men. Treatment options include topical 5 fluorouracil, photodynamic therapy and surgical excision. If left untreated, it may develop into a squamous carcinoma or a basal cell carcinoma.
6 **Drug reactions** can present as any lesion, from eruptions to purpura. Pathological thinning of the skin secondary to chronic steroid use is another common example.
7 **Ulceration** can be secondary to trauma complicating other pathology.
8 **Rosacea** typically occurs in older women with fair skins; characterized by erythema, telangiectasia and pustules on nose, cheeks and forehead. Occasionally men develop a severe form with hypertrophy of sebaceous glands and skin of the nose producing disfiguring rhinophyma. It seems to be triggered by stress, high temperatures, hot drinks and alcohol. Treatment includes oral tetracyclines, topical metronidazole or topical permethrin. Laser therapy can reduce the appearance of telangiectasia and rhinophyma.

Malignant diseases of the skin

The major predisposing factor in fair-skinned people is excessive exposure to sunlight.

Basal-cell carcinoma (BCC)

BCC is the most common skin malignancy (accounts for 80% of skin cancers) and it usually occurs in sun-damaged skin. It arises as a pearly papule, usually on the upper face, ears or scalp. It slowly, but inexorably, enlarges. Typically it is scaly and erythematous with a rolled edge with telangiectasia and a central ulcerated area. Metastatic spread is extremely rare. A BCC is easily removed in early stage by curettage. It is preferable to remove BCCs when they are small to preserve nearby organs such as the eyes, ears and nose. If the BCC is close to the eye it is better to surgically excise the lesion to determine the margin of the tumour. Larger lesions may require radiotherapy. If they are ignored, they can cause significant local destruction, hence the common name 'rodent ulcer'.

Bowen's disease: intraepidermal epithelioma

These lesions appear as single scaly, erythematous plaques, usually in sun-exposed areas. They are squamous-cell carcinomas (SCCs) that have not invaded beyond the epidermis. They are treated with cryotherapy, surgical excision or radiotherapy.

Squamous-cell carcinoma (SCC)

SCC is less common than BCC. It presents as a reddened, indurated ulcer, nodule or plaque. SCC often arises in sun-exposed areas, e.g. in a solar keratosis or patch of Bowen's disease, but also in other situations where the skin has been damaged, such as chronic venous ulcers of the lower leg. SCC is becoming more common, perhaps secondary to greater sun exposure of the general public. It may metastasize to lymph glands. Once the diagnosis is confirmed by biopsy, it should be excised or treated with radiotherapy.

Malignant melanoma

These are expanding pigmented lesions, again usually, but not always, arising in sun-exposed skin. They require early wide excision because of high risk of metastases.

Hair and nails

Age changes

1 *Hair* – becomes thinner and more brittle and loses its natural colour. Baldness may occur in both sexes but with differing distribution. Body hair is lost in the same order as its acquisition. Facial hair increases in women.
2 *Nails* – become thicker and harder; onychogryphosis when extreme.

Pathological changes

1 Retention of hair colour is said to indicate hypothyroidism. If the hair is especially dry, this also may be a sign of hypothyroidism.
2 Exaggerated hair loss may indicate hypopituitarism or Addison's disease, or be a consequence of cytotoxic therapy.
3 Toe nails may be neglected because of difficulty with maintenance due to visual impairment, arthritis or stroke disease.
4 Brittle and deformed nails may indicate systemic disease, e.g. deficiencies such as calcium or iron. Clubbing, pitting and white bands may indicate disease elsewhere.
5 Discomfort due to toe nail deformity and neglect can seriously impair mobility.
6 Extra care is needed in nail maintenance in patients with peripheral vascular disease and neuropathy, especially diabetics.

➔ FURTHER INFORMATION

Action on Hearing Loss charity: www.actionon-hearingloss.org.uk/.

Cavallotti CAP, Cerulli L (eds) (2008) *Age-Related Changes of the Human Eye*. Humana Press, New York.

Finlay AY (ed.) (2000) *Dermatology Parts 1 & 2. Medicine*, Vol. 28: 11 and 12. The Medicine Publishing Group, New York.

Harvey PT (2003) Common eye diseases of elderly people: identifying and treating causes of vision loss. *Gerontology* 49: 1–11.

Macular degeneration website useful for patients: www.macula.org/.

NICE Guidelines for Pressure Ulcer Prevention: http://guidance.nice.org.uk/CG29/QuickRef-Guide/pdf/English.

NICE Guidelines on Treatment of Wet AMD: http://guidance.nice.org.uk/TA155/QuickRef-Guide/pdf/English.

RNIB information regarding registration as being blind/partially sighted: http://www.rnib.org.uk/livingwithsightloss/registeringsightloss/Pages/vision_criteria.aspx

RNIB patient information on AMD: http://www.rnib.org.uk/eyehealth/eyeconditions/conditionsac/Pages/amd.aspx.

Sprinzl GM, Riechelmann H (2010) Current trends in treating hearing loss in elderly people: a review of the technology and treatment options – a mini-review. *Gerontology* 56: 351–358, doi: 10.1159/000275062

16

Legal and ethical aspects of medical care of elderly people

Most elderly patients pose no more ethical or legal problems than other adults. In a few cases, particularly where there is mental as well as physical frailty, problems are numerous. Some ethical issues have recently been under the spotlight, with accusations of 'ageism' and 'medical paternalism' being hurled at anyone who dares to suggest that it is sometimes in a patient's best interest to be a little economical with the truth or less than heroic in efforts at resuscitation. Some legal aspects are straightforward, others less so. Ethical problems are often resistant to dogmatic resolution. Remember the four common, basic moral commitments:

1 Respect for autonomy (informed consent, confidentiality).
2 Beneficence.
3 Non-maleficence.
4 Justice:

- Fair distribution of scarce resources (distributive justice – particularly relevant to ageism).
- Respect for people's rights (rights based justice).
- Respect for morally acceptable laws (legal justice).

(Source: Gillon 1994.)
For any ethical issue a framework can help you consider the issues. One example is:

The Ethics Grid (Seedhouse 1998, see discussion by Green).

1 Describe the details of the case.
2 List the possible options for management and, for each, consider the practicalities including:
- any disputed facts or evidence,
- the degree of certainty around the facts,
- likely effectiveness of the action,
- the risk,
- resources available,
- wishes of others,
- codes of practice,
- the law.
3 Look at the consequences to find the most beneficial outcome for:
- yourself,
- a particular group,
- the individual,
- society.
4 Remember duties:
- tell the truth,
- keep promises,
- do most good,
- do least harm.
5 Remember core ethical concepts:
- respect/create autonomy,
- serve needs first,
- respect persons equally.

Lecture Notes Elderly Care Medicine, Eighth Edition. Claire G. Nicholl and K. Jane Wilson.
© 2012 John Wiley & Sons, Ltd. Published 2012 by John Wiley & Sons, Ltd.

Driving in later life

UK *law* obliges everyone to surrender their driving licence at the age of 70. A new licence is issued, which is valid for 3 years but can be renewed every 3 years on completion of a declaration of good health. The *insurance company* may insist on a medical examination. It is a person's duty to inform the Driver and Vehicle Licensing Authority (DVLA) of any change in health status. Certain conditions will render the individual unfit to drive and the patient must be informed:

- Episodic impairment of consciousness (e.g. epilepsy, hypotension, severe vertigo, poorly controlled diabetes).
- Paroxysmal symptomatic cardiac arrhythmia and severe coronary artery disease (e.g. angina at the wheel).
- Severe PD.
- Fluctuating or declining cognitive function.
- Uncorrectable visual impairment, particularly significant field defects.
- MI, pacemaker insertion, stroke with good recovery or TIA (for at least a month).

Always check details of the length of driving restrictions on the DVLA website. Advice for older drivers includes:

- Avoid distractions such as chatty passengers and changing CDs.
- If a long journey is unavoidable, take adequate breaks.
- If the route is unfamiliar, make advance preparations and allow plenty of time.
- Avoid rush hour and night driving.

Two ethical dilemmas are common:

1 A patient with one of the disorders listed above refuses to accept advice to stop driving.
2 A patient without a proscribed condition, but with a degree of cognitive impairment such that the doctor is convinced they are unsafe.

When advising someone to stop driving, suggest that 'the other drivers on the road ... so much more traffic, drivers are less courteous these days, if someone else did something silly it might take longer for you to weigh up the options', etc. If you fail to persuade them to give up driving, a family member may be prepared to try, particularly if they have experienced a terrifying ride as a passenger. Suggest seeking the opinion of a professional driving instructor or a session at a driving assessment centre (e.g. www.rdac.co.uk, staffed by therapists, fee for assessment, but enabling where appropriate).

If a patient continues to drive after being advised to stop, it becomes the doctor's duty to the public to inform the DVLA (tell the patient also).

Confidentiality

Older people have the same rights as everyone else to confidentiality. If older people are dependent on others, the family will need to be informed, but do discuss this with the patient first.

The Mental Capacity Act (MCA) 2005

This came into force in 2007 and is a statutory framework:

- To empower and protect vulnerable adults who are not able to make their own decisions ranging from the daily, e.g. what to eat, to the occasional but serious, e.g. consent to surgery.
- To enable people to plan for a time when they may lack capacity.

Who needs to know about the MCA?

If you have a patient who lacks capacity, this may affect how they are managed in a number of ways:

1 If they are to be discharged from hospital to different accommodation.
2 If decisions are to be made about serious medical treatment, e.g.:
   - Decisions about surgery.
   - Medical investigation.
   - Cancer treatment.
   - Dialysis.
   - Feeding tubes.
3 If they are to be included in drug trials.

The MCA will affect how you consult family and friends and the patient may need an advocate.

Serious medical treatment

This is defined as providing, withdrawing or withholding treatment where:

- There is a fine balance between benefits/burdens and risks, e.g. deciding whether to amputate a gangrenous foot in a patient who has just had a stroke.
- Choice of treatments is finely balanced, e.g. type of chemotherapy in advanced breast cancer.
- What is proposed would have serious consequences for the patient.

Five principles underpinned by the MCA

1 There is presumption of capacity, unless demonstrated otherwise.
2 Individuals should be supported to make their own decisions.
3 People retain the right to make an eccentric or unwise decision.
4 Others must act in the best interests of the patient.
5 If an intervention is needed, it should be the least restrictive.

Assessment of capacity

This is only considered if the patient has impairment of brain function. Capacity is decision and time-specific, i.e. a person may be able to decide what to eat and to make a will, but may not be able to decide about returning home. However, the situation may be different tomorrow.

In order to have capacity, the person must be able to:

1 *Understand* information relevant to the decision (consequences of deciding one way or another or failing to make the decision).
2 *Retain* that information for long enough to decide (even though they may then forget a decision had been made).
3 *Use* that information as part of the process of making the decision.
4 *Communicate* the decision (any method including sign language, squeezing the hand).

Advance decisions

The MCA puts the status of advance decisions on a statutory footing. A person:

1 Can specify what treatment they would not want and under what circumstances.
2 Cannot demand treatment.

The advance decision must have been made when the person had capacity to be valid. It only applies to the circumstance described, e.g. 'I do not want resuscitation if I cannot speak after a stroke' will not influence treatment after a heart attack. To refuse life-sustaining treatment, the advance decision must be in writing, signed and witnessed and specify 'even if life is at risk'. If the person is detained under the Mental Health Act (MHA), this takes precedence over the MCA.

Lasting power of attorney

This is the method by which a person with capacity can choose who will look after his or her affairs in the future if capacity is lost.

1 Replaces Enduring Power of Attorney (EPA), which only looked after property and affairs.
2 The donor confers on the *attorney* (a person of their choice, usually a relative or friend) authority to make decisions about all or any of:
   - The donor's health and personal welfare.
   - The donor's property and affairs.
3 Lasting Power of Attorney (LPA) must be registered (Office of the Public Guardian).
4 If your patient lacks capacity and has a personal welfare LPA, the attorney will discuss the patient's treatment with you.

A patient who has a moderate estate but does not have capacity to take out an LPA should be referred to the Court of Protection. Application may be made by a relative, the solicitor or the doctor. A medical certificate is required and the court will usually appoint an interested relative or other suitable person as a deputy, to act as the patient's agent, but not to dispose of assets. Where the assets only consist of social security benefits, the Department of Social Security can nominate an *appointee* to deploy them for the person's benefit.

Court of protection (2007)

This is a specialist court that:

1 Declares whether a person has capacity if there is dispute.
2 Makes decisions about health care/treatment.
3 Makes decisions about property/financial affairs.
4 Appoints deputies (previously receivers) to have ongoing authority.
5 Makes decisions in relation to LPA and EPAs.

The court can issue a declaration that a proposed treatment would be lawful. In considering the patient's best interests, the court will be guided by the *Bolam test*, which simply asks whether the treatment would be supported by a responsible body of medical opinion. An approach to the court is best made through the hospital's legal services manager or, in an emergency, through the duty manager. One source of uncertainty is whether a refusal to be treated reflects a depressive illness where it would be necessary to seek a psychiatric opinion. People are allowed to make unusual decisions: the judgement in the highly publicized case of 'Miss B' in the UK (2002) gives a strong steer to the profession that, providing the patient is competent, the stated wishes should be respected however apparently irrational. The public guardian and his office run the affairs of the court. It is now a criminal offence to mistreat a person lacking capacity.

Independent mental capacity advocates (IMCA)

1 Most people who lack capacity have support from family and friends (or an attorney or deputy).
2 If there is no such person (or they are 'not practicable or appropriate' to consult) and a decision is needed about serious medical treatment (not emergency) and change of accommodation, there is a duty to instruct an IMCA. They will need access to and be able to copy health/ social care records.

The duties of an IMCA

1 Support the person who lacks capacity and represent their views and interests to the decision maker.
2 Obtain and evaluate information.
3 Ascertain the person's wishes, feelings, beliefs and values.
4 Ascertain alternative courses of action.
5 Obtain a further medical opinion if necessary.
6 Challenge a decision if necessary in the patient's interests.

Consent

Consent must be sought for all medical interventions, although this will often be a very informal process and sometimes only implied. Without it, the health care professional has committed the crime of *battery*. Written forms are highly desirable for surgical procedures and research involving drug trials or other interventions, although oral consent is equally valid in law. Consent must be *informed*, which means that the doctor must provide the necessary information, and ambiguities can arise concerning just how much information has been imparted and whether it was couched in appropriate and readily assimilable terms. Consent must also be voluntary, i.e. no undue pressure must have been exerted on the patient.

Testamentary capacity

Testamentary capacity means mental competence in the single connection of drawing up (or revoking) a will. In order to be capable of this act, a person needs to:

• Understand the nature of such an act.
• Have a reasonable grasp of the extent of their assets, so an assessing doctor has to have at least a vague idea of the patient's circumstances.
• Be aware which persons have some claim on their property.
• Be free of delusions which might distort their judgement.

Emergency symptomatic treatment of the incompetent patient

In practice, this implies the parenteral sedation of the acutely confused, disturbed patient whose restlessness or aggressive behaviour is a danger to themselves or, less commonly, to others. It is permissible under common law to hold the patient down to administer an injection as a last resort and for their own protection, if other physicians would regard it as appropriate and if reasonable people would want the treatment themselves. The procedure is deeply distressing to one and all and can usually be avoided (see also Chapter 4).

Restraints

Sedation is a form of chemical restraint and has been termed a 'pharmacological straitjacket' but may be temporarily necessary in the acutely confused, ambulant patient until investigations and treatment rectify the condition. Patients may fall while trying to get out of bed, so fitting bedrails only ensures that the fall occurs from a greater height. Nursing them on a very low bed or even a mattress on the floor may be preferable but this can be seen as a form of physical restraint. Frail subjects may receive some protection from bedrails, which remind them to ask for help to go to the toilet and prevent them from slithering from the side of the bed to the floor. Tilting or 'bucket' chairs should be avoided where possible, but poor staffing levels and a rising tide of complaints and litigation has made the prevention of falls by any means a higher priority for management than respect for autonomy.

Environmental restraints

Environmental restraints include doors that, although not locked, are difficult to open, or a barricaded kitchen in the home, both occasionally necessary for the individual's protection. The gas supply to the cooker may be disconnected and hot meals delivered instead. A controversial restraint is the *electronic tag*, which triggers an alarm if the patient leaves the hospital ward. This may infringe civil liberties but less so, perhaps, than having your life support systems switched off as you lie in ITU by a disorientated patient who wanders in and wants to plug a toaster into an inconveniently occupied socket! Whatever type of restraint is used, the method, the reasons and the arrangements for review should be documented.

Deprivation of liberty

The Deprivation of Liberty Safeguards (DOLS) were introduced into the MCA 2005 by the MHA 2007 and have been operative since April 2009. The aim is to provide legal protection for vulnerable adults (mainly with learning disabilities and dementia), who are not detained under the MHA but are restricted in their freedom due to their inability to consent to care or accept treatment. The safeguards apply to patients in hospitals and care homes and are designed to ensure compliance with the European Convention of Human Rights which first highlighted the human rights infringement in the Bournewood case (HL v UK). The care of such individuals should be the least restrictive possible and contact with family or friends should be encouraged. If hospitals and care homes are depriving people of their liberty, this needs to be minimized and registered.

The Mental Health Act (Table 16.1)

The MHA 2007 amends the MHA 1983 and the MCA 2005 and is an Act of the Parliament of the UK that applies to people in England and Wales.

It introduced significant changes which include:

- Introduction of Supervised Community Treatment which enables a person to be forcibly medicated.
- The patient may appoint a civil partner as nearest relative.
- A new definition of mental disorder throughout the Act.

Most people in psychiatric hospitals are informal patients who have agreed to admission. Twenty-five percent are formal patients, compulsorily detained under a section of the MHA.

Ethical issues relating to life-supporting interventions

Cardiopulmonary resuscitation (CPR)

CPR is the issue that ferments the most emotion. This is because of massive publicity in the media, which has led to a widespread misconception by the public that the 'do not attempt cardiopulmonary resuscitation' (DNACPR) decision by hospital staff is the major determinant of life or death during the admission. There is a great deal of pressure on staff to introduce this topic at their first encounter with the patient. Yes, it is

Table 16.1 Sections under the Mental Health Act

Section	Use	Applicant	Signatory	Duration
Section 2	Admission for assessment	Nearest relative or AMHP	Two doctors: a Section 12 approved doctor (trained in MHA) and (usually) patient's GP	28 days
Section 3	Admission for treatment		As above	Up to 6 months, unless consultant discharges the patient, renewable
Section 4	Emergency admission	As above, but must have seen patient in last 24 h	Any doctor	72 h
Section 5	Holding power	A doctor can detain a patient needing treatment (including for physical illness). A psychiatric nurse can detain an informal patient for 6 h until the clinician in charge arrives	Hospital manager is informed by the doctor that an application for a compulsory admission 'ought to be made'	72 h
Section 7	Guardianship, more often used in the USA and Canada than the UK. A guardian is appointed to direct the affairs of an incapacitous person	As above	Two registered practitioners. Guardian is local authority social services or their appointee	Up to 6 months, renewable
Section 135	Warrant to search for and remove a person	A magistrate issues a warrant on sufficient grounds of mental illness and being unable to care for themselves	Doctor and AMHP (accompanied by police can enter any premise where the person is believed to be)	72 h maximum
Section 47; National Assistance Act (1948, amended 1951)	Removal to place of safety, e.g. geriatric or psychogeriatric ward or care home, rarely used	GP, social worker or police apply to director of public health for compulsory removal of older person from a life-threatening situation	Requires authority of magistrate. Specialist advice required in view of human rights legislation; Section 135 preferred.	3 weeks

AMHP, Approved Mental Health Professional.

important, but it only applies to cardiorespiratory arrest, and except in the setting of ACS in coronary care, CPR has a very low success rate. In studies, which are always of patients selected for CPR, about 20% of patients survive resuscitation, but only about 14% will leave hospital, and only 4% of those will be over the age of 75. It is a procedure about which patients, relatives and hospital staff harbour unrealistic expectations.

A DNACPR decision should be taken by the most senior doctor available, ideally after discussion with the patient, the team and, with the permission of the competent patient, the relatives, regularly reviewed, and recorded in the notes, together with the reason. A DNACPR order is appropriate:

- Where CPR is not in accordance with the sustained wishes of the patient.
- Where successful CPR would be followed by a quantity and quality of life that would be unacceptable to the patient.
- Where the patient already has a poor quality of life they do not wish to have prolonged.
- Where effective CPR is unlikely to be successful, e.g. the treatment is futile. This applies to patients with:
  o Terminal cancer (death expected in days or weeks).
  o Sepsis.
  o Pneumonia on admission.
  o Kidney failure.
  o Hypotension.
  o Severe disability.
  o Deteriorating consciousness, e.g. severe stroke.
  o Arrest due to GI haemorrhage.

However competent the patient, no discussion needs to be held in this situation. The General Medical Council (GMC) advises: 'While some patients may want to be told, others may find discussion about interventions that would not be clinically appropriate burdensome and of little or no value'. If a patient lacks capacity, you should **inform** any legal proxy and others close to the patient about the DNACPR decision and the reasons for it.

A DNACPR decision is not a proxy for other decisions and does not imply 'not for treatment'; the patient must continue to receive appropriate treatment for their condition.

The intensive therapy unit (ITU)

The usual reason for considering admission to ITU is to access respiratory support, e.g. by ventilation,

for life-threatening respiratory failure due to airway obstruction, pneumonia, neurological disorders or drug overdose. The dilemma is to avoid deaths when the cause is reversible (asthma, Guillain–Barré syndrome) but also avoid prolongation of life when the outlook is hopeless (end-stage emphysema, motor neuron disease). Other considerations are similar to those governing CPR: the patient's and relatives' wishes and the previous quality of life. Unlike cardiac arrest, one of the commonest causes of respiratory failure, COPD, is predictable and will end in respiratory failure; so the patient's wishes can, ideally, be ascertained while they are well. Age *per se* is not a bar to ventilation.

Invasive methods of nutrition and hydration

- Nasogastric (NG) or percutaneous gastrostomy (PEG) feeding and intravenous or subcutaneous fluids are considered to be medical treatment [GMC and British Medical Association (BMA)].
- If a patient lacks capacity and cannot eat or drink enough to meet their needs, the doctor must assess whether providing clinically assisted nutrition or hydration would be of overall benefit.
- As with other treatments, the patient's wishes are the key issue. Discuss what the patient would have wanted if known or their best interests with input from the family, friends or an IMCA. If after discussion the doctor still considers that the treatment would not be of benefit, there is no obligation to provide it. However, as well as a full explanation a second opinion should be offered.
- Even food and drink by mouth (basic care rather than treatment) may lead to choking and aspiration.
- NG tubes look unsightly to the family, are often pulled out by patients (even when bridled) and are associated with reflux and aspiration. Placing a PEG tube in a frail patient has risks including death. Skin infections, tube blockage and aspiration occur and patients may also pull these out.
- Stroke, terminal cancer and advanced dementia are common situations where feeding and hydration issues arise. In stroke, except where the prognosis looks hopeless, it should initially be assumed that recovery is possible so hydration and nutrition are generally provided. Many cancer patients are able to express their wishes and in the later stages the clear trajectory of the illness may make the timing of decisions easier.

Patients with advanced dementia are perhaps the most difficult. Oropharyngeal dysphagia and aspiration are common. Eating and drinking, even small amounts, may be a last remaining pleasure. The drive to eat and drink is very basic. Keeping a patient 'nil by mouth' and tube feeding them when they cannot understand why they are not offered food or drink may be both unkind and futile as tube feeding does not prevent aspiration. Speech and language therapists and dieticians can provide useful input. Generally the best approach is to offer the safest texture of food (usually puree) and thickened fluids, when the patient is alert and well-positioned, pausing if aspiration is suspected. This is time consuming and requires skill. If the patient does not take a sufficient amount it is unlikely they are experiencing hunger or thirst. It can be distressing to watch a visibly dehydrating terminal patient. However, it may be considered that 'the ethical situation is not that the patient is failing to drink and therefore will die, but that the patient is dying and therefore does not wish to drink'. In England, Wales and Northern Ireland, the withdrawal or withholding of artificial nutrition and hydration (ANH) from a patient in a persistent vegetative state needs to be subject to court review, but this is rarely encountered in old age.

(See p. 000 for evidence that tube feeding in advanced dementia is not beneficial.)

Age discrimination

Ageism is another hot topic and is said to remain widespread throughout the NHS, despite the measures outlined in the National Service Framework (NSF) for Older People. In a book on geriatric medicine, the easy option would be to make a sweeping condemnation of it as an evil similar to racial or gender discrimination. When based upon blind prejudice, this may be so. But age discrimination is often based on three rational and humane, if misconceived, principles:

- Older people are denied access to high-tech interventions on the basis that they do much less well than younger ones. There are usually studies available that indicate just how beneficial each intervention is for elderly subjects; to use chronological age as a proxy for cardiorespiratory, functional and cognitive assessment is lazy.

- The potential quantity and quality of life are too low to justify the procedure under consideration. Life expectancies for otherwise well elderly people are surprisingly high, and quality of life can only be assessed by that person and is consistently underestimated by doctors and others.

- To make such interventions available to older patients is to deny them to younger ones. It is not the role of physicians to compare how deserving their patients are. Politicians should accept responsibility for rationing when resources are inadequate. If asked, older people are often very altruistic about resource allocation but this may change as the baby boomer generation reaches old age.

Elder abuse

Old age abuse is difficult both to define and to detect. It takes many forms:

- Physical – pushing, punching, slapping, overdosing or withholding medication.
- Psychological – verbal abuse, shouting, swearing, blaming, humiliating.
- Financial – 'asset-stripping'.
- Emotional.
- Neglect – withholding food, drink and warmth.

Risk factors

Victim

- Heavy dependency, communication difficulties.
- Dementia.
- Behavioural problems, aggression.

Shared

- Poor housing.
- Poor long-term relationship.

Carer

- Excessive alcohol consumption.
- Changed lifestyle due to caring role.
- Divided loyalties, e.g. elderly parent and child.
- Health problems, including psychiatric.
- Role reversal, ageing child and aged parent.
- Isolation, real or perceived.

- Sexual.
- Cultural – e.g. forcing a vegetarian to eat meat.
- UK and USA studies suggest the prevalence of elder abuse is 5–10% of dependent older people. As countries such as India experience marked demographic change, abuse is now being reported as an issue.

Detection

Although the diagnosis is difficult to substantiate, there are some warning signs:

- Recurrent falls and accidents, unexplained fractures.
- Multiple bruising, especially clear thumbprint bruises to arms sustained while being shaken, or bruises or burns to unusual areas such as flexure surfaces.
- Injury similar in shape to an object.
- Patient tries to hide a part of the body from examination.
- Patient withdrawn, frightened (especially of carer), anxious, makes effort to please.
- Carer complaining of 'nerves' or of being under stress.
- Difficulty gaining access to patient.
- Isolation of patient in one room of home or care setting.
- Refusal by patient and/or carer to accept necessary support services.

Action to be taken

A competent older person has the right to choose to remain in a setting where there is risk of or actual abuse, if they wish to do so. They may be very reluctant to admit to what is going on and support must be offered to make the situation as safe as possible. Vulnerable patients without capacity must be protected. Any discussion must be held in private and, if there are grounds for suspicion, the matter must be pursued through interdisciplinary channels; there should be a local lead agency.

Euthanasia

Euthanasia, the active and intentional termination of a person's life, remains illegal in the UK. If euthanasia were taken in its literal sense of 'a good death', all would be in favour, but most are opposed to the practice of the more generally accepted definitions:

- *Voluntary euthanasia:* the deliberate and intentional hastening of death at the request of a seriously ill patient. This is legal in Belgium, Luxembourg and the Netherlands.
- *Involuntary euthanasia:* ending a person's life without seeking their opinion.
- *Non-voluntary euthanasia:* ending a person's life for their benefit, when they cannot possess or express views whether they should live or die.
- *Physician-assisted suicide:* the patient takes a lethal cocktail that has been prescribed or provided by the physician at the patient's request. Assisted suicide is legal in Switzerland and the US states of Oregon, Washington and Montana.

It is perfectly acceptable morally and legally to administer increasing doses of sedative and analgesic drugs that may, incidentally, shorten life (which they actually seldom do), if the doctor's intention is to provide effective pain relief – the so-called double effect.

To withhold potentially life-prolonging treatment is sometimes called *passive euthanasia* and some ethicists regard it as morally indistinguishable from active euthanasia. But, as we have seen, no doctor is obliged to initiate or continue treatment that they consider futile.

While suicide or travelling abroad to receive assisted suicide are not illegal, facilitating suicide is a criminal offence. As yet, no doctor providing a report nor any accompanying person has been prosecuted for helping patients to travel abroad to end their lives, but this remains a contentious area.

Death certification and the role of the coroner

After a death at home, the GP should see the body to confirm and certify death. In hospital, deaths are commonly confirmed by the nursing staff. The certificate is then completed by a hospital doctor, except in those cases where the coroner needs to be informed. The Department of Health (2010) has produced a useful summary on improving death certification.

Her majesty's coroner

Doctors must exercise their judgement in individual cases, but when in doubt, ring the coroner's office. The following deaths should be reported:

- Death of a person not attended by a doctor during their last illness.
- Death of a person not seen by a doctor either within 14 days before death or after death.
- Cause of death unknown.
- Deaths after accidents including falls, misadventure, starvation, severe deprivation (neglect) including hypothermia, poisoning.
- Drugs, whether therapeutic or of addiction, or abuse, including alcohol.
- Anaesthetic, surgical or medical mishap or when relatives express serious dissatisfaction or allege neglect.
- Deaths within 24 h of an operation.
- Deaths within 24 h of emergency admission should be discussed.
- Industrial diseases, even if not a cause of death.
- Septicaemia of possible unnatural cause.
- Those with disability pensions from service with the Crown.

- Prisoners and anyone in the custody of the police.

Following the Shipman scandal, reform of death certification and the coronial system was promised. Although an Act was passed this is to be partly revoked because of costs. However, some proposed changes are currently being piloted (see Figure 16.1).

Coroners and death certification bill

The main elements of the Bill are to:

- Create a new system of secondary certification of deaths that are not referred to the coroner, covering burials and cremations.
- Establish a new group of medical examiners to scrutinize the causes of death on death certificates.
- Introduce new powers of investigation for coroners, including improved procedures for post mortems and inquests.

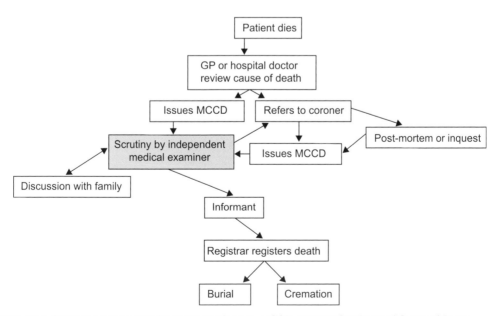

Figure 16.1 Proposed new system for death certification. MCCD, Medical Certificate of Cause of Death.

REFERENCES

Department of Health (2010) *Improving the Process of Death Certification in England and Wales 2010.* http://www.dh.gov.uk/en/Publication-sandstatistics/Publications/PublicationsPolicy AndGuidance/DH_111252.

Gillon (1994) Medical ethics: four principles plus attention to scope. *BMJ* 309: 184, doi: 10.1136/bmj.309.6948.184.

Green B (undated) *Medical Ethics.* Priory Lodge Education Ltd. http://priory.com/ethics.htm.

 ## FURTHER INFORMATION

Action on elder abuse: www.elderabuse.org.uk/.

BMA ethics advice: www.bma.org.uk/ethics/index.jsp.

BMA summary of the Mental Capacity Act: www.bma.org.uk/images/MentalCapacityToolKit %20July2008_tcm41-175571.pdf.

BMA view on end of life decisions: www.bma.org.uk/images/endlifedecisionsaug 2009_tcm41-190116.pdf.

DOLS summary for Greenwich council – a clear summary and early case law: www.greenwich.gov.uk/NR/rdonlyres/2763E986-75BB-45B5-927F-F11A4D994C2F/0/FinalDraftCareHomes-DOLSGuidanceJan2009.pdf.

Driving: www.dft.gov.uk/dvla/medical.aspx.

Example of an agency providing IMCAs in Cambridge: www.voiceability.org/.

GMC guidance on end of life issues, 2010: www.gmc-uk.org/End_of_life.pdf_32486688.pdf.

GMC guidance on ethical issues: www.gmc-uk.org/guidance/ethical_guidance.asp.

HM Coroner, Manchester: www.manchester.gov.uk/download/6147/death_certification-guidance_for_doctors_certifying_cause_of_death. Good summary of what to write in death certificates.

Mental Health Act: www.mind.org.uk/Information/Factsheets/. Type in Mental Health Act.

National Assistance Act: www.healthprotection.org.uk/. Type in National Assistance Act.

Royal College of Psychiatrists: www.rcpsych.ac.uk/mentalhealthinfo.aspx. Information leaflets.

17

Palliative care

Death is a fact of life which is shied away from by most people, including doctors and health care workers who may see death as a failure of treatment. However, it is essential to face the inevitable to plan for a 'good death' for every patient (see box below). Older people tend to be philosophical about dying, but their families sometimes have unrealistic expectations. Ensure that patients and families understand what is happening and why; this reduces dissatisfaction with medical and nursing care and complaints.

In the UK, there is a national drive to make death less of a taboo so that people know more about what to expect. The goal is provision of hospice level of care in all settings including home, with privacy and dignity, optimal symptom control plus spiritual and psychological support. For this to happen, there has to be excellent communication between patients and carers, primary, secondary and social care and the development of coordinated services.

Age and place of death

- In the UK 500,000 people die annually.
- In the UK 80% of deaths occur in people aged over 65.
- Sixty-five percent of women die aged 75 or over.
- Seventy percent of people would choose to die at home, but most deaths occur in institutions, as Table 17.1 shows.
- People over 80 are more likely to die in nursing homes.
- People under 65 are more likely to die at home.

Aspirations for a 'good death'

- Understanding that death is imminent and what is likely to happen.
- Feeling in control.
- Being free of pain and other symptoms.
- Dying at home or place of choice.
- Being with family and friends.
- Resolving personal conflicts and unfinished business (e.g. funeral planned and paid for) and having time to say goodbye.
- Making sense of the universe within personal beliefs and values system.
- Having privacy and dignity.
- Confidence that life will not be prolonged unnecessarily when futile.
- Access to appropriate spiritual and religious support.
- Access to information and expertise of whatever kind is necessary.
- Knowing that one's wishes, including advance statements, are and will be respected.

Table 17.1 **Place of death (based on Office for National Statistics for 2009)**

Percentage of deaths	Location
55%	NHS hospitals
18%	Private hospitals, nursing homes and residential care homes
5%	Hospices
22%	Own home or elsewhere (e.g. public places)

Lecture Notes Elderly Care Medicine, Eighth Edition. Claire G. Nicholl and K. Jane Wilson.
© 2012 John Wiley & Sons, Ltd. Published 2012 by John Wiley & Sons, Ltd.

Recognizing the last year of life

In the UK, 1/3 of general practices now use the Gold Standards Framework (GSF). This aims to improve early identification of patients who are deteriorating. The patient's GP is prompted to consider:

- Would you be surprised if this person were to die in the next 6–12 months?
- Do you think the person is aware?
- Can they be approached to talk about likely trajectory?

If the GPs can identify this group, they can explain the significance of their condition to the patient and their family, provide information, reduce fear of the unknown and offer better planning of supportive and palliative care.

Possible warning signs:

- Recurrent hospital admissions.
- Weight loss > 10% over 6 months, serum albumen < 25 g/L.
- Exhaustion.
- Needing more help with activities of daily living.
- Already on maximal therapy.
- Cardiac cachexia, breathlessness at rest in heart failure.
- Oxygen dependency, right heart failure in COPD.
- Worsening renal failure with nausea, pruritus, fluid overload.
- Deterioration of speech, swallow and aspiration in neurological conditions.

There is a danger that in insisting on observing the patient's right to know, we may neglect the patient's right not to know. It is usually sensible to take some notice of a relative's plea, 'For Heaven's sake don't tell him – it would kill him', but not to be bound by it. If a patient makes it clear that they do not wish to be burdened with diagnostic and prognostic information it is only humane to continue to offer the opportunity but do not force the issue. Remember your duty of confidentiality and do not inform relatives without the explicit consent of a competent patient. The health care team is different because they are all bound by a similar ethical code, but this may not apply to the manager of a care home, so bear this in mind.

Breaking the bad news

There are a few generally accepted guidelines:

- Suggest that the patient asks a family member or friend to be present at an appointed time – this warns them that the situation is serious.
- If possible, take a nurse with you.
- Pre-plan the discussion: check your information, make sure that you have time and ensure privacy.
- Sit beside the patient, signalling that you are willing to spend time.
- Identify the relatives and introduce yourself.
- Start by finding out what the patient already understands. Often the patient will have insight that their dramatic weight loss must be due to a cancer.
- Use a warning shot: 'I am afraid I have some bad news for you.'
- Avoid jargon. Explain in simple terms what the diagnosis is and what that is likely to mean.
- Break the news into small sections and check the patient understands what you have said so far.
- Do not be afraid of eye contact, physical contact or silence.
- If you are ordering more tests explain what they are for.
- Try not to remove all hope or to give a precise prognosis. Offer a second opinion, if wanted.
- Do not be afraid to speak of dying, but only give as much information as they can cope with, and agree to meet again.
- Do not strive for too much detachment – patients and relatives often appreciate it if they see that the doctor or nurse is affected emotionally.
- Undertake to continue support and to relieve symptoms.
- If treatment is palliative explain how the palliative care team, Macmillan nurses, etc. will be involved, as appropriate.
- Ask if the patient or relative has questions.
- If you are asked something you do not know, say you will find out and get back to them.
- Record what was said, and to whom, in the notes.
- When giving relatives the news that the patient is in their last few days/hours, it is helpful to be able to offer the Liverpool Integrated Care Pathway for the Dying (LCP), so that you are actively managing symptoms.

Advanced care planning (ACP)

Although 68% of people asked say they are comfortable talking about death, only 29% have discussed their wishes with their families and only 4% have an advance statement.

ACP has been defined as a process of discussion between the patient, their care providers and often those close to them about their future care. It may lead to:

- An advance statement.
- An advance decision to refuse treatment (ADRT).
- Appointment of a personal welfare LPA.

ACP should be considered in patients with long-term conditions and in the broad context of end of life planning, for example after a person has settled into a care home. A helpful approach is to acknowledge that the person is well at the moment, but ask whether they have views on what they would like to happen in the future. ACP is important in conditions where cognitive deterioration is likely, such as early dementia or PD, but should be encouraged in everyone as 'none of us has a crystal ball'. An advance statement of wishes may be hard to draw up because of the huge number of variables and in English law a person cannot demand treatment, for example tube feeding. A general discussion may benefit the family and at least ensure that a will is made and there is some discussion about funeral arrangements. However, it may be easier to specify what is not wanted.

Advanced decision to refuse treatment (ADRT)

Competent patients may choose to refuse treatments such as PEG tubes, dialysis and antibiotics. Usually patients draw up these forms with their family and GP. The decisions are legally binding and doctors should respect them. Refusing treatment may result in an earlier death, and the patient must be made aware of this and specifically include this on their form. If a patient no longer has capacity but has an LPA the attorney must be involved in discussions about the person's health care.

Hospice care

- Still regarded as the gold standard provider of palliative and end of life care.
- Offers short in-patient admissions to control difficult symptoms with a view to getting the patient home to die, if that is their choice.
- Day care facilities for symptom control.
- Opportunities to address emotional and spiritual needs.
- May provide outreach to a wider group of patients dying at home.

Symptom control

Pain

Whereas acute pain which lasts for 2–4 h is treated with analgesia as needed, chronic pain, which is common in advanced disease, is better managed with longer acting analgesics given in anticipation of pain. The dose will require titration to the individual patient. The principles are the same whether the cause is malignancy or an inoperable gangrenous leg. The usual concept is that of the 'analgesic ladder'. This implies a long and weary climb to the top, whereas in practice the number of steps is usually only two or three.

1 Paracetamol, given regularly, has been proven to reduce even severe pain. NSAIDs are generally avoided in old age but have a role in bone secondaries.
2 The next step is a 'weak' opioid. Many avoid high dose codeine in older people as the side-effects of nausea, constipation and confusion are often disproportionally high for the additional analgesia. A synthetic opioid analogue is often used. Meptazinol seems to cause less confusion and constipation than tramadol (although this is much cheaper).
3 Strong opioids are usually given regularly, with additional doses as needed for breakthrough pain. Oral, rectal, transdermal and injectable preparations are available. In the UK, the principal drugs are morphine and diamorphine, although the latter is illegal in other countries, notably the USA, where hydromorphone is used instead. Diamorphine is more soluble than morphine, permitting the injection of smaller

volumes, making it comfortable to administer subcutaneously and it may cause less nausea. In addition to analgesia, some gain benefit from the euphoriant effect of these drugs, but others find this distressing.

The main problems associated with strong opioids are:

- *Drowsiness,* may be unacceptable, but it usually wears off within a few days.
- *Constipation* is universal. Prescribe a strong laxative such as Movicol or co-danthramer (restricted to terminally ill patients because of its carcinogenic risk), which combines lubricant and stimulant properties.
- *Nausea.* Co-prescribe regular anti-emetics initially, but again nausea usually wears off (see Table 17.2).
- *Respiratory depression, cough suppression and hypotension* seldom limit use of these agents in end of life care.
- *Tolerance and addiction.* These are not issues in end of life care, but explain this to the patient so they don't ration themselves.

Causes of pain requiring specific treatments

1 *Neuropathic pain:* responds better to tricyclic antidepressants, anticonvulsants (e.g. pregabalin, gabapentin or valproate) or transcutaneous electrical nerve stimulation (TENS) than conventional analgesics. Nerve blocks and other specialist interventions may be required.
2 *Bony metastases:* NSAIDs with a proton pump inhibitor (PPI); avoid if serious risk of GI bleeding] or intravenous bisphosphonates are often helpful. Hormonal treatment usually relieves the pain of prostatic secondaries, and a single bony deposit will respond well to a palliative dose of radiotherapy.
3 *Headache due to raised intracranial pressure:* dexamethasone 16 mg in divided doses at breakfast and lunch-time (not at night as it increases alertness) is given for a week and then reduced by 2 mg a week to 4–6 mg daily.
4 *Nerve compression:* dexamethasone 8 mg orally a day can help; consider local anaesthetic infiltration.

Table 17.2 Causes and treatment of nausea and vomiting

Symptoms	Clinical pattern	Causes	Drug treatment
Persistent, severe nausea, little vomiting	Chemical/ metabolic	Uraemia Hypercalcaemia Opioids Chemotherapy	Haloperidol Granisetron
Early satiety. Intermittent mild nausea, large volume vomiting	Gastric stasis/ outflow obstruction	Drugs including opioids, anticholinergics Local tumour Hepatomegaly	Metoclopramide
Dysphagia with little nausea relieved by vomiting	Regurgitation	Oesophageal or mediastinal disease	Dexamethasone
Intermittent nausea, completely relieved by vomiting Large volume vomiting, may be faeculent, sometimes with little warning May be associated abdominal pain, distension, constipation	Bowel obstruction	Malignant; tumour in lumen, within bowel wall or pressing on bowel wall Benign: post-op adhesions, secondary to radiotherapy Oedema of bowel wall secondary to inflammation Faecal impaction	Metoclopramide only if no colic Hyoscine butylbromide if colic present Cyclizine and/or haloperidol Octreotide
Headaches, nausea, worse in the mornings	Intracranial disease	Intracranial tumour Cranial radiotherapy Raised intracranial pressure	Dexamethasone Cyclizine
Mixture of above symptoms	Multiple causes	Combination of above	Levomepromazine

Using morphine

1 Start with oral morphine sulphate solution or tablets, e.g. 5 mg regularly 4 hourly. Oramorph® solution contains 10 mg/5 mL and there is a concentrated solution containing 20 mg/mL.
2 Titrate up until pain relief is adequate. Note the total dose used over the last 24 h.
3 Convert to morphine sulphate modified-release tablets, capsules or suspension: using the same total amount of morphine in two equal doses. The MXL preparation lasts for 24 h. Prescribe immediate-release morphine as needed for breakthrough pain.
4 To convert to morphine injections, use half the oral dose of morphine. To convert to diamorphine injections, use one-third the oral morphine dose. Usual route is subcutaneous, by syringe driver if needed regularly.
5 Fast-acting fentanyl 'lolly pops' provide a boost of analgesia to cover incident pain from dressing changes and personal care.
6 Fentanyl and buprenorphine are available as transdermal patches across a wide dose range and provide analgesia for 72 h to 7 days. Conversion tables from oral morphine are available. They are not suitable for titration but have the advantage of allowing free mobility and reducing tablet burden.
7 In renal failure, use low dose tramadol, oxycodone and alfentanil subcutaneously.

5 *Stretching of liver capsule by metastases:* prednisolone up to 25 mg a day.
6 *Intestinal colic due to partial bowel obstruction:* try loperamide and hyoscine hydrobromide as Kwells® sublingually (see later for parenteral management).

Restlessness and confusion

Look for physical causes, e.g. a distended bladder or rectum, or a respiratory or urinary tract infection. Oxycodone may cause less confusion and agitation than morphine. If restlessness and agitation persist, try midazolam 2.5 mg subcutaneously or haloperidol 0.5 mg.

Nausea and vomiting

These are unpleasant symptoms, especially early in the dying process, and may prevent the patient from preparing food, eating with their family or enjoying their daily routine. In hospital, boredom may make the symptoms seem even worse.

Identify any precipitating causes and treat those that are reversible.

- Always prescribe anti-emetics and laxatives when commencing opioids.
- Treat constipation.
- Treat hypercalcaemia; rehydrate with intravenous fluids or give intravenous pamidronate.

If there are no reversible precipitants:

- Identify the cause to choose the most appropriate anti-emetic. See Table 17.2.
- All causes of nausea and vomiting produce gastric stasis, so use parenteral preparations until symptoms are controlled.
- Metoclopramide is prokinetic (muscarinic agonist) in gastric and small intestinal smooth muscle and a D2 blocker (and 5HT3 blocker in higher doses) at the chemoreceptor trigger zone (CTZ).
- Cyclizine is an antihistamine (H1 blocker) and central antimuscarinic.
- Do not use metoclopramide with cyclizine as they counteract each other.
- Haloperidol is another option for chemically induced nausea as it blocks D2 and 5HT3 receptors in the CTZ.
- Granisetron has superseded ondansetron as the 5HT3 receptor antagonist of choice (once daily, and oral and subcutaneous preparations available). It is second line to haloperidol because of cost and its constipating effect. However, 5HT3 antagonists are usually only needed for vomiting due to chemotherapy.

Anorexia and malaise related to hepatic metastases

Prednisolone 20 mg a day is often extremely successful.

Breathlessness

Seventy-five percent of all dying patients suffer from breathlessness, not just those with end-stage heart failure or lung disease. Where possible, identify and treat the cause in the usual way. The following types of dyspnoea require specific management:

1 *Superior vena cava obstruction.* This is an oncological emergency presenting with increasing breathlessness and facial oedema. Treat with

radiotherapy. Dexamethasone 16 mg a day can be used if there is any delay.

2 *Lymphangitis carcinomatosis.* Dexamethasone is sometimes of value.

3 *Pleural effusions.* Fluid usually reaccumulates after drainage. Consider pleurodesis.

4 *Intractable breathlessness* of any cause can be treated using opioids, diazepam and/or oxygen, whichever gives the best relief. A battery-operated hand-held fan can reduce the associated claustrophobic fear.

5 The '*death-rattle*' occurs as secretions are inadequately cleared by dying patients. The patient is generally unconscious by this stage, but it is upsetting for relatives who need reassurance that the patient is not distressed. Glycopyrronium 0.6–1.2 mg/24 h subcutaneously will help dry up the secretions. Avoid suctioning as this will not remove secretions in the lower respiratory tract but will agitate the patient and family.

Offensive fungating tumours

Radiotherapy is often helpful. Topical metronidazole and charcoal dressings may reduce odour and exudate.

Bowel obstruction

Depending on the progress of the patient, this might be best managed by palliative colostomy. If surgical intervention is no longer appropriate avoid the 'drip and suck' regime and allow the patient to take small sips and talk to the family without a nasogastric tube. The pain can be relieved by a diamorphine infusion. Colicky pain should be alleviated by means of subcutaneous hyoscine butylbromide (Buscopan®) 60–240 mg over 24 h (this higher dose is sometimes needed in dying patients). As vomiting is likely to be a problem, strong parenteral anti-emetics and octreotide (300–600 mcg subcutaneously) may well be required. A phosphate enema can be used to try to relieve the associated constipation, and patients who respond to these measures can be permitted small quantities of food and fluid.

Other problems and some solutions

- *Hiccough:* use metoclopramide or chlorpromazine.
- *Dysphagia:* consider stent or laser treatment for oesophageal carcinoma.

- *Dry or painful mouth* (poor oral hygiene or thrush): good mouth care, artificial saliva such as Biotene Oral Balance; quarter of a vitamin C tablet, treat thrush with fluconazole.
- *Diarrhoea:* treat cause. Don't forget overflow secondary to constipation.
- *Constipation:* treat cause. If very severe, may need manual evacuation.
- *Cough:* oxygen, opioids, local anaesthetic lozenges and hyoscine.
- *Insomnia:* treat cause, e.g. pain, depression, fear.
- *Hypercalcaemia:* treat if symptomatic.
- *Ascites:* drain if causing discomfort.
- *Spinal-cord compression:* radiotherapy if diagnosed early.
- *Lymphoedema:* pressure device, support.
- *Pruritus*: attention to hygiene, use soap substitutes and emollients.

Diagnosing dying

In a perfect world, doctors would always recognize this time, but it can be notoriously difficult. The trajectory of metastatic cancer is more predictable than for heart failure, stroke disease and respiratory failure, all of which are leading causes of death in developed countries. It is particularly challenging to recognize the final dip in function of frail, elderly patients who have frequent admissions with pneumonia, 'off legs', etc. Often the nurses, who have more hands-on time with the patients, are better at predicting imminent death.

Signs of impending death:

- Lack of interest in eating and drinking.
- Poor swallow, not taking medicines.
- Bed bound.
- Drop in level of consciousness.
- Patient distress.
- Cheyne–Stokes breathing.

Advantages of recognizing dying:

- Establishes trust between patient, family and team.
- Enables family to gather and say goodbye.
- Can follow the wishes of the patient and family regarding end of life care, place of death, spiritual and emotional support, etc.
- Enables the team to focus on good symptom management.

Ethical and legal aspects of 'end of life decisions' are considered in Chapter 16. At this point, spend time with the patient (if they are conscious) and their family and explain that death is imminent. It is helpful to have something positive to offer in terms of care, and this is where the LCP comes into its own. Explain that the LCP is so-called because it was developed in Liverpool, not because you plan to move the patient there!

The Liverpool integrated care pathway for the dying patient (LCP)

- Promotes the ethos of a good death, aiming to enable all patients to die with dignity.
- Supports the family and others by making it explicit that the patient is dying and that the focus of care is symptom relief.
- Enables ward staff to explain that some symptoms such as the 'death rattle' are more distressing to relatives than to the patient.
- Explains that eating and artificial nutrition will not cure the patient and may cause distress.
- Encourages pre-emptive prescribing for symptom control.
- Reduces unnecessary disturbance of the patient, by stopping observations and using that time to provide comfort and mouth and skin care.
- Prompts team to address the patient's emotional, psychological, spiritual and religious needs.
- Provides educational support to relatives and the medical and nursing staff.

How a patient is managed in their last few days of life affects the way their relatives think about them afterwards and impacts on their grieving. Good symptom control, good communication between the family and the care team and the opportunity to work through family issues to reduce anger, guilt and desire to blame reduce complaints.

Syringe drivers

When patients are unable to take medications orally but are distressed, a subcutaneous syringe driver is an excellent method of providing symptom control. Use 'as needed' subcutaneous doses until the pump is set up and to gain control of symptoms, which can then be maintained without interruption.

- Diamorphine for pain and severe distress.
- Anti-emetic: consider cyclizine, haloperidol or methotrimiprazine.
- Midazolam to control fits and for terminal restlessness.
- Glycopyrronium to reduce respiratory secretions.

Spiritual and religious support

Spiritual care for a dying patient is centred on their need to find a meaning for their life, their illness and their impending death. It may include helping the patient find self-worth and just helping them to express themselves. Spiritual support should be available for people of all faiths or none. Religion is a mode of spirituality but does not necessarily encompass the whole of it. Patients may find great comfort in religious support, rites, prayer and the sacrament.

It may be difficult to assess the spiritual needs of patients. Ask open and general questions such as 'How do you usually make sense of things?' and 'How do you cope?' These questions may reveal a specific religious need or a more nebulous desire to talk things through. All care professionals can provide some spiritual care, but avoid projecting one's own beliefs on the patient. More specialist spiritual help can be delivered by the chaplaincy service or a faith leader.

The chaplaincy service has evolved to provide for a more secular society. The role of the chaplain might include counselling, help with ethical decisions, supporting the family and the ward team and education, as well as worship and liaison with the community and church to which the patient belongs.

Considerations for people of different faiths

Ask the patient/family what they want, as people may be more or less strict in adherence to their faith. The following list gives examples only and is by no means exhaustive.

- Patients of Anglican or Free Church faiths may wish a chaplain to visit.

- Buddhists prefer to be mentally alert at the time of death, so avoid sedatives where possible.
- Hindu patients often wish a Hindu priest to perform the last rites. Approach the family sensitively if a coroner's post mortem is needed as this is felt to be disrespectful to the dead.
- Jehovah's Witnesses will refuse blood transfusions and blood derivatives.
- Jewish patients would often wish their own Rabbi to be summoned. The body should not be undressed. The family will need careful support if a coroner's post mortem is needed. The funeral must occur as soon as possible after death, so timely completion of the death certificate is appreciated.
- A Muslim patient's family will traditionally stay with the patient. After death, the body should not be washed, and the head is turned toward the right shoulder to enable the body to be buried facing Mecca. Traditionally, the body is carried out by Muslims of the same sex and washed. The funeral should be as soon as possible.
- Roman Catholic patients derive comfort from the priest performing the Sacrament of the Sick and the Last Rites.
- A Sikh patient's family or priest may read from the Adi Granth. A few drops of holy water will be placed in the patient's mouth at the time of death. Usually, families choose to wash and dress the body. Cremation is preferred as soon as possible after death.

Emotional support

Support the family and carers and encourage them to talk with and listen to the patient. Enable them to work through feelings of grief, loss and fear. Explain that it is entirely normal for the patient to feel sad, angry, guilty and depressed about their illness and impending death. The patient may be anxious and fearful about what will happen to their spouse or family. Talking things through and bringing them into the open will help the patient find some resolution of their emotions. Encourage discussions regarding the last few days and the patient's wishes for their funeral.

Enabling people to die at home

In most cases, it is possible to achieve good symptom control. The pain service and community palliative care nurses can offer specialist expertise in difficult cases. Usually, care for older people will comprise a care package from social services, plus support from the district nurse to manage syringe drivers, etc. In 90% of cases where dying patients are admitted to hospital the reason is inadequate community support or distress of the relatives.

Additional support may be available from the following:

- Marie Curie cancer nurses provide hands-on care for the patient including personal care, dressing changes and emotional support for the family. They can visit during the day or night, to allow the family to rest.
- Macmillan nurses are trained to provide good symptom control. They also have an educational role so they can answer questions. They work 9–5 and do not offer emergency support.
- An outreach team from the local hospice may provide advice and offer short-term admission if symptom control is not optimal.
- Patient support groups may provide practical advice and support.

Care after death

See Chapter 16 for information regarding death certification and informing the coroner.

Bereavement

After the age of 75, 30% of men and 64% of women are widowed. Four main phases of grief have been described, but the stages vary enormously between individuals and few people progress steadily through each stage in a logical way.

1 *Shock and disbelief:* characterized by numbness and an inability to accept what has happened.
2 *Yearning:* may be characterized by acute pangs of severe loss and pining and a restless searching for the dead person, who often appears in

dreams and hallucinations. Periods of guilt and anger are directed at oneself, the dead person or other family members, friends and hospital staff.

3 *Depression and apathy:* a time of hopeless despair, with periods of joyless monotony. It is often associated with profound depression and loss of self-confidence. Guilt and anger are again common features. This emotional turbulence may continue for a year or more.

4 *Acceptance:* of the reality that the loved person is dead and that life has changed. The bereaved person resumes a lifestyle that, to a greater or lesser extent, has become adapted to his or her new status. This phase enables the bereaved person to let go of the dead loved one and to start a new sort of life.

The first of these phases may last for days and the second for weeks. The third phase is likely to last for a number of months, but most people adjust to a major bereavement within 1–2 years. Hallucinations, in which the dead person is vividly seen, may continue for a prolonged period. Mourning is associated with a number of 'tasks', which include acceptance of the reality, experiencing the pain, adjusting to the new environment and redirecting energy towards new relationships and activities.

Inability to work through the phases of grief is sometimes called a pathological grief reaction and is particularly likely to occur following sudden or untimely deaths. There is a high incidence of ill health and death in the surviving spouse following bereavement. Most areas of the UK now have a branch of the charity Cruse Bereavement Care, which offers help of many different kinds to bereaved people ranging from talking to a trained volunteer to meeting up with other bereaved people to share their feelings. There is a very helpful leaflet called 'Bereavement Advice for Older People: Coping with Death' which contains advice on registering the death and arranging the funeral (http://www.crusebereavementcare.org.uk/ Booklets.html).

→ FURTHER INFORMATION

British Geriatrics Society guidelines on advanced care planning: www.bgs.org.uk/index.php?option=com_content&view=article&id=1218:gpgadvancecare&catid=157:advancedplanning&Itemid=146.

British National Formulary (Current Edition) *Palliative Care*. BMJ Publishing Group, London.

Conroy S, Fade P, Fraser A, et al. (2010) Advance care planning: concise evidence-based guidelines. *Clinical Medicine* 9: 76–79.

Cruse Bereavement Care: www.crusebereavementcare.org.uk.

Department of Health End of Life Care Strategy: www.dh.gov.uk/en/Publicationsandstatistics/Publications/PublicationsPolicyAndGuidance/DH_086277. Promoting high quality care for all adults at the end of life.

Dying Matters: www.dyingmatters.org.

Gold Standard Framework (GSF): www.goldstandardsframework.nhs.uk.

Liverpool Care Pathway for the Dying Patient: www.lcp-mariecurie.org.uk.

Macmillan Cancer Support: www.macmillan.org.uk/Home.aspx.

Marie Curie Cancer Care: www.mariecurie.org.uk/.

Murray Parkes C (2010) *Bereavement*, 4th edn. Studies of Grief in Adult Life. Penguin, London.

Palliative care adult network guidelines: http://book.pallcare.info/index.php.

Spiritual care at the end of life: a systematic review of the literature: www.dh.gov.uk/en/Publicationsandstatistics/Publications/PublicationsPolicyAndGuidance/DH_123812.

Index

Page numbers in *italics* denote figures, those in **bold** denote tables.

Lecture Notes Elderly Care Medicine, Eighth Edition. Claire G. Nicholl and K. Jane Wilson.
© 2012 John Wiley & Sons, Ltd. Published 2012 by John Wiley & Sons, Ltd.

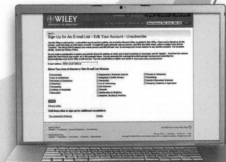
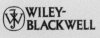